Qualitative Health Research

This accessible text supports health practitioners undertaking qualitative research to inform clinical practice, guiding readers through the decision-making process from planning and proposing, through data collection, to dissemination and impact. Qualitative research makes an important contribution to the health evidence base, including improving service provision, practitioner communication, and patient safety, as well as informing policies, generating important knowledge about health, and providing populations with a voice in the health context.

Balancing the need for practitioners to operate in an evidence-informed way, the increasing role of a research culture in the health service, and the everyday clinical demands faced in practice, this book includes strategies for managing the reality of undertaking qualitative research while working in clinical practice and includes a wide range of "bite size" chapters on topics such as:

- Quality improvement.
- Evidence-based practice and practice-based evidence.
- Managing dual roles.
- Planning a project.
- Working with stakeholders.
- Ethics.
- Data collection methods.
- Conducting digital research.
- Recruitment and sampling.
- Data management.
- Analytical approaches.
- Thematic approaches.
- Research with vulnerable groups.
- Dissemination.
- Translating research into practice.

This book is a practical resource for clinical researchers, designed to support the application of learning. Each chapter opens with learning objectives, and ends with a reflection on the chapter, integrating case examples and highlighting core issues. Practitioner experience boxes and reflective activities bring an invaluable real-world perspective to each chapter.

Qualitative Health Research is the ideal text for all healthcare practitioners and trainees new to qualitative research, including those from medicine, nursing, midwifery, psychology, allied health, and public health.

Michelle O'Reilly is Associate Professor of Communication in Mental Health at the University of Leicester and a Research Consultant and Quality Improvement Advisor for Leicestershire Partnership NHS Trust. Michelle is also a Chartered Psychologist in Health and a Visiting Lecturer at the Tavistock and Portman NHS Foundation Trust.

Philip Archard is a Senior Lecturer in the Department of Education and Training at the Tavistock and Portman NHS Foundation Trust, where he works on two doctoral courses: a qualifying programme in child, community, and educational psychology, and a programme in advanced practice and research for experienced social work and health and social care professionals. He is also an Honorary Fellow in the School of Criminology, Sociology and Social Policy at the University of Leicester.

Nikki Kiyimba is a Clinical Academic, who works in private practice as a Chartered Consultant Clinical Psychologist in Aotearoa New Zealand. She is also an academic with extensive experience in tertiary education, and of postgraduate programme leadership. She is a Journal Editorial Member, Guest Editor, and Peer Reviewer for several international journals.

Qualitative Health Research

A Practical Guide for Clinical Practitioners

Michelle O'Reilly, Philip Archard and Nikki Kiyimba

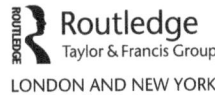

LONDON AND NEW YORK

First published 2025
by Routledge
4 Park Square, Milton Park, Abingdon, Oxon OX14 4RN

and by Routledge
605 Third Avenue, New York, NY 10158

Routledge is an imprint of the Taylor & Francis Group, an informa business

© 2025 Michelle O'Reilly, Philip Archard and Nikki Kiyimba

The right of Michelle O'Reilly, Philip Archard and Nikki Kiyimba to be identified as authors of this work has been asserted in accordance with sections 77 and 78 of the Copyright, Designs and Patents Act 1988.

All rights reserved. No part of this book may be reprinted or reproduced or utilised in any form or by any electronic, mechanical, or other means, now known or hereafter invented, including photocopying and recording, or in any information storage or retrieval system, without permission in writing from the publishers.

Trademark notice: Product or corporate names may be trademarks or registered trademarks, and are used only for identification and explanation without intent to infringe.

British Library Cataloguing-in-Publication Data
A catalogue record for this book is available from the British Library

ISBN: 978-1-032-39475-6 (hbk)
ISBN: 978-1-032-39467-1 (pbk)
ISBN: 978-1-003-34990-7 (ebk)

DOI: 10.4324/9781003349907

Typeset in Sabon
by Deanta Global Publishing Services, Chennai, India

We dedicate this book to the staff working in Leicestershire Partnership NHS Trust (LPT). All three of us work (or have worked) for LPT, and in so doing have been privileged to work alongside many clinical practitioners, clinician-researchers, and staff in other roles. Our time in this Trust provided us with a learning environment and facilitated the development of our expertise to write this book and therefore we dedicate it to all in LPT.

Contents

About the authors		ix
Acknowledgements		x
Abbreviations		xii
1	Introduction – the clinician-researcher	1
2	Quality improvement: Differentiating audit, service evaluation, and research	11
3	Theory in qualitative research	29
4	Evidence-based practice and practice-based evidence	51
5	Planning a project	68
6	Types of qualitative research	94
7	Working with gatekeepers, stakeholders and experts by experience	129
8	Ethics and integrity	150
9	Dual roles – the clinician and researcher roles	170
10	Sampling and recruitment	191
11	Sensitivity, vulnerability, and barriers to participation	210
12	Managing researcher safety	225
13	Methods of data collection	251

CONTENTS

14	Interviews and focus groups	275
15	Qualitative health research and digital technologies	302
16	Transcription and data management	319
17	Using clinical skills in research	332
18	Thematic approaches and coding data	346
19	Common analytic approaches	368
20	Dissemination and translating research into practice	389
Index		411

About the authors

Michelle O'Reilly is Associate Professor of Communication in Mental Health at the University of Leicester and a Research Consultant and Quality Improvement Advisor for Leicestershire Partnership NHS Trust. Michelle is also a Chartered Psychologist in Health and a Visiting Lecturer at the Tavistock and Portman NHS Foundation Trust. Michelle has research interests in mental health and social media, self-harm and suicide, neurodevelopmental conditions, and child mental health services, such as mental health assessments and family therapy. Michelle recently won the Anselm Strauss Award for Qualitative Family Research for her co-authored contribution to discursive psychology in this area (with Nikki Kiyimba and Jessica Lester). Michelle has expertise in qualitative methodologies and specialises in discursive psychology and conversation analysis and has written several books about research methods for different audiences.

Philip Archard is a Senior Lecturer in the Department of Education and Training at the Tavistock and Portman NHS Foundation Trust, where he works on two doctoral courses: a qualifying programme in child, community, and educational psychology; and a programme in advanced practice and research for experienced social work and health and social care professionals. Philip is also a Honorary Fellow at the University of Leicester School of Criminology, Sociology, and Social Policy. A social worker by background, Philip's research interests are in the areas of qualitative research, child and adolescent mental health, and child welfare. Until recently, Philip was working as a mental health practitioner in a specialist child and adolescent mental health service team.

Nikki Kiyimba is a Clinical Academic, who works in private practice and a Chartered Consultant Clinical Psychologist in Aotearoa New Zealand. She is also an academic with extensive experience in tertiary education, and of postgraduate programme leadership. She is a Journal Editorial Member, Guest Editor, and Peer Reviewer for several international journals. She has co-authored three textbooks on research methods and has an extensive publication history at the intersection of the fields of mental health, spirituality, trauma, discursive practice, and research methodology.

Acknowledgements

We are grateful to those who have shared their practical experiences of being clinician-researchers and their voices are represented in boxes throughout the book. We therefore thank:

- Dr Tina Adkins
- Dr Sewanu Awhangansi
- Dr Dave Clarke
- Dr Leanne Chrisostomou
- Professor Nisha Dogra
- Dr Alison Drewett
- Linda Homan
- Dr Sarah Hunt
- Dr Sam Little
- Dr Pallab Majumder
- Dr Isobel Moore
- Tala Noweisser
- Dr M. Farhad Peerally
- Dr Massimiliano Sommantico
- Dr Calvin Swords
- Dr Samuel Tromans
- Professor Panos Vostanis

We are also grateful to our own participants who have given up their time over the years to be part of our research projects. They have taught us so much about qualitative health research by sharing their experiences and views. We also thank the funding bodies who provided us with the resources to undertake those projects.

We thank Routledge and the supportive editors who have been behind the scenes in publishing this book.

Finally, we are grateful to our families and colleagues for supporting us in the many hours we dedicated to writing this book.

Abbreviations

CAMHS	Child and Adolescent Mental Health Service
COPE	Committee on Publication Ethics
COREQ	COnsolidated criteria for REporting Qualitative research
CQC	Care Quality Commission
EPB	Evidence-Based Practice
GDPR	General Data Protection Regulation
GMC	General Medical Council
HRA	Health Regulation Authority
ICT	Information and Communication Technologies
IM	Instant Messaging
NHS	National Health Service
NICE	National Institute for Health and Care Excellence
NRES	National Research Ethics Service
NSPCC	National Society for the Prevention of Cruelty to Children
PAR	Participatory Action Research
PDSA	Plan, Do, Study, Act
PPIE	Public Patient Involvement and Engagement
PR	Participatory Research
PRN	Practice Research Networks
QI	Quality Improvement
RCT	Randomised Controlled Trial
SMS	Short Message Service
SNS	Social Networking Services
TCU	Turn Construction Unit
TRP	Transition Relevance Place
UK	United Kingdom

CHAPTER 1

Introduction – the clinician-researcher

> **Learning objectives**
>
> This chapter enables the reader to:
>
> - Identify the focus of the book and its contents.
> - Appreciate the ways in which different concepts and ideas will be used throughout the book.
> - Understand the way the book is structured.
> - Identify the main contents of the book.
> - Use the book to help develop a research project.

Introduction

Qualitative Health Research: A Practical Guide for Clinical Practitioners is a pedagogical textbook. The book is intended to be a resource for healthcare practitioners who are undertaking a qualitative research project in the field or considering doing so. Our aim is to provide a useful guide that is relevant to all areas of physical and mental health and is designed to be especially helpful for early career practitioners, trainees on clinical courses, professionals working to develop a clinical academic career, as well as academics working in areas of health.

The focus of this book is on qualitative health research only, and throughout our writing we refer to qualitative health research when we are being specific to health, and qualitative research when we are referring to the qualitative approach more generally. Whilst randomised controlled trials, surveys/questionnaires (with a quantitative focus), experiments, and other forms of quantitative research have significant value for the field, qualitative research is growing in popularity across health and related disciplines. Qualitative research differs from quantitative research theoretically, in design, methods, and analysis. The defining criteria of this approach vary considerably, as it is not an approach that is easily categorised (Hammersley, 2012). However, as Hammersley also pointed out, there is a common set of features that unite qualitative approaches, including the flexibility of the approach, being data-driven, recognition of the role of the researcher, reflexivity, smaller samples, verbal/textual data, and theoretical heterogeneity. Our standpoint is that doing qualitative health research well requires attention to detail; recognition of a multitude of influencing factors; knowledge of theory, method, methodology, and practice; and specific practical skills to implement research.

To improve service provision, practitioner communication, and patient safety and to inform policies and generate knowledge about health, it is necessary to undertake research. Qualitative research makes a vital contribution to the health evidence base and helps provide recipients of health services with a voice. We have argued previously that this growth of the health evidence base benefits from the integration of science and practice, and partnerships between clinical practitioners and academic scholars (O'Reilly and Kiyimba, 2015). Qualitative research is rarely, if ever, a straightforward endeavour and requires careful planning and thought regarding methodological rigour and quality.

This book seeks to provide a practical benchmark for clinical practitioners who want to undertake qualitative health research, offering guidance through the decision-making process, from planning and proposing a research project to dissemination and impact. The book does this by providing guidance and strategies for managing the reality of undertaking qualitative health research whilst also working or training in clinical practice. Thus, we are writing this book for clinical practitioners interested in research as a vehicle for improving care and the work they do, whether this be individually or with their teams and organisations. With this in mind, we take the value of research for improving practice as a foundational assumption.

Terms used

There is some terminology we use consistently throughout this book. Some terms are straightforward, whilst others are debated regarding their usage, and we acknowledge those challenges here to illustrate the rationale for why we are favouring certain language. We recognise that language is constantly evolving, and the meanings of words and the value of concepts change over time and according to context. We also recognise that some concepts are used by some groups and not others. In a pedagogical text like this, there is not space to go into those broader critical debates in detail, and so we do some work here to illustrate our choices.

Our style of writing also bears acknowledging. As reflexive writers, we have opted to adopt a more personal writing style over a strongly "scientific" or formal academic style. This means the text may read as more conversational in places, but it enables us to situate ourselves in the arguments and claims made.

■ **You – the reader**

In opting to use a style of writing in this text which is reader-friendly, we write directly in various places to our audience, i.e. the reader. Consequently, throughout, we predominantly use the pronoun "you" to refer to the reader. At other times, we use the broader term "researcher" where the point being made is more general.

- Us, we, I – the authors

In our writing we use the personal pronouns "us" and "we" to refer to ourselves as the three authors of this book. There are occasions throughout the text where we will use the personal pronoun "I". In so doing, we will differentiate which of the three of us is writing. This will be done reflexively and with case examples. Each of the main chapters contains a contribution from a clinical or health expert who may also elect to use the personal pronoun "I" to refer to themselves and their experiences.

- Experts by experience and service users

There are various terms used in the methodological literature to refer to individuals who provide support to a research team and have lived experiences of the phenomena being researched, particularly when occupying support roles, consultation roles, and sitting in an advisory capacity, as well as participants recruited for a project. It is difficult to use language that is entirely acceptable to everyone and reflects how valuable it can be to include these people. Historically in health research, "patients" was the conventional way to refer to individuals receiving care, and in many areas of clinical practice, this term is still used. However, this is viewed by some as signifying an overly paternalistic stan, and not all healthcare providers use the term, with some using the term client instead. In some literature, these individuals are referred to as service users. We use this phrasing when referring to those who use a service where appropriate, and sometimes we use the terms patient/client where it is more aligned with a point we are making. Thus, in the book you will see that we ourselves grapple with the language of participants, as patients in a health service, clients (a term preferred by some groups), and those who use a service - the service user. When referring to those who support a research project by being part of a stakeholder group, a steering group, a rights-holder group, an advisory board, or by co-design/co-production, we align with the literature that refers to them as "experts by experience". This helpfully foregrounds lived experience (which may equally apply to carers, family members, and other stakeholders who live through something), as well as recognising their equal footing with health practitioners. In this way, there is recognition of the value of the contribution of these groups to the design, planning, and undertaking of qualitative research.

- Clinician-researcher

Most often, a clinician-researcher is someone who has a primary career as a healthcare professional and, as part of that role (or in addition to it), also engages in empirical research. It can also be the case that a person will have completed a PhD and have a first career as a researcher and then choose later to undertake clinical training, subsequently combining the two identities. When we refer to the clinician-researcher throughout this book, we refer to a practitioner who is primarily a health practitioner, such as a nurse, physician, speech and language therapist, dentist, occupational therapist, social worker, or psychologist, and is also involved in academic research and writing. Depending on the training a clinician has received during (or prior to) their vocational qualification, clinician-researchers have varying skills in research when they begin to engage seriously with the academic research world in conjunction with their clinical practice.

This book is designed to support clinicians to develop their research skills and engage in quality, ethically robust, and publishable research projects connected with or related to their clinical work. The advantage of the clinician studying the published research evidence is that the lessons learnt from those studies can be applied in their own clinical work. This is usually referred to as evidence-based practice. In a similar and complementary way, research engaged in by the clinician in their professional context is usually referred to as practice-based evidence. There are many advantages to having a dual role as a clinician and researcher, including developing the ability to see from the experience of providing care and everyday professional encounters where the gaps are in our current knowledge and, in turn, what a useful research project might be. Additionally, when research data have been collected and the findings are examined, the clinician-researcher is well placed to be able to speak to what the implications of the findings might be for practice, as well as identifying future research that may be needed in that area.

■ Children and young people

There are occasions in the book where we refer to younger populations and some of the specific methodological adaptations that may need to be made. It is necessary to be reflective about the terms used, however. For example, in developmental psychology, children are typically positioned as progressing through different childhood stages and meeting a series of developmental milestones. In sociology, there is a view that children and childhood are socially constructed entities, and there are a range of different conceptualisations that capture the various stages of childhood (neonate, toddler, young child, pre-teen, tween, young adolescent, older adolescent). Whilst these distinctions and disciplinary differences are notable, we have chosen to use the terms "children" and "young people" to distinguish younger children from adolescents.

■ Older adults

There are also occasions in the book where we refer to older populations. Again, for this demographic group, there are a few recommendations we offer as methodological adaptations to consider. Definitions of this category tend to vary somewhat between cultural groups, but generally refer to senior members of a community who are chronologically older in years. Often in Western settings, older adults are those who have reached the end of their working careers and have entered retirement. They may have age-related physical impairments such as hearing loss or reduced mobility, and taking these considerations into account is important in the data collection stage.

■ Where in the world

We acknowledge that we are academics, clinicians, and researchers living in Western Europe and Australasia. Our research and clinical experience are therefore largely in that context. Notably, also, much of the methodological literature regarding qualitative research has been written by authors living in those global regions. However, our commitment to inclusion and diversity means that we will draw on references and case examples where research has taken place across different geographical spheres. On this basis, we use the terms "majority world" and "minority world" when we are differentiating between global locations. Again, whilst there are some arguments around these terms, they are largely the more accepted concepts, as the term "developing countries" has been criticised for lacking nuance, and "Global North/South" for its inaccuracy. Thus, "majority world" denotes areas where most of the world's population resides, and these historically refer to those areas that are "developing" economically (see O'Reilly, Dogra, Levine, and Donoso, 2021). Minority world by contrast refers to those that historically possess greater economic wealth.

■ Mental health

In a text focusing on health and health services research, we also attend to issues around doing research in the field of mental health. This is another area where some of the language has been subject to debates about the most appropriate terminology. Broadly, when we refer to a person's overall psychological well-being, we use the term mental health. We acknowledge that physical and mental health are intrinsically linked, and any dichotomous positioning can be linked to different Western philosophical ideas. We appreciate that in many cultures there is no distinction between physical, emotional, mental, social, spiritual, and physical well-being. These boundaries are largely starting to be dissolved even in Western medical contexts, where more scientific research is showing the interconnectedness of well-being across these dimensions. However, for the purposes of this text, when we talk about mental health, we are typically referring to individual thoughts and feelings. A person who is mentally healthy, therefore, would be someone who for the most part is not struggling with thoughts or feelings that are harmful or overwhelming. Conversely, when we refer to people who have mental health difficulties, we mean people whose difficulties either meet the criteria for a mental health diagnosis or have significant difficulties in their daily living.

■ Practitioner perspective

We greatly value the views, experiences, case examples, and research perspectives of clinical practitioners from across the globe. We believe that the practitioner voice is central to pedagogy in practitioner-led research and have sought to ensure that a wide range of practitioners are represented throughout this text. We refer to these as "practitioner perspectives", and these are written from the viewpoint of an individual clinician working in the field.

Contents
This book is designed to be a practical and pedagogical text that you can refer to as you progress with a research project. It accounts for the multiple competing pressures on clinical practitioners to operate in an evidence-informed way, the growing emphasis on

a research culture in health services, and the everyday clinical demands faced in practice. In other words, we have written each chapter in a way that recognises the value of research undertaken by clinical practitioners, but also acknowledge that this is realised in an environment where there are many demands on practitioners' time. In this spirit, we include our first practitioner voice here and present the view of Dr Pallab Majumder on being a clinician-researcher in Box 1.1.

Box 1.1

Being a clinician-researcher – practitioner perspective of Dr Pallab Majumder

Dr Pallab Majumder is a Consultant Child and Adolescent Psychiatrist, Nottinghamshire Healthcare NHS Foundation Trust, and an Honorary (Clinical) Associate Professor at the University of Nottingham. At the time of writing, he is the Clinical Director (Interim) for CAMHS.

I have been actively involved in health research from the beginning of my career in psychiatry and later as a Consultant Child and Adolescent Psychiatrist. I think that being a clinician, we are in a privileged position to have firsthand experience and knowledge of the challenges, the blind spots, and the gaps of knowledge in providing the optimum service to our patients. Therefore, it is easier for practising clinicians like us to come up with a research question that is the most clinically relevant and has the most impactful service implications. A clinician is also positioned very well to involve other stakeholders in the health economy in the research process, such as the patients, the carers, health service managers, other gatekeepers, commissioners, health leaders, decision- and policymakers, and regulatory bodies. Without this connection and effective involvement of all the stakeholders, research findings may be treated in isolation, regardless of what research question is being answered. In that way, the whole endeavour can become disjointed from effective clinical application and as a result may fail to bring about meaningful change to clinical practice or beneficial change to the lives of patients, families, and the overall health and well-being of the society.

There are, nevertheless, some challenges being an actively involved researcher whilst also carrying on with the regular job of a full-time clinician. The clinical commitments can, particularly in the current overall situation of the NHS [UK National Health Service], become overwhelming. This leaves very little diary space and headspace for the clinician to effectively and meaningfully engage in envisaging a research project, coming up with the right research question, planning the project, preparing, executing and succeeding in applying to procure research grants, delivering the research project on time, and during the whole process of the research project, continuing to successfully liaise, collaborate and co-produce with what can be a very extensive network of researchers, clinical professionals, service users, and other stakeholders. What has helped me in this endeavour was to have well protected time agreed with my line manager, support from the organisation, presence of a well-functioning research network embedded within the service framework, and the culture of a research-active service provider NHS Trust.

The chapters of this book are organised around "chunks" of information so that it can be a "pick-up-put-down" text to fit around busy schedules. Each chapter addresses a different part of the research journey. The book is designed to guide you through the complete qualitative health research process. We have constructed the book to help you plan your project, attend to the ethical governance process adequately, choose methods of data collection and analysis, select appropriate channels of dissemination, and manage pathways to impact. To complement those decision-making practices, we also highlight areas of concern and debate and encourage reflective thinking.

Being a reflective reader and researcher
As a practitioner you are probably familiar with the professional skill of reflection as part of your daily work. It is also likely that, during your professional training, you were encouraged to reflect on your practice and think about how your personal beliefs, values, attitudes, and worldview shape the way you approach your work. We recognise that not all our readers work in an area of clinical practice, and you might be a trainee, an academic, a student, a policymaker, or from some other relevant discipline. In that case, you may be less familiar with the process of reflecting on practice. Through reading this book, there is the opportunity to develop this skill. Within each chapter, we encourage you to think about your own role, your practice, the people you work with, your thoughts, feelings, and lived experience. During the research process, you will also need these skills to strengthen the credibility of your research. The quality of your research will be greatly enhanced by engaging in what is referred to in qualitative research as "reflexivity".

We deal with qualitative researcher reflexivity and practitioner reflection later in the book when addressing the topics of research quality and translating knowledge. However, so you have some sense of what these terms mean, we provide a definition of each here.

Reflexivity
Reflexivity refers to the recognition by the researcher of the intersecting relationships between themselves and their participants (and the topic of study), including their race, gender, age, cultural background, and socio-economic status. Reflexivity specifies how an understanding of the self can influence the development of new knowledge (Berger, 2015).

Reflection
Through reflection one learns from one's experience. Reflection, or reflective practice, can also be defined as a process whereby the practitioner becomes consciously aware of the influence of ideological and societal assumptions, especially their own moral and ethical beliefs, that underpin their thinking and professional practice (Yip, 2006).

> **Key point!**
>
> Being reflective is a process that takes time and effort, and is a professional practice underpinned by guidelines, codes of conduct and training shaped by an individual's personal belief system.
>
> (Yip, 2006)

There are different kinds of reflection. Schőn (1983) distinguished:

- **Reflection-in-action** – refers to when you reflect in the moment on an event or incident as it occurs.
- **Reflection-on-action** – refers to when you reflect on an event or incident after it has occurred.

The importance of a research diary

From this point onwards we recommend you keep a research diary. This is essential for qualitative research to maintain a document that tracks your thoughts, beliefs, decisions, and emotional experience as you work through your project. Whilst it may feel like a time-consuming addition to your research project, it is a beneficial activity as, among other things, it will function as an aid to your memory and allow you to reflect further on aspects of your research.

We have previously outlined three general formats for keeping your diary (O'Reilly and Parker, 2014):

- Some people like to keep an electronic diary, which they can synchronise across their devices. There are different types of software available that allow you to import images, text boxes, and diagrams into the diary.
- Other people prefer a simple pen and paper format. Again, there are different options on the market, but one recommendation is a notebook style that has colour-coded dividers in it so you can separate and organise your different kinds of diary entries.
- Another option is the traditional diary, either a diary notebook or diary pages that can be printed or saved to a computer. This way, entries correspond to specific dates within the diary.

There are different kinds of entries that you will want to include as you work through your project. There are two types of diary entries that figure in tracking your research process we have highlighted (O'Reilly and Parker, 2014):

- **Factual information** – a log of facts relevant to your project. These might be the reference of a published article, the dates of research events or seminars, appointments with researchers and academic staff, participants, gatekeepers, and so on.

- **Decisions** – during your research project, you will make many decisions. Some of these will be minor, and others will be more impactful on the process. All decisions you make will need a defensible rationale, and ideally, one you can support from the literature. It is helpful to document any discussions you have with mentors, supervisors, gatekeepers, and participants, as well as any reading you did that helped to shape that decision.

Keeping your research diary is not only a valuable organisational tool and a helpful aid to memory but is also fundamental to "doing" reflexivity as a researcher (O'Reilly and Parker, 2014). To help strengthen your project, you can use your diary to document your reflections, thoughts, emotions, and personal reactions to events, data collection, and analysis, as well as noting down how your positionality, personal factors, sense of self, and so forth are shaping the production of knowledge. In this way, the diary becomes an anchor for your thoughts and feelings and can function as a catalyst for dialogue, which will help you to become more aware of how knowledge is created (Gerstl-Pepin and Patrizio, 2009).

Keeping your diary is also beneficial as a learning tool. Engin (2011) observed that the opportunity to re-read and interact with your own thoughts and feelings can be a mediator in helping you to understand your role as the researcher and your influence on the research process. Ultimately, keeping a research diary will help you to stay organised and reflective as you undertake your research project. Whatever modality you choose, you should seek to make regular entries as you go along. To get you started, we invite you to complete the activity in Box 1.2.

Box 1.2

Time to start your research diary – reflective activity

Before you go any further, it is time to start your research diary. Take a few minutes now to set this up, whether it be the pen and paper approach or an electronic file. Your first entry is to answer the following questions:

- Why am I engaging in research?
- What do I want to understand by undertaking my research project?
- What do I hope or intend to write about in my research diary?

Author reflections and concluding remarks

Rather than end each chapter with the usual conclusion and summary style, we will close with author reflexivity, where one or all of us will provide a clinical/academic reflection on the chapter contents and issues. Thus, the second author, Philip, closes this introduction with a reflective message.

From Philip

Starting out in qualitative research can be daunting – full of abstract concepts and complicated language. If one goes into the field of healthcare with a desire to work with – and help – people, research activity can seem somewhat detached from the real work: at worst, something irrelevant to one's daily work and, at best, something that is interesting, but nevertheless a matter for which one has limited time. The mindsets of the clinician and researcher can also be different. The clinician, by necessity, must focus on how they can specifically help someone. This involves complex ways of viewing things but is based on an, ultimately, circumscribed field of vision. Conversely, the researcher holds a very wide field of vision before narrowing this and focusing their energies on a very specific problem or area of investigation they can say something meaningful about.

And yet, my own experience is that there is considerable space for cross-fertilisation between research and clinical practice, and that building experience and skills in qualitative research can help one to be a better clinician (and I hope the potential for this becomes apparent as you read this book). By the same token, as a professional, one brings something unique to research, not least in identifying areas for research that, with diligence, may yield findings that are meaningful for one's practice and organisation. As a clinician-researcher, I have also found that research is, or can be, most fulfilling when engaged in alongside others. Research is very much a team game. Working on a project together with interested colleagues can be a very rewarding experience, especially as a clinical team or service, and can lead to improvements in clinical care.

References

Berger, R. (2015). Now I see it, now I don't: Researcher's position and reflexivity in qualitative research. *Qualitative Research*, 15(2), 219–234.

Engin, M. (2011). Research diary: A tool for scaffolding. *International Journal of Qualitative Methods*, 10(3), 296–306.

Gertstl-Pepin, C., and Patrizio, K. (2009). Learning from Dumbledore's pensieve: A metaphor as an aid in teaching reflexivity in qualitative research. *Qualitative Research*, 9, 299–308.

Hammersley, M. (2012). *What is qualitative research?* London: Bloomsbury Academic.

O'Reilly, M., Dogra, N., Levine, D., and Donoso, V. (2021). *Digital media and child and adolescent mental health: A practical guide to understanding the evidence*. London: Sage.

O'Reilly, M., and Kiyimba, N. (2015). *Advanced qualitative research: A guide to contemporary theoretical debates*. London: Sage.

O'Reilly, M., and Parker, N. (2014). *Doing mental health research with children and adolescents: A guide to qualitative methods*. London: Sage.

Schön, D. (1983). *The reflective practitioner*. New York: Basic Books.

Yip, K.-S. (2006). Self-reflective practice: A note of caution. *British Journal of Social Work*, 36, 777–788.

CHAPTER 2

Quality improvement

Differentiating audit, service evaluation, and research

> **Learning objectives**
> This chapter enables the reader to:
> - Recognise the core domains of quality improvement.
> - Identify the value of quality improvement in health.
> - Appreciate the steps involved in quality improvement.
> - Critically assess different ways to do quality improvement.
> - Differentiate clinical audit, service evaluation, and research.
> - Recognise which is most suitable of these approaches for the goals of your own work.

Introduction
Quality improvement (henceforth QI) is an umbrella term that captures activity within healthcare organisations to advance knowledge, improve quality of care, and promote safety. This includes clinical audits, service evaluations, and research. While there are connections across these different approaches, there are also important differences. The aim of this chapter is to guide you through these different ways of working on a problem so that you have a foundational knowledge of what kind of work you want to do.

Differentiating audit, service evaluation, and research – in brief
There are different ways of improving services, promoting better health outcomes, advancing our knowledge of health and healthcare, and generating new theoretical perspectives. To improve quality in healthcare, practitioners may choose to do a QI

project, or they might choose to do a clinical audit, a service evaluation, or a piece of research. You might find it a bit confusing to ascertain whether you are planning to do some QI and in what format, or whether it is a research project you are planning (Varkey, Reller, and Resar, 2007). This is because there are some similarities across QI, service evaluation, audit, and research. However, there are differences.

For simplicity, you can think about research as involving a search for answers to questions about improving health and care where findings are generalisable or transferable across contexts; audits as examining what is being done by a service against a baseline requirement; and service evaluation as examining the effect of care on the service user's experience and outcomes (Twycross and Shorten, 2014). Whereas service evaluation and clinical audit tend to address a local service need, a local problem, and a local population to meet the needs of a specific organisation, research aims to address problems in a way that is more transferable, representative, or generalisable of wider services, populations, or problems (Varkey et al., 2007). Thus, service evaluations and clinical audits tend to be concerned with assessing whether predefined standards are met by a local service. Conversely, research is about generating new knowledge, testing or developing theory, and understanding phenomena (O'Reilly and Parker, 2014).

We now invite you to reflect on your own plans and think about what you want to accomplish by engaging with the reflective activity in Box 2.1.

Box 2.1

Reflective activity on the scope of your own project

Using your existing knowledge, experience, and what you have learnt so far, we invite you to think about what you are doing and why. In other words, consider whether you believe your project is QI, audit, service evaluation, or research. In a few sentences, write down what kind of project you plan to do, what you want to achieve, and whether it can be defined as a research project. As you work through the rest of the chapter, your confidence should build, and you should have a stronger idea about which category your project fits into.

Quality improvement

The aim of QI is to make a difference to patients/clients by making changes that improve the effectiveness, safety, and experiences of care. To achieve this, QI has two core elements: 1) *change*, i.e. an improvement and 2) *method*, i.e. the techniques and tools to achieve it (Atkinson, Ingham, Cheshire, and Went, 2010). The core domains of QI are outlined in Table 2.1.

If you decide to engage in some QI work within your healthcare organisation, you will benefit from working with a team (Jones, Lyle, Brunero et al., 2015). Ideally, this team should be multi-disciplinary, with different skills and representing different health expertise and care roles (Silver, Harel, McQuillan et al., 2016). When you plan your team composition, bear in mind you will need to fill different project roles. We provide a practical overview of how to assemble a team in Box 2.2, based on guidance by Silver et al. (2016).

Table 2.1 Domains of quality improvement

Safety
Patient experience
Efficiency
Equity
Effectiveness
Timeliness
Sustainability

From Royal College of Physicians (2010)

Box 2.2

Practical steps to compose your QI team (Silver et al., 2016)

There are several key roles that need to be filled when you assemble your team, and we advise you appoint one of each of the following as recommended by Silver et al. (2016):

- **Team Lead**: The person who is responsible for leading the QI project.
- **Technical Experts**: The people who have knowledge and understanding of different components of the QI problem.
- **Clinical or System Leader**: The person who takes on the role of manager. This person should have an understanding and overview of the implications of the changes on other parts of the system and how the QI problem intersects with the organisation. They need sufficient authority to implement and test the changes that are recommended by the project.
- **Improvement Adviser**: This is an expert in QI methods who will act as an adviser during the process. You might choose to have more than one of these advisers on your team to represent different types of expertise.
- **Executive Sponsor**: This is the person who has power and leadership skills within the organisation who can support access to resources and help you navigate any resource barriers.

Remember that some of these team members will have more involved roles than others, and if you are leading the project, you will need to delegate responsibilities, manage tasks, keep a log of activities, and consult with others where their support may be beneficial.

Planning a QI project

QI projects require careful planning, collaboration, and time and effort. Once you have your multi-disciplinary team in place, you can start to think about the project itself and how you might begin to carry it out in practice. To help you do this, we outline the main steps of planning a QI project as proposed by Jones et al. (2019) in Box 2.3.

> **Box 2.3**
>
> **The practical steps of planning QI (Jones et al., 2019)**
>
> Here we outline the steps to help you get started with your own project.
>
> - **First** – assemble a collaborative team and identify knowledge or expertise gaps.
> - **Second** – alongside your main team, if you are new to doing QI, it can be helpful to seek out a colleague who has experience of doing QI to provide mentoring and advice.
> - **Third** – identify the nature of the problem to be addressed. It is useful to understand what might be leading to the problem and the contributing contextual factors.
> - **Fourth** – develop clear aims and objectives for the project.
> - **Fifth** – map out the stakeholders who are likely to be impacted by your QI project, and, as appropriate, engage them in the QI process. We will give you more information on how to do this shortly.
> - **Sixth** – it can be helpful to have clarity about the project's value. We recommend you spend time with your team together and map this out.
> - **Seventh** – be mindful that there are likely to be iterative changes in response to false starts and obstacles; indeed, it may be necessary to refine your project.
>
> In addition to these steps, we also recommend that you keep a log or record of the steps you take, the methods you use, and the findings produced so that you can track your progress as you move your QI work through the different stages.

You will see that in the fifth step of planning it is highly recommended that you complete a stakeholder mapping exercise. This activity enables you to identify any gaps in your current team before you go too far with the process and consider the role of any additional contributors that might be helpful (Silver et al., 2016). Stakeholders are a vital resource in QI projects (Jones et al., 2019). In Box 2.4, we outline some practical ways to do a stakeholder mapping exercise, drawing on suggestions made by Silver et al. (2016).

> **Box 2.4**
>
> **How to do stakeholder mapping (Silver et al., 2016)**
>
> There are several practical ways to create a stakeholder map for your QI project, as outlined by Silver et al. (2016):
>
> - Effective stakeholder mapping techniques include brainstorming activities, listing a range of stakeholders, and mapping them into clusters.
> - It is helpful to reference the relationships between your included stakeholders.
> - Creating a visual map helps you see the connections among your stakeholders.
> - You can use lines or arrows to connect the stakeholders to the quality problem, which is defined at the centre of the map.

QUALITY IMPROVEMENT

> - Undertake some analysis of your map to identify which people should be approached. To achieve this, you will need to create a prioritisation hierarchy of stakeholders with memos about the feasibility and/or value of their involvement.
> - When mapping, keep in mind the possible motivations of different stakeholders that may act as facilitators or barriers to success.

For more depth and a helpful visual representation of stakeholder mapping, we suggest you read the Silver et al. (2016) article.

Doing a QI project

There are different ways you can do your QI project, and if you explore the literature you will see that there are three main ways:

- The Model for Improvement approach.
- The Lean approach.
- The Six Sigma approach.

We provide you with a general overview of these three different ways of doing a QI project but encourage you to read more about them if you decide to undertake a project of your own.

> **Key point!**
>
> When doing any kind of project, QI, or research, background reading is key: engage with the seminal and recent literature on the methodology, methods, and techniques you use.

- The Model for Improvement approach (referred to as a PDSA cycle approach)

This is arguably the most common way by which healthcare practitioners carry out QI work. Although originating outside healthcare, the focus of this approach resides in what the project is aiming to accomplish, establishing that the change leads to improvement, and ascertaining what changes are necessary to establish that improvement (Silver et al., 2016).

When undertaking a QI project based on the Model for Improvement approach, you need small cycles of work. These have been identified in the literature as the PDSA cycle (Varkey et al., 2007) and the four letters each represent a practical step in the process:

- **Plan** – the team provides clear objectives and develops a plan to carry out their test cycle.
- **Do** – carry out the test and document the process, problems, unexpected observations, and analyse the data.

- **Study** – create a summary of what was learned.
- **Act** – identify and implement changes to be made.

> **Key point!**
>
> The PDSA cycle approach to improvement is typically most suitable when the QI problem has a clear cause and/or evidence-based solution.
>
> (Scoville and Little, 2014)

You may need to go through this cycle several times before you conclude your project, so take care to document decisions and outcomes in an iterative fashion along the way. Do not forget to engage your team as you work through the four elements of the cycle and consult the literature to support your work.

- **The Lean Model**

The Lean Model approach arose in commercial fields outside of health (Scoville and Little, 2014). The main aspect of this approach to QI is a reliance on continuous improvement and refers to distinguishing value-added activities from those that fail to add value (Silver et al., 2016).

> **Key point!**
>
> The Lean Model approach to QI is viewed as the most suitable for problems that are directly observable and where waste might be eliminated, as well as in situations where speed, flow, and efficiency are a priority.
>
> (Bercaw, 2022)

If you decide to use a Lean Model approach to QI, be mindful that this places staff at the centre of change, and those staff are actively involved and engaged in the process of improvement due to their knowledge and expertise in identifying areas for change (Silver et al., 2016).

- **The Six Sigma approach**

This approach to QI was developed in commercial environments and is credited to the company Motorola in the 1980s (Chassin, 1998). The Six Sigma method is a project-driven business strategy approach to managing the improvement of services, products, or processes by seeking to reduce organisational defects (Kwak and Anbari, 2006). It has become popular in times of economic recession, when organisations are seeking ways to limit expenditure and maintain cost-effectiveness; for example, to streamline healthcare delivery processes (Ettinger, 2001), and improve reimbursement claims to be timelier and more accurate (Lazarus and Butler, 2001). The design for the Six Sigma (DFSS) method has several steps, as outlined by Varkey et al. (2007):

- **Define** – create a project charter that defines the customer needs, scope, goals, success criteria, and team members while setting clear deadlines.
- **Measure** – create a data collection plan and collect data from appropriate sources.
- **Analyse** – data analysis.
- **Improve** – develop creative solutions and implement plans.
- **Control** – control the process by implementing guidelines, policies, and error-proofing strategies.

Some researchers (Senapati, 2004) also add an additional step at the end:

- **Report** – report the benefits of the change in process.

Healthcare services are a key area where Six Sigma has been adopted, and it is a good match due to factors including the importance of reducing the possibility of medical errors. However, researchers who have used Six Sigma principles point out that the value of this approach is not just to ascertain and identify defects or problems, but primarily to improve overall management performance (Wang, 2008).

Doing QI within your organisation

As we noted earlier, to do your QI project effectively you will need a team, where different members occupy specific roles. However, that is only part of the picture, as successful QI activity relies heavily on the structure, commitment, and ethos of your healthcare organisation. In the UK, many National Health Service (NHS) trusts have a dedicated part of the service committed to QI because it is part of the national agenda through the Care Quality Commission (CQC, 2024). Your organisation may already have one of these services, but if not, you might be instrumental in helping your organisation create one.

Limitations of QI

While we advocate the value of QI in healthcare and have illustrated some of the benefits of doing a QI project, we note there are limitations. This is because the overall impact of QI in healthcare remains mixed, which may reflect poor fidelity to established QI methods (Dixon-Woods and Martin, 2016), and because many QI projects fail to lead to improvement interventions (Jones et al., 2019). As you continue to read this book, we hope to help you develop some critical thinking skills, so you can critically appraise the literature you read. So, we start here in helping you think critically about QI. We provide a list of some of the possible limitations, as noted by Dixon-Woods and Martin (2016):

- A lot of QI work is undertaken as time-limited, small-scale projects and as part of professional accreditation requirements. It can lack "buy-in" from organisational leadership and decision-makers. Trainee professionals do not have the resources or power to promote the kind of change necessary.
- There are risks related to the perceptions of QI, with some staff seeing it as a "series of bounded, time-limited events rather than a continuous commitment, and overly focused on 'innovation' rather than replication" (p. 192). Treating QI as a series of small local projects can lead to different solutions to the same problem.
- The accumulation of knowledge and learning through QI work is not always shared across the service or similar organisations. If a QI project does lead to change, then the learning should be shared in an accessible way.
- Frequently, QI interventions are viewed in a narrow way, like checklists, thus overlooking the impact of context in intervention implementation. It is helpful to have an appreciation of the wider social and cultural context for improvement to work. The solution does not lie with individuals alone but with structural change, initiated and sustained through leadership and advocacy.

Clinical audit

Clinical audits are a form of QI, and these are used to assess clinical effectiveness (Jones et al., 2019). An audit typically involves a QI process designed to measure care against a predetermined standard (a benchmark) to enable services to act to improve care and monitor ongoing sustained improvement against those standards (Gerrish and Lacey, 2010). In other words, you might choose to undertake an audit to investigate whether a service, or service activity or intervention aligns with agreed standards so you can identify any improvements that need to be made (Health Foundation, 2015). The aim of an audit, therefore, is to determine whether current practice meets best standards so that actions might be taken if necessary (Moule, Armoogum, Dodd et al., 2016). Audits often follow "cycles": data are collected on one occasion, action is then taken depending on what it shows (for example, the need for staff training), and further data is collected to evaluate changes that occurred.

Audits can be conducted at a local level but can also be conducted regionally or nationally (Health Foundation, 2015). The Health Foundation notes that knowledge generated by the audit, however, is usually only applicable to the context in which it was conducted, and the results generated from one are not necessarily generalisable beyond that. If you do decide you want to conduct a clinical audit, then you will need to involve your organisational governance structures. The need for an audit is typically identified via your organisation's "clinical audit plan", which is part of the broader clinical governance and quality monitoring processes (Moule et al., 2016).

Service evaluation

A service evaluation is an evaluation that can be conducted before, during, and after an intervention or activity and examines the quality of the content, the delivery process, and the impact to assess the worth or value of it (Research Councils UK, 2011). Service evaluations are a common approach to examining the quality of a service in a healthcare setting and of ascertaining the usefulness of healthcare interventions. Indeed, evaluations have become an important contributor to healthcare provision and reflect a growing trend among healthcare providers to determine the quality and effectiveness of services and frontline care delivery (Moule et al., 2016). In this way, evaluation is a valuable aspect of QI, as it can help to solve problems, inform decision-making, and build knowledge, with the improvement of care as the guiding concern (Health Foundation, 2015). A service evaluation is concerned with assessing whether the service offered is delivering what it is expected to offer and to establish the standards under which that service operates (Health Regulation Authority, 2013).

The purpose of a service evaluation is to rigorously review a specific aspect of an existing service and to form an appraisal of how well the service is meeting its aims and objectives (Healthcare Quality Improvement Partnership, 2011), determining aspects of a service that are effective and where improvement may be required (Moule et al., 2016). As such, evaluations capture useful insights and generate local knowledge which can help steer the development of new ways of working (Health Foundation, 2015).

If you are going to conduct a service evaluation, you need to ascertain what kind suits your needs. There are different types of evaluation, and these are referred to in slightly different ways depending on which literature you engage with. We provide two tables that describe the different types of evaluation, Table 2.2. and Table 2.3.

There are different methods you can use to conduct your service evaluation, and these can be quantitative, qualitative, or mixed methods, with your choice depending on what it is you are intending to measure or explore (Moule and Goodman, 2014). As is the case when you are doing empirical research, you need to select methods and sources of data that will address your service evaluation questions (Health Foundation, 2015). Ultimately, the results of your service evaluation can be used to inform local decision-making (Twycross and Shorten, 2014).

Qualitative research
We have deliberately kept this section of the chapter brief, as the rest of the book from this point onwards is devoted to providing you with a foundation for doing qualitative research in the context of health and illness, including signposting to specialist literature. This short section is therefore designed to simply introduce you to the concept of research as it relates to QI, service evaluation, and audit, and how it is different from them, while giving you some context as to what qualitative research is and what its benefits are.

If you choose to do a qualitative research project, it will be because you are probably interested in the perspectives, beliefs, opinions, views, perceptions, feelings, and lived experiences of certain stakeholders relevant to the field of health. These may be the colleagues you work with, specific professional groups, wider professionals working in related areas, advocates or political representatives, or the populations experiencing the health phenomenon of interest. Typically, as a qualitative researcher, you will be asking "how" and "why" questions to generate data that will provoke insights and ideas, raise further questions, inform change, or generate theories (LaDonna, Artino, and Balmer, 2021).

Table 2.2 Four types of evaluation (identified and described by Health Foundation, 2015)

Type	Description
Summative	This has the function of summing up the overall effect of an intervention and is conducted at the end of its implementation when data are available. *An example of this was conducted by Nazar, Nazar, Simpson et al. (2016) to assess whether community pharmacists in the UK were able to manage out-of-hours patient requests for emergency repeat prescriptions for medication. Results showed that pharmacists were content to provide the service, patients were happy, and the cost was substantially lower than emergency prescriptions being filled by other services in the NHS.*
Formative	This type is designed to help form or shape an intervention and is used as the intervention evolves so that modifications can be applied. *An example of this was conducted by Henderson, Hess, Mehra, and Hawke (2020) to understand the facilitators and barriers to the implementation of community-based service hubs for youth. Focusing on the YouthCan IMPACT project, this formative service evaluation identified the importance of previous positive working relationships and that investment of resources from partnering organisations is essential to consider in developing the work of the service hubs.*
Rapid cycle	This is a type of formative evaluation that uses "single loop learning" wherein goals are relatively fixed but details on how to obtain them may be refined. Methods are utilised to decide whether an intervention is effective, and the aim is continuous improvement by experimenting with different adaptations. *An example of this was conducted by Kathuria, Herbst, Seth et al. (2021) using two rapid-cycle evaluations over the first six months of an inpatient Tobacco Treatment Consult service to address cigarette smoking at Boston Medical Centre. The quick loop learning approach helped clinician-researchers to understand the hospital's priorities, gain leadership buy-in, and recognise implementation challenges early to make real-time adaptations and create an acceptable clinical workflow.*
Developmental	This involves a "double loop learning". Innovation theories and assumptions become revised over time during the evaluation, and the goals of the intervention may also require change. This is also a type of formative evaluation that facilitates real-time (or close to it) feedback to the team. During this kind of evaluation, activities should be documented with the short-term consequences, and processes and outcomes should be identified. There should be the development of intervention, theory of change, and occasionally the aims of the initiative should be modified. This is well-suited to complex environments looking for innovative solutions or social change. *An example of this was conducted by Jones et al. (2015) where the authors argued that a community-centred developmental evaluation approach was required to evaluate service innovation in healthcare provision for remote communities in Australia. For these communities, fixed interventions and predetermined programme deliverables were not considered to be meeting the complex needs of service users. With higher levels of health risk and disease burden, these communities also had limited access to health services. These had contributed to children having speech and motor skill delays. The developmental evaluation design enabled researchers to evaluate how to effectively respond to these complexities and led to the development of a new approach to providing essential health services that was aligned to community need.*

Table 2.3 Two further types of evaluation

Type	Description
Process	This reviews the implementation of changes made to your practice and evaluates how the activities are enacted so that you can explore whether this was intended in your original plan (Moule et al., 2016).
Impact	This type of evaluation has its focus on the short-term and long-term outcomes of the service or the project and ascertains if that service or project is meeting its intended aims and goals (Billings, 2000).

There are three broad types of qualitative research as described by Hesse-Biber (2017) and we outline these in Table 2.4.

In the context of health, it has been argued that there is a sub-discipline referred to as qualitative health research that is distinguishable from other forms of qualitative inquiry (Morse, 2010). We use the term "qualitative health research" for our book to capture this. Qualitative health research has been defined by Rolfe, Ramsden, Banner, and Graham (2018, p. 1) as being "the collection and systematic analysis of non-quantitative data about peoples' experiences of health or illness and the healthcare system". They argue that qualitative health research should incorporate the perspectives and experiences of key stakeholders (including patients/service users) into the design and process of the project, should be inclusive and diverse, and should treat participants as equal partners in the process.

We argue that qualitative health research, while maintaining many of the general aspects of all forms of qualitative inquiry, is distinctive for several reasons:

Table 2.4 Types of qualitative research (Hesse-Biber, 2017)

Type	Overview
Exploratory	When there is a limited research literature regarding a certain topic, it can be useful to explore this under-researched area to gain some preliminary insights about the issues that can refine a focus and shape future directions.
Explanatory	Based on prior knowledge or assumptions, an approach may be used that asks specific questions that relate to what is known to explain that issue further. This kind of work investigates the how or why of phenomena and to analyse patterns that might guide further work.
Descriptive	This type of work focuses on developing "thick descriptions" about the experiences and lives of participants. The focus is on describing situations, problems, and experiences rather than relationships or associations.

- In most cases health research is applied, in the sense that there is often a practical goal of the project to inform, shape, or support an area of healthcare practice, or to improve the lives of those with health conditions.
- Health research often involves healthcare professionals as gatekeepers, co-researchers, or, in some cases, leading the research, and therefore the role of these individuals will heavily shape the knowledge produced.
- Health research frequently explores "sensitive" research topics and is likely to involve populations who are "vulnerable". We are not taking these terms for granted, as they should be critically questioned, and we do return to these later in the book. Nonetheless, health research will have ethical issues and potential safeguarding concerns that need a great deal of attention.

We now encourage you to reflect on why you are doing qualitative research and what you want to learn from reading this book. Please consult the reflective activity in Box 2.5 and, in your research diary you started earlier, try to answer the questions.

Box 2.5

Reflective activity on choosing qualitative research

Try to answer these questions as honestly as you can and document your answers in your research diary.

1. What do you think is the main value of qualitative approaches to research?
2. What is the main motivation for you to undertake your research project?
3. What do you think the value of your project will be?

To help support your thinking we also asked a clinical practitioner, Dr Isobel Moore, to reflect on her motivations and experiences of getting started in qualitative health research. Her response can be seen in Box 2.6.

Box 2.6

The practitioner perspective of Dr Moore

Dr Isobel Moore is a Clinical Psychologist working in adult community mental health teams (CMHTs) in the UK National Health Service. She is interested in conceptual issues in psychology and clinical practice, relational dynamics in mental health care, and service user voice and participation.

I developed my interest in qualitative research during my clinical doctorate. I identify with the "reflective practitioner" model and value the questions and answers qualitative research enables. For example, while on a training placement in a community mental health team, I conducted a service evaluation on the perspectives of members of the multi-disciplinary team on ending work with service users, which helped inform considerations of how the clinical psychology service could support the wider team in handling endings and the discharge process. My thesis research took a critical, conceptual orientation, exploring professionals' constructions of "female autism" as a concept and individuals' identity narratives at the intersection of autism and gender: one intention was to encourage critical reflection on how we as healthcare professionals position ourselves in relation to concepts of "autism" and "gender" and the clinical, ethical, and political ramifications of this.

I have been fortunate to have opportunities to collaborate on both academic research and practice-based service evaluation projects with more established researchers from different clinical and academic disciplines, and these partnerships helped me to build my understanding of the practicalities of how to do qualitative research and quality improvement activity in healthcare. I have seen how qualitative and interdisciplinary approaches can add value to services as well as to individual job roles (in terms of task variety, continuing professional development, opportunities to carve out areas of special interest, to develop projects, and to build partnerships and connections within and across services). Qualitative research offers a means to engage with meaning-making, stories, language, ideas, and how we conceptualise experiences: this is relevant to seeking and amplifying the voices of people accessing our services, understanding their perspectives and needs, gathering their feedback, and creating opportunities for involvement, collaboration, and co-production; it also helps us in understanding how we and our colleagues think about and approach the work in healthcare, and how this shapes how services operate.

Interdisciplinary research

We advocate that many research problems are best addressed by research teams with a range of skills and expertise, which involve collaboration between individuals from different disciplinary backgrounds. The more complex the problem, the more beneficial interdisciplinary working may be. A blended team will bring different disciplinary knowledge, methodological preferences and skills, and multiple research vocabularies. The ways in which a researcher explores and interprets data are influenced by their disciplinary background (Alvesson and Skölberg, 2000), and thus taking an interdisciplinary approach to a research problem is helpful because mono-discipline approaches are not able to fully account for all the parts of the puzzle (Tobi and Kampen, 2018). Indeed, there are calls from various fields to recognise the need to find solutions to critical questions by integrating different disciplinary knowledge and skills (Lakhani, Benzies, and Hayden, 2012), while recognising that interdisciplinary teams may find it challenging to reconcile theoretical and disciplinary tensions and consequently need to talk openly about these aspects of the research and recognise the lack of a common disciplinary language (Massey, Alpass, Flett et al., 2006).

If you plan to be part of an interdisciplinary research team, then you will play a role in ensuring that your team has purpose, clear goals, and acts with mutual respect, which relies on strong leadership, reflection, and good communication (Lakhani et al., 2012). It is argued that interdisciplinary research provides a collaborative foundation to address a research problem and provides for accountability within institutions (Huutoniemi, 2016). To accomplish addressing a research problem, therefore, it is essential to work on breaking down barriers to interdisciplinary working by managing paradigmatic differences and tensions in collaboration (Fischer, Tobi, and Ronteltap, 2011), otherwise there will be challenges to provide translatable messages for application (Kvarnström, 2008).

We would like to point out that in the literature, this interdisciplinarity within qualitative research (and within mixed-methods research more specifically, as discussed later) is sometimes referred to as bricolage. Technically, the French concept of *bricoleur* refers to the creative use of available tools to complete a task (Kincheloe, 2005), but in the research context this has been adapted. Bricoleurs recognise that the production of monological knowledge, that is, unilateral perspectives and single methods, fails to account for the complex relationship between material reality and human perspectives or perceptions (Kincheloe, 2005). Hence, the idea of bricolage indicates the significance and importance of interdisciplinary working, and yet in itself does not indicate an absence of disciplinarity (Pinar, 2001). Rather, the bricoleur attempts to identify and develop strategies that go beyond the dimensionality of an individual method or an individual discipline (Kincheloe and Berry, 2004). In this way, "bricoleurs move beyond the blinds of particular disciplines and peer through a conceptual window to a new world of research and knowledge production" (Kincheloe, 2005, p. 323).

As a clinician-researcher, you may be working in a professional context where you work alongside people from different professional disciplines. Depending on the focus of your planned research project, it may be very valuable to create a research team that includes people from other disciplines. For example, a research project in the community may be developed through the partnership of nurses and social workers, or in an inpatient setting medical doctors and occupational therapists may work together. Whatever combination of people you recruit for your research team, consider the value that each professional perspective might bring in both the data collection and analysis phases. Additionally, if you are applying for funding for research, often funding bodies appreciate that your research team is interdisciplinary, as they can appreciate the value of multiple perspectives for the outcomes of the research project. If you place a strong value on the input of the people who will benefit from the research to decide on the research focus and the way that the data are collected, you may also want to include members of the participant population in your research team.

Who is research for and who benefits?
Research conducted by clinicians working in the field of physical and/or mental health has great benefit to those experiencing health conditions, their families, and wider society. Health research is subject to public and government scrutiny, as there are potential risks as well as possible multiple benefits. Much of the discussion regarding the benefits of qualitative research has been in relation to the perceived "trade-off" between the risk to the individual (such as a possible lack of privacy) and the wider societal benefits (Aitken, Jorre, Pagliari et al., 2018). When examining public attitudes towards health research, there has been a general perception that health research should have public benefits or at least potential benefits (Aitken et al., 2016). We return to the issues of risk and benefit when we discuss research ethics later in the book.

The benefits of qualitative health research are important for you to think about. This is because much of the qualitative health research conducted tends to be motivated by practical or applied goals rather than being conceptually driven (Chafe, 2017). Indeed, in the qualitative methodological literature a distinction has been made between "pure" and "applied" research, whereby applied research has a set of aims that reflect the goal of solving practical problems (Green and Thorogood, 2009). Evidently, qualitative health researchers can manage the applied implications of their studies but also work at the conceptual level (Morse, 2012).

Notably, some participant groups that have been heavily researched strongly argue that researchers ought to move away from a position of researching "on" populations and instead take a lead from those groups, asking them first what questions they might be interested in finding out more about. As researchers, our relationship with participants is important to consider in terms of the ethics involved at the outset of the research project. Arguably it is unethical to start a research project without a clear vision of how the findings from the project will be of practical benefit – particularly to the population sampled. A population-led research position acknowledges the privileged position that the clinician-researcher has in terms of knowledge and access to resources. By partnering with participants, we can support these groups of people to join with us in establishing research goals and priorities.

Author reflections and concluding remarks

In closing, we recognise that there has been a lot of information to absorb from this chapter. By this point, you should be able to see how you, as a practitioner, have an instrumental role in driving the development of new knowledge and promoting changes to practice via QI activity or research. As we conclude, we provide you with some points to remember as you go forward with reading this book in Box 2.7.

Box 2.7

Things to remember about QI, audit, service evaluation, and research

From your reading should now be able to differentiate QI, clinical audit, service evaluation, and qualitative research. There are some points we have made, and we draw your attention to these here:

- QI is fundamental for changing healthcare practice and developing new local knowledge.
- QI projects involve a team of practitioners and stakeholders. They must be carefully planned to ensure their effectiveness.
- Clinical audits measure current practices against predefined standards. Service evaluations can be national, regional, or local and evaluate a practice, intervention, or service in a specific context. Research aims to generate new knowledge, theories, and inform practice and policy development.
- There are different types of service evaluation: summative, formative, rapid cycle, developmental, process, and impact.
- As a qualitative researcher you need to consider how you can work in partnership with your participants and key stakeholders for your project.

To close this chapter, Nikki reflects on the value of clinician-researchers being involved in QI activity, service evaluations, and audits and how these are important in healthcare settings.

From Nikki

As a Clinical Psychologist, I have been involved in several mental health service evaluations and clinical audits in different places where I have worked. It can be helpful to have a baseline assessment of where the organisation is currently performing on a particular measure, whether it is demographic (i.e. how well the service is reaching certain target demographics in the population), or whether the outcome measures of success for each client are analysed to see where there are areas for improvement. Where there is a need for time and/or funding to be released, pragmatically, it is often easier to obtain the resources needed to conduct a QI project because managers and commissioners of services can easily see where the benefits may lie. Where the focus is on improving the quality, efficiency, and cost-effectiveness of the service, providing the finances, time, or other requirements is usually understood as an investment rather than a drain on resources. QI is a good place for the clinician-researcher to get involved and is usually conducted on a small scale locally compared to larger-scale qualitative research projects that involve interviews or focus groups, for example. Because QI tends to use existing information and documents, access to data is often relatively straightforward, and there may be an administrator in the organisation who can also be released for some time to help with the project.

Although QI has a lot of benefits and will increase the efficiency and quality of the service provided, it is still important not to rush the planning stages. Make sure that you have consulted widely in the first instance to make sure that you are targeting your energy in the right place. Take time to think about who needs to be involved and when, and what resources you need. Think about what time of year is the best time to do it and what other pressures or demands there might be at certain times. When you are clear about your focus, your team, and your resources, collect your data systematically. The end results will only be as good as the information you have collected. When decisions are being made about changes to implement within the organisation, ensure that people are clear about why and what the benefits will be. Ideally you will also have a service user involved at the stage where you plan what the improvements will be as an outcome of the study.

References

Aitken, M., Jorre J., Pagliari C., Jepson, R., and Cuningham-Burley, S. (2016) Public responses to the sharing and linkage of health data for research purposes: A systematic review and thematic synthesis of qualitative studies. *BMC Medical Ethics*, 17(1), 73.

Aitken, M., Porteous, C., Creamer, E., and Cunningham-Burley, S. (2018). Who benefits and how? Public expectations of public benefits from data-intensive health research. *Big Data & Society*, 5, 1–12.

Alvesson, M., and Sköldberg K. (2000). *Reflexive methodology: New vistas for qualitative research*. London: Sage.

Atkinson, S., Ingham, J., Cheshire, M., and Went, S. (2010). Defining quality and quality improvement. *Clinical Medicine*, 10(6), 537–539.

Bercaw, R. (2022). *Taking improvement from the assembly line to healthcare: The application of Lean within the healthcare industry* (2nd ed.). Boca Raton, FL: Taylor and Francis.
Billings, J. (2000). Community development: A critical review of approaches to evaluation. *Journal of Advanced Nursing, 31*(2), 472–480.
Care Quality Commission. (2024). Guidance for NHS trusts and foundation trusts: Assessing the well-led key question. https://www.cqc.org.uk/guidance-regulation-nhs-key-question-well-led-learning
Chafe, R. (2017). The value of qualitative description in health services and policy research. *Healthcare Policy, 12*(3), 12–18.
Chassin, M. (1998). Is health care ready for Six Sigma quality? *The Milbank Quarterly, 76*, 565–591.
Dixon-Woods, M., and Martin, G. (2016). Does quality improvement improve quality? *Future Hospital Journal, 3*(3), 191–194.
Ettinger, W. (2001). Six sigma adapting GE's lesson to health care. *Trustee, 54*(8), 10–16.
Fischer, A., Tobi, H., and Ronteltap, A. (2011). When natural met social: A review of collaboration between the natural and social sciences. *Interdisciplinary Science Reviews, 36*(4), 341–358.
Gerrish, K., and Lacey A. (2010). Research and development in nursing. In K. Gerrish and A. Lacey (Eds.), *The research process in nursing* (6th ed., pp. 3–11). Oxford: Wiley-Blackwell.
Green, J., and Thorogood, N. (2009). *Qualitative methods for health research* (2nd ed.). Thousand Oaks, CA: Sage.
Health Foundation (2015). *Evaluation: What to consider commonly asked questions about how to approach evaluation of quality improvement in health care*. London: Health Foundation.
Health Research Authority (HRA). (2013). *Defining research*. London: HRA.
Healthcare Quality Improvement Partnership (2011). HQIP guide for clinical audit, research and service review. https://www.hqip.org.uk/resource/hqip-guide-for-clinical-audit-research-and-service-review/
Henderson, J., Hess, M., Mehra, K., and Hawke, L. (2020). From planning to implementation of the YouthCan IMPACT project: A formative evaluation. *The Journal of Behavioral Health Services & Research, 47*, 216–229.
Hesse-Biber, S. (2017). *The practice of qualitative research* (3rd ed.). London: Sage.
Huutoniemi, K. (2016). Interdisciplinarity as academic accountability: Prospects for quality control across disciplinary boundaries. *Social Epistemology, 30*(2), 163–185.
Jones, D., Lyle, D., Brunero, C., McAllister, L., Webb, T., and Riley, S. (2015). Improving health and education outcomes for children in remote communities: A cross-sector and developmental evaluation approach. *Gateways: International Journal of Community Research & Engagement, 8*(1), 1–22.
Jones, B., Vaux, E., and Olsson-Brown, A. (2019). How to get started in quality improvement. *British Medical Journal, 364*, k5408.
Kathuria, H., Herbst, N., Seth, B., Clark, K., Helm, E. D., Zhang, M., O'Donnell, C., Fitzgerald, C., Itchapurapu, I., Waite, M., Wong, C., Swamy, L., Olson, J., Mishuris, R., and Wiener, R. (2021). Rapid cycle evaluation and adaptation of an inpatient tobacco treatment service at a US safety-net hospital. *Implementation Research & Practice, 2*.
Kincheloe, J. (2005). On to the next level: Continuing the conceptualization of the bricolage. *Qualitative Inquiry, 11*(3), 323–350.
Kincheloe, J., and Berry, K. (2004). *Rigour and complexity in educational research; Conceptualizing the bricolage*. Maidenhead: Open University Press.
Kvarnström, S. (2008). Difficulties in collaboration: A critical incident study of interprofessional healthcare teamwork. *Journal of Interprofessional Care, 22*(2), 191–203.
Kwak, Y., and Anbari, F. (2006). Benefits, obstacles, and future of six sigma approach. *Technovation, 26*(5–6), 708–715.
LaDonna, K., Artino, A., and Balmer, D. (2021). Beyond the guise of saturation: Rigor and qualitative interview data. *Journal of Graduate Medical Education, 13*(5), 607–611.

Lakhani, J., Benzies, K., and Hayden, A. (2012). Attributes of interdisciplinary research teams: A comprehensive review of the literature. *Clinical & Investigative Medicine, 35*, 260–265.

Lazarus, I., and Butler, K. (2001). The promise of six sigma. *Managed Healthcare Executive, 11*(9), 22–26.

Massey, C., Alpass, F., Flett, R., Lewis, K., Morriss, S., and Sligo, F. (2006). Crossing fields: The case of a multi-disciplinary research team. *Qualitative Research, 6*(2), 131–149.

Morse, J. (2010). How different is qualitative health research from qualitative research? Do we have a subdiscipline? *Qualitative Health Research, 20*(11), 1459–1468.

Morse, J. M. (2012). *Qualitative health research: Creating a new discipline.* New York: Routledge.

Moule, P., Armoogum, J., Dodd, E., Donskoy, A.-L., Douglass, E., Taylor, J., and Turton, P. (2016). Practical guidance on undertaking a service evaluation. *Nursing Standard, 30*(45), 46–51.

Moule, P., and Goodmand, M. (2014). *Nursing research: An introduction* (2nd ed.). London: Sage.

Nazar, H., Nazar, Z., Simpson, J., Yeung, A., and Whittlesea, C. (2016). Summative service and stakeholder evaluation of an NHS-funded community Pharmacy Emergency Repeat Medication Supply Service (PERMSS). *BMJ Open, 6*(1), e009736.

O'Reilly, M., and Parker, N. (2014). *Doing mental health research with children and adolescents: A guide to qualitative methods.* London: Sage.

Pinar, W. (2001). The researcher as bricoleur: The teacher as a public intellectual. *Qualitative Inquiry, 7*(6), 696–700.

Rolfe, D. E., Ramsden, V. R., Banner, D., and Graham, I. D. (2018). Using qualitative health research methods to improve patient and public involvement and engagement in research. *Research Involvement & Engagement, 4*, 1–8.

Research Councils UK (2011). Evaluation: Practical guidelines. https://www.ukri.org/publications/evaluation-practical-guidelines/

Scoville, R., and Little, K. (2014). *Comparing lean and quality improvement.* IHI White paper. Cambridge, MA: Institute for Healthcare Improvement.

Senapati, N. (2004). Quality and reliability corner: Six Sigma: Myths and realities. *The International Journal of Quality & Reliability Management, 21*(6/7), 683–690.

Silver, S., Harel, Z., McQuillan, R., Weizman, A., Thomas, A., Chertow, G., Nesrellah, G., Bell, C., and Chan, C. (2016). How to begin a quality improvement project. *Clinical Journal of American Society of Nephrology, 11*, 893–900.

Tobi, H., and Kampen, J. (2018). Research design: The methodology for interdisciplinary research framework. *Quality & Quantity, 52*, 1209–1225.

Twycross, A., and Shorten, A. (2014). Service evaluation, audit and research: What is the difference? *Evidence Based Nursing, 17*(3), 65–66.

Varkey, P., Reller, K., and Resar, R. (2007). Basics of quality improvement in health care. *Mayo Clinic Proceedings, 82*(6), 735–739.

Wang, H. (2008, October). A review of six sigma approach: Methodology, implementation, and future research. In *2008 4th International Conference on Wireless Communications, Networking and Mobile Computing* (pp. 1–4). IEEE.

CHAPTER 3

Theory in qualitative research

> **Learning objectives**
>
> This chapter enables the reader to:
>
> - Appreciate the meaning of core theoretical and philosophical concepts associated with qualitative research.
> - Identify the importance of theory.
> - Recognise the meaning of ontology, epistemology, and axiology.
> - Differentiate methodology and method.
> - Critically assess the value of interdisciplinary research.
> - Critically assess the benefits of qualitative research.

Introduction

In our work as lecturers and research supervisors, when we broach the subject of the philosophy of research to students or clinical trainees it tends to send them into a slight panic. Understanding theory in research can be a challenge and the theoretical literature can be complex. Nonetheless, if you are going to do a piece of qualitative research, then you need to be mindful of the theories related to your work. When we talk about *theory*, we mean all the ways researchers formulate and express their findings (Risjord, 2022). Theory is essential to research as it provides a "lens" through which the researcher can explore problems and social issues and provides a framework of ideas for a research project (Reeves, Albert, Kuper, and Hodges, 2008). In this chapter, our discussion is designed to help you to understand more about the choices you will need to make in your own project. We will guide you through common theoretical concepts associated with qualitative research and some of the wider debates that are useful for you to know about in the context of health research. We will address epistemology, ontology and explanatory theory, looking at how different schools of thought (at least in broad terms) to support you to meaningfully underpin your own work with theory.

Paradigmatic considerations

The concept of a "paradigm" will be relevant for you as a clinician-researcher doing qualitative research. A paradigm is a set of basic beliefs or a worldview that defines how someone, or indeed a discipline, perceives the nature of the world and a person's place within it. It has been noted that in the natural sciences, awareness of anomalies leads scientists to question the established paradigm, and as a new one becomes accepted, a paradigm shift occurs (Kuhn, 1970). Researchers use different labels for paradigms which sometimes overlap; so, paradigms can be thought of as related schools of thought rather than rigid frameworks (Glesne, 2015).

There are two elements of paradigms, as noted by Paul and Elder (2020). The first is that paradigms differ in their assumptions about reality, the nature of the relationship between the knower and what is known, and how knowledge is constructed. The second is that paradigms shape, restrict, and promote aspects of inquiry. The research paradigm, in turn, relates to the ontological question about the nature of reality, the epistemological question about what can be known, and the methodological question about techniques to construct what can be known (Guba and Lincoln, 2004). As such, when thinking about theory in research, we need to consider:

- What do we believe about what can be known about the nature of the world?
- What do we believe about how we can produce knowledge about that world?
- What are the appropriate techniques to generate knowledge about the world?

In terms of assumptions regarding what can be known about the nature of the world, these questions refer to *ontology*, or the nature of things (Hollis, 1994). Hollis further noted that, regarding the production of knowledge about the world, these questions refer to *epistemology*, which is about the nature of knowledge and its relationship with the knower. Hollis argued that appropriate ways to generate knowledge about the world refer to *methodology*, which denotes the processes and techniques through which we acquire knowledge. It is helpful for you to understand, then, that your ontological and epistemological position within your research paradigm will, in different ways, determine the entire direction of your project (Hussey and Hussey, 1997).

Thus, one of the first choices researchers face is whether to take a quantitative approach or a qualitative one. Some scholars have argued that it is problematic that quantitative and qualitative methods are pitched as "being in competition with each other" (Onwuegbuzie and Leech, 2005, p. 267). Onwuegbuzie and Leech argued this creates an unhelpful polarisation where researchers position themselves in one camp or the other. The two approaches view the nature of reality differently, with quantitative theorists contending (or working from the assumption that) there is a single objective reality that can be measured via scientific principles, and qualitative theorists promoting a stance that there are multiple constructed realities with different meanings for different people, with the interpretation of those realities being dependent upon the researcher (Onwuegbuzie and Leech, 2005). As such, Onwuegbuzie and Leech proposed we stop thinking in this binary way and select approaches based on the research question, the type of knowledge needed, and the best methods to arrive at that knowledge. In determining a suitable paradigm, there are several dichotomies to consider.

- Inductive versus deductive

It is generally agreed among researchers that you can choose between a deductive or an inductive paradigm (Hussey and Hussey, 1997). Hussey and Hussey argued that research within a deductive paradigm is when the conceptual and theoretical structure is developed first and then tested via empirical observation. Thus, deductive research moves from the general to the specific. They described research within the inductive paradigm as one in which theory is developed by observing an empirical reality and inferences are induced from specific circumstances. In other words, the deductive researcher does their work in a "top-down" manner, starting with theory, to hypotheses, to data (Creswell and Piano-Clark, 2007). In terms of paradigms, quantitative research tends to be deductive in style and qualitative research tends to be inductive, although there are variations (Soiferman, 2010).

- Empiricist/naturalist versus rationalist

As a foundation for research, science can be construed in terms of how knowledge is acquired, how knowledge is tested, and how knowledge of the world is deepened. In this way, research has been influenced by naturalist ideas which envision research in social and health sciences as (needing to be) influenced by the natural sciences. Rationalism refers to the idea that humans can acquire knowledge due to their capacity to reason and is grounded in the work of Plato (Bernard, 2011). From this position, researchers take the perspective that there is a concrete reality that exists *a priori* or before we engage in research to discover what that reality is (Bernard, 2011). Rationalism is therefore a top-down approach (Hjørland, 2005).

The opposing position to rationalism is empiricism, which argues that what we know is because of the accumulation of experiences that, when added together, allow us to make generalisations (Bernard, 2011). This thinking is grounded in the work of Hume and Locke and is a bottom-up approach (Hjørland, 2005). Empiricism argues that knowledge is not present prior to experience and that knowledge of the world cannot be acquired through reasoning alone. Thus, empiricism is central to the naturalist conception of science (Bernard, 2011). Note, however, that whilst the terms naturalism and empiricism are frequently used interchangeably, empiricism has a narrower meaning than naturalism, and we encourage you to read further on this if it is pertinent to your project.

- Objective versus subjective

Objectivism is a position that considers that reality exists independent of human contact with it. Objectivism claims that a researcher can obtain objective knowledge, and thus scientific methods are needed that are replicable and reliable (Diesing, 1965). Alternatively, subjectivism takes a position that there is no underlying reality that exists independent of our perception of it. Thus, subjectivism considers that different viewpoints are alternative ways of approaching things (Ratner, 2002), advocating that the unique characteristic of human behaviour is its subjective meaningfulness (Diesing, 1965). So, as a clinician-researcher, think about the extent to which you are happy to embrace subjectivism in research, that is, the extent to which you influence the research process and outcome; or objectivism, a preference to try to eliminate any subjective interpretation or influence over the research findings.

- Etic versus emic

These two concepts are pertinent in research as they refer to two different approaches. Initially, the concepts were developed by Kenneth Pike, who coined the terms from the suffixes of the words phonetic and phonemic (Harris, 1976). The etic approach, which is also known as an outsider perspective, a deductive approach, or a top-down position, starts from the point of theory or hypotheses and promotes analyses that are expressed in terms of scientific categories (Lett, 1990). An emic approach, which is also known as an insider perspective, inductive approach, or bottom-up position, starts with the perspectives of participants and promotes analyses of accounts that are expressed as meaningful by members of a group or culture (Lett, 1990). An advantage of the etic approach is that researchers can compare contexts or populations, whereas the advantage of an emic approach is that it allows a focus on participant perspectives (Lett, 1990).

- Idiographic versus nomothetic

The philosopher Windelband proposed the concepts of idiographic and nomothetic in relation to different types of knowledge, using idiographic to refer to experiences of events as unique and not generalisable, and nomothetic as a kind of knowledge that locates generalities within a class of particulars from which theories can be derived (Robinson, 2011). Simply stated, idiographic methods focus on the individual, and nomothetic methods seek to provide explanations through discerning patterns in social phenomena. Although these may be complementary, they are often pitched as dichotomous categories (Robinson, 2011). The debates that dichotomise these concepts are rooted in psychology, as different branches of the field began to favour one over the other (Florell, 2019).

Before we go into more detail about qualitative theory, we encourage you to identify the gaps in your knowledge and think about how confident you feel about this aspect of research. We outline an activity in Box 3.1.

THEORY IN QUALITATIVE RESEARCH

> **Box 3.1**
>
> **Reflective activity on theory in qualitative research**
>
> We invite you at this point in the chapter to make a list of the knowledge you feel you need about philosophy, theory, and other related concepts in relation to qualitative research.
>
> How confident do you currently feel about being able to critically assess and formally decide which theories are underpinning your research project? Please write a few lines of reflection in your research diary.
>
> We hope that by the time you have finished reading this chapter, your confidence level will have increased.

An awareness of theory and an ability to critically assess it will sharpen your inquiry (Risjord, 2022), as the quality of your research project can depend greatly on how theory is integrated into your research design (Pope and Mays, 2020).

> **Key point!**
>
> These theoretical concepts and the practicalities of the research process that emanate from them apply across disciplines and different fields of clinical practice. They are relevant to both social and health sciences and remain pertinent in qualitative health research.

The role of theory in qualitative research

As a researcher who is also a clinician, understanding some of the arguments within the field will help you to make informed decisions for your own project. As we have already noted, when we discuss theory we are not referring to explanatory theories (for example, like those that seek to explain health behaviours or learning). Instead, we are referring to the broader ideas about the nature of reality, what research might allow you access to, the determination of what constitutes meaningful knowledge, and issues around language and how it operates (Braun and Clarke, 2022). Within the qualitative research community, there are two broad positions regarding to the role of theory:

1. Because of the inductive nature of qualitative research, there is an absence of theory during the early phases of the research process (Freshwater and Cahill, 2013). Qualitative research seeks an understanding of phenomena through the exploration of the lived experiences of the participants (Nguyen, Whitehead, Demody, and Saunders., 2022), and therefore care needs to be taken to ensure that the use of theory does not impose meaning or alter the understanding of that phenomenon (Bendassolli, 2014). According to this first perspective, to truly appreciate the multiple meanings that individuals construct about their social worlds, it is helpful to start without a theory (Creswell and Creswell, 2018).
2. Other qualitative researchers argue that intersubjectivity (the exchange of thoughts and feelings) and transparency (making all decisions visible) are central to qualitative

research, and because all knowledge is theory-laden, it is not possible for research to be fully inductive. Therefore, theory will always inform the research design (Pope and Mays, 2020). From this perspective, a failure to be clear on theoretical positions at the beginning of the research process might lead to purely descriptive information rather than the level of interpretation needed to answer "how" and "why" questions (King and Brook, 2017). Thus, drawing on theory in research is necessary to achieve rich description (Nguyen et al., 2022).

Notably, both positions appreciate the value of theory but differ in the extent to which they allow theory to inform the research process, at what point theory matters, and how theory is applied during the process. Nonetheless, all qualitative approaches contain theoretically embedded assumptions, and it is theory that gives the approach its analytical power (Braun and Clarke, 2022).

We suggest it will be beneficial for you to engage in further reading around research theory so you can arrive at a place where you feel comfortable with the theories inform your work. There are some practical strategies for the application of theory in qualitative research that we previously outlined (O'Reilly and Kiyimba, 2015) and we replicate these in Box 3.2. Note that the concepts of axiology, ontology, and epistemology are explained in more detail later in this chapter.

Box 3.2
Practical steps for the application of theory

We have previously recommended that in applying theory in your qualitative research project, you should (O'Reilly and Kiyimba, 2015):

- Try to have clarity about ontological, epistemological, and axiological positions in your research from the outset and continue to be transparent throughout your work.
- Read. It is necessary that you engage with the wider literature on theory in qualitative research and build your knowledge and understanding.
- Use your research diary to track your decisions related to theory and to make a note of useful references.
- Be consistent in your theoretical approach. Do not claim to be informed by a theoretical perspective and then write in ways that are inconsistent with it.
- Be reflexive and reflective throughout the research process (there is more on this in Chapter 9).

Research philosophy

Whilst we will not delve too deeply into the field of philosophy, some understanding of this will be useful to you when you are considering the role of theory in your qualitative health research project. Philosophy as a discipline tends to be divided into three domains (Risjord, 2022):

1. **Value theory** – this is concerned with issues regarding the source and justification of social values, norms, and rules.
2. **Epistemology** – relates to human knowledge, questioning what constitutes knowledge and how it is justified.
3. **Metaphysics** – is concerned with fundamental characteristics of the world, questioning whether humans have free will, what causes things, and rationality.

In the context of research, we are primarily concerned with the nature of knowledge and how it is produced. For any qualitative research project, there should be congruence theoretically across your work which is appropriately tied to the decisions you make as a researcher. In simple terms, the methods you choose need to be mapped against your research question, theory, design, and methodology (Ormston, Spencer, Barnard, and Snape, 2014). In this way, it is helpful to recognise that essentially qualitative research is an interpretative process, and data collection and analysis are the main mechanisms for *making* rather than discovering meaning (Ravitch and Riggan, 2012).

By this point in the chapter, we have already introduced several concepts and ideas about research philosophy and the role of theory in qualitative research. We encourage you to pause for a moment and reflect on what you have learnt so far and consolidate your learning in relation to your own work. We outline some things for you to remember based on the chapter so far in Box 3.3.

Box 3.3

Things to remember about philosophy and theory in qualitative research

- A paradigm is the overarching worldview within which your approach to research sits. Often this is implicit, but taking time to reflect on your contextual paradigm explicitly will improve the quality of your research by enabling you to be more transparent about your relationship with the object of study.
- The next thing to reflect on is whether you will approach your research to generate new knowledge from a "top-down" or "bottom-up" perspective. Put differently, do you wish to start with a theory and look for specific examples of it, or start with specific examples in what you observe and seek to understand what these instances might tell us about how things work in more general terms? Is it about developing a theory from the observation of specific instances rather than looking to evidence a theory by finding specific examples that support that theory?
- Each of these decisions is philosophical in nature. By this, we mean it is not already decided for you; you will need to engage with your own reflective process to decide what you believe and then approach your research from that philosophical position.
- All research is based on an underlying philosophical premise, which may be implicit or explicit. Identifying your philosophical standpoint before starting your research project and being explicit about what it is and why will make your research more robust.

Now that you have had an opportunity to remind yourself of some of the core concepts from the chapter, we encourage you to try the activity in Box 3.4 as a way of facilitating your engagement with the material.

> **Box 3.4**
>
> **Reflective activity on core concepts in research**
>
> One of the best ways to test your understanding is to write it out in your own words. We encourage you to try the activity below:
>
> - In your research diary, create your own glossary of concepts that are relevant to your project. Take each concept and define it in your own words. You can also cite articles or book chapters for future reference.
>
> As you read through this book, we encourage you to maintain this glossary and add new concepts as you develop your learning.

Axiology

Broadly, the concept of axiology is tied to philosophy and is embedded in ethics, aesthetics, and religion, which, when translated into a research context, relates to the researcher's beliefs about what is ethical and valuable (Killam, 2013). In that sense, axiology can be thought of as relating to normative judgements about what is "good" or "bad", or what is "beautiful" or "ugly" (Hart, 1971). As a researcher with clinical skills, you may not adopt these values, but there will be ethical principles and values that you hold to, either personally or culturally, that are drivers in how you approach the research process. For qualitative research, axiology is pertinent as it recognises the researcher is an instrument in the process of inquiry, and that the researcher influences all aspects of the process and decisions. Thus, the values the researcher brings to inquiry inevitably shape the project, and the researcher's personal ethical standpoint will affect their perspective on the world, which influences the ways they conduct research (Ponterotto, 2005).

> **Key point!**
>
> Note that your values and worldview are interconnected, and this will influence decisions you make about your research project.
>
> (Hill, 1984)

Qualitative research is clear that it is not possible for research to be neutral and will always inevitably be influenced by the researcher (Arneson, 2009). In doing your qualitative project, then, you need to be aware of your values and how they shape and influence your project. Maintaining your axiological integrity means a retention of values in transferring, translating, or synthesising research evidence (Kelly, Ellaway, Reid et al., 2018). One way to facilitate this is by using your reflexive research diary to capture your reflections and perspectives throughout the project (Zaidi and Larsen, 2019).

Ontology

A fundamental aspect of your research will be your ontological position, that is, the reflexive consideration of your own ontology as a starting point. Ontology refers to how the nature of reality and existence is understood, and ontological questions relate to what can be known about the world (Hesse-Biber and Leavy, 2004). The concept of ontology is linked to questions about whether reality exists independently from human interpretation (Ormston et al., 2014).

> **Key point!**
>
> Ontological assumptions are typically framed in terms of a dichotomy; on one hand, an objective reality exists independent of the researcher, and on the other, reality is subjective and negotiated.
>
> (Bryman, 2016)

There are slight differences in the literature about ontology but significant similarities in their meanings. Snape and Spencer (2003) outlined three main ontological positions:

- **Realism** – presupposes there is a reality existing independent of human thought or observation.
- **Idealism** – claims it is only possible to understand reality via the human mind or socially constructed meaning.
- **Materialism** – claims the real world does exist, but it is only the material (physical) world that can be thought of as real, whereas beliefs, values, and experiences come from the material world but do not shape it.

Other literature (see, for example, Hesse-Biber, 2017) have posited that the three ontological positions are:

- **Positivism** – claims the social world consists of patterns and that it is possible to establish causal relationships that can be tested through reliable methods.
- **Interpretivism** – claims the social world is continuously being constructed via social interaction, and social reality can only be understood through the perspectives of social actors.
- **A critical position** – claims social reality is constructed through discourse; discourse creates shifting fields of social power, and these discourses shape reality and our study of it.

To simplify, we differentiate realism and relativism, as, very broadly, these are the two main ways to think about reality. In (very) simple terms, in research, researchers tend to adopt either a realist or relativist position, in the sense that facts are accepted as real and independent (that is, objective) or that reality is relative (that is, subjective in nature). Realism proposes there is an independent reality that is separate from individuals' beliefs about it (Bryman, 2016), whereas relativism contests that reality is dependent on human construction and no reality can exist independently from it (Smith, 1983). The distinction is more complicated as realism has several variants which we outline in Table 3.1.

Like realism, relativism is not a single doctrine, but there is a common theme regarding the central aspects of experience, thought, and reality as relative to something else.

For relativists, reality does not exist independently of human experience, and therefore it is not possible to access things that are only accessible to us via our representations of them (Chen, Shek, and Bu., 2011).

> **Key point!**
>
> Relativism refers to the idea that there is no shared reality; rather, what we experience is a series of social constructions.
>
> (Edwards, Ashmore, and Potter, 2003)

Table 3.1 Variants of realism

Type	Description
Naïve realism	Claims that reality can be accurately and directly observed (Madill, Jordan, and Shirley, 2000).
Critical realism	Claims that reality is made up of different levels; first is the empirical domain of experiences encountered through the senses, second is the domain which exists regardless of observation, and third is the domain of underlying mechanisms and processes (Ormston et al., 2014).
Subtle realism	Claims that an external reality exists, but it is only possible to know this realism through the human mind and socially constructed meaning (Ormston et al., 2014).
Materialism	Recognises only material features, such as the physical features of the world. It holds that there is a reality, and experiences, values, and beliefs arise from the material but do not shape it (Ormston et al., 2014).

Epistemology

Tied to your ontological position will be your epistemological perspective. As we noted at the outset of the chapter, epistemology is concerned with the theory of knowledge and refers to the relationship between the knower and what can be known (Guba and Lincoln, 2004). It relates to the theories of knowledge (Harding, 1987) and the methods through which knowledge is produced (Soini and Kronqvist, 2011). Within the qualitative approach there are a range of epistemological positions that researchers can occupy in their endeavours. Before we provide an overview of the main ones, we first offer a brief introduction to positivism and post-positivism, typically associated with quantitative research, and the positions against which qualitative epistemologies are usually pitched.

Auguste Comte, the founder of positivism, was one of the first scholars to develop the idea that society moved through an evolution from the theological, to metaphysical, to the positive (Smith, 1983). Positivism refers to the idea that there is a direct relationship between the world and the researcher's perception of it, which is accessible via research that draws upon the natural sciences in a value-free and objective way (Willig, 2008). Researchers who operate from a positivist epistemology work on the basis that it is possible to discover a single truth because reality is observable and measurable (Glesne, 2015). However, post-positivism proposes that measurement is fallible, researchers can be biased, and thus absolute objectivity is not possible (Glesne, 2015). Such an objectivist epistemology of positivism and post-positivism has typically been contrasted against the alternative epistemologies, and this distinction has been one of the major contributors to the quantitative/qualitative divide (Staller, 2013). Staller pointed out that this distinction has also contributed to the misconception of qualitative research being treated as a homogenous approach when in fact there is considerable diversity.

> **Key point!**
>
> Recognise that some scholars claim that some of the key theories in qualitative research, like interpretivism and phenomenology, are epistemologies (e.g. Padgett, 2008) and others position them as paradigms (e.g. Crotty, 2003).
>
> Also, some scholars take the concepts of hermeneutics, symbolic interactionism, and phenomenology as theories, while others refer to them as epistemologies (e.g. Staller, 2013).

As you can see, which literature you read will make a difference in the terminology applied. We encourage you to engage in further reading around the specific theories, ontologies, and epistemologies that are fundamental to your own project. In the meantime, we treat these as epistemologies and provide you with a basic definition of each as a starting point for your understanding. We introduce each one in turn in alphabetical order and recognise our list is not comprehensive and limited to the more common positions in qualitative research.

- **Critical theory**

The premise of critical theory is that there is no such thing as an objective world, and therefore knowledge can never simply be a mirror of reality, as there is always a value-determined nature to inquiry (Guba and Lincoln, 2004). The concern for critical theory is to challenge prevailing power structures. In that sense, "critical theory" is an umbrella term covering certain movements, including neo-Marxism, critical race theory, queer theory, feminism, and the social model of disability (Ormston et al., 2014).

- **Dialectical pluralism**

A dialectic refers to the two polarities of seemingly opposite positions that can be simultaneously held, such as thesis and antithesis. When a researcher takes a dialectical approach, it means they welcome more than one paradigmatic tradition simultaneously and typically use more than one methodological approach or more than one method of data collection or analysis (Greene and Hall, 2010). Thus, dialectical pluralism is a theoretical position often taken by mixed method researchers or by interdisciplinary teams of researchers using more than one qualitative method or methodology for their research. Because of its pluralism, researchers taking a dialectical position make a commitment to the potential for genuine discovery and sense-making (Cronenberg and Headley, 2019). As such, dialectical pluralism is a meta-paradigm for mixed methods research, whether mixing quantitative and qualitative, or mixing within qualitative. This means that dialectical pluralism is a theoretical mechanism for researchers, stakeholders, policymakers, practitioners, and clients/patients to work in collaboration to produce new "wholes" simultaneously whilst developing intellectual tensions (Johnson, 2017). Johnson observed that to accomplish this effectively, the team needs multiple members who reflexively contribute to the project and bring different perspectives to the problem, whilst working through disagreements and tensions to collaboratively find solutions.

- **Empiricism**

Empiricism assumes that observations and sensory experiences are methods for the acquisition of knowledge and assumes claims can be verified through observation (Hjørland, 2005). Hjørland argued that empiricism is premised on certain assumptions about the world, in that it posits the mind, concepts, and languages form the basis of empiricism. Thus, empiricism relies on observation of and experimentation with data that can only be accessed through the senses (Borman, Lecompte, and Goetz., 1986). For empiricism, there is an assumption that knowledge about the world is derived from facts, and knowledge acquisition relies on methods of data collection where the knowledge claim is grounded in the data (Willig, 2008).

- **Existentialism**

Kierkegaard is credited with being the first existentialist philosopher (Law, 2007) with the belief that individuals did not see a need to struggle with the direction of their existence (Moss, 2001). The existentialist philosophy emphasises the free agency of the individual, who can determine their own course in life through decisions of the will.

It was, however, Sartre who coined the phrase "existentialism" (Law, 2007), which is also described as a "humanism" (Kaufmann, 1975). Humans are not understood as beings with fixed essences, nor are they beings who interact in a world of objects (Crowell, 2010). Simply put, existentialism advocates that "existence precedes essence" (Law, 2007) and begins with the idea that humans exist because they think, act, feel, and live (Macquarrie, 1972).

■ Feminism

There is ambiguity regarding feminism as an epistemology, as there is no specific feminist epistemological position. Instead, feminism is typically thought to be a movement which developed during the 20th century (Friedman, Metelerkamp, and Posel, 1987). The ideology of feminism focused on women seeking equality with men (Fiss, 1994). This position tends to posit that research should not be conducted *on* women but *with* them and *for* them (Doucet and Mauthner, 2006), and feminist research tends to be concerned with issues related to broader social change and social injustice (Friedman et al., 1987). Be mindful that there are different types of feminism and different forms of feminist theory, and you will need an awareness of these if your research is going to be informed by feminist theory.

■ Hermeneutics

In the context of qualitative research, hermeneutics refers to processes of interpreting data that emphasise accounting for the context in which it was collected. As Braun and Clarke (2022, p. 160) explain, "(h)ermeneutics refers to the philosophy of interpretation – the assumptions that underpin how we make sense of and interpret data". Thus, when understanding an action, it is necessary to understand the context in which that action took place (Smith, 1983). Hermeneutics arose because of a critique of objectivity which claimed there will always be a subjective influence of ideology, language, expectations, culture, and assumptions (Rennie, 1999). It is therefore argued that a hermeneutic approach is useful to achieve an interpretive understanding of human activity (Smith, 1983).

■ Humanism

Humanism has its roots in phenomenological philosophy with subjectivity as a source of knowledge (Bernard, 2011). In that sense, Bernard argued that the uniqueness of humanity calls for non-scientific approaches to research. Humanism has a place in psychology as, within that discipline, it is an approach concerned with the whole person, accounting for the unique individual (Moss, 2001) and is also associated with the work of Carl Rogers in humanistic (i.e. person-centred) psychology and psychotherapy (Moreira, 2012).

■ Idealism

There are different types of idealism, including classical idealism, objective idealism, subjective idealism, absolute idealism, transcendental idealism, actual idealism, conceptual idealism, pluralistic idealism, ontological idealism, and relativism. Thus, idealism is a cluster of philosophical ideas with a foundational assertion that reality is mentally constructed and immaterial (Smith, 1983). Idealism is connected to hermeneutics, in that understanding is a hermeneutic process and human experience is context-bound rather than context-free (Smith, 1983).

■ Interpretivism

Interpretivism is rooted in the work of Kant, who claimed there are ways of knowing about the world other than via direct observations. Kant argued that perception relates to the human senses, but also to human interpretation of what those senses tell us, and our understanding of the world is based on reflections of what happens, not just experience (Ormston et al., 2014). Interpretivists thus claim that we need to understand individuals' subjective interpretations of reality (Chen et al., 2011).

■ Materialism

Materialism recognises only material or physical features of the world, whereby values, beliefs, and experiences are features that arise from, but do not shape, the material world (Ormston et al., 2014). Thus, the fundamental principle of materialism is a set of theoretical positions that propose that all entities and processes are composed of, or are reducible to, material forces or physical properties (Stack, 1998). Materialism has been challenged by those who focus on mental phenomena like reason, values, and consciousness, who critique the reductionist proposition that all can be reduced to basic biological processes (Jaworski, 2016).

■ Phenomenology

Phenomenology is a movement led by Husserl, who emphasised the intentionality of human mental activity (Moss, 2001). Phenomenologists argue that researchers need to understand the worlds of their participants from the participants' perspective. Thus, the aim of phenomenology is to facilitate a more in-depth understanding of the lived experiences of individuals (Starks and Trinidad, 2007). Husserl claimed that perception is influenced by assumptions, anticipations, expectations, and sensory experience (Rennie, 1999). Phenomenology has been combined with existentialism by Heidegger (Moss, 2001) with reality understood through embodied experience (Starks and Trinidad, 2007).

■ Post-modernism

Post-modernism is a philosophical movement capturing a range of phenomena and representing an array of theoretical frameworks that include the foundational theories of Nietzsche and Heidegger (Rosenau, 2004). Post-modernism wrestles with the idea of absolute truth and can be considered a reaction against intellectual assumptions that characterised the modern period, particularly faith in science as an instrument of enlightenment and progress (Lucy and Mickler, 2008). Fundamental to post-modernism is the idea that researchers seek to locate meaning rather than discover it (Rosenau, 2004).

■ Post-structuralism

Post-structuralism builds upon but also moves away from structuralism, which focuses on structural linguistics where human culture is seen as a structure modelled on language (Harcourt, 2007). Post-structuralism, also referred to as neo-structuralism (Peters, 2001), is associated with the theorists Derrida and Foucault (Harcourt, 2007). The basis of post-structuralism is that all knowledge is contingent, or that knowledge is located within communication, and people construct knowledge together socially (Fraser and Robinson, 2003). This position focuses on the explanations of how we fill gaps in knowledge and how people hold true to their beliefs (Harcourt, 2007).

■ Pragmatism

Pragmatism is an intellectual movement that is seen as a mediation between empiricism and philosophy, which is argued to be essential for the science of truth, and in that sense is an epistemology that returns to common sense and experience (Shook, 2023). Shook argued therefore that pragmatism is a systemic worldview that views reality, knowledge, and truth as coordinated with approaches to morality, value, and justice. Pragmatism is based on the principle of usefulness and workability, stressing the priority of action over ideas and experience over principle (Rosenthal and Thayar, 2024). Rosenthal and Thayar argued that existence, if concerned with action and change, is part of the condition of life. They argued that pragmatists are critical of moral and metaphysical doctrines and focus on more concrete philosophy.

■ Symbolic interactionism

This is a sociological approach grounded in the work of Blumer, Mead, and Weber. Blumer (1969) laid out three core principles: 1) that individuals act based on the meanings they ascribe to an object or event, 2) that those meanings are derived via social interaction, and 3) those meanings are modified through an interpretive process. Thus, symbolic interactionists see individuals first as members of society (Ashworth, 2003). Ashworth argued that in the context of qualitative research, researchers consider the symbolic systems in society, including those that are linguistic.

■ Social constructionism

In the tradition of social constructionism, human experience is viewed not as not a fixed aspect of the person, but rather as something that is mediated culturally, linguistically, and historically. Indeed, the critical "turn" to language is a crucial moment in the history of academic social science as it signalled a change in how humans are studied (O'Reilly and Lester, 2017). Broadly, social constructionism is an assembly of diverse approaches and is a rubric for a range of research efforts with similar theoretical and empirical foundations (Gubrium and Holstein, 2008). Qualitative research underpinned by social constructionism is concerned with identifying the ways of constructing social reality (Willig, 2008). There are different types of social constructionism, but the most common are macro- and micro-. Macro-social constructionism is concerned with the role of social and linguistic structures that shape the social world, whereas micro-social constructionism is concerned with the micro-structures of language, focusing on situated interaction and interactional order (Gubrium and Holstein, 2008).

- **Social constructivism**

Social constructivism is often conflated with social constructionism, but it is a different epistemological position. This position argues that the world is independent of the human mind (Crotty, 2003) and derives from cognitive and developmental psychology that emphasises the role of culture in cognitive development, influenced by psychologists, notably Piaget, Vygotsky, and Bruner (Young and Collin, 2004). Social constructivism is concerned with the way the world is constructed by individuals; thus, the focus is on how individuals cognitively shape the construction of knowledge (Young and Collin, 2004).

We now draw your attention to a list of things to be mindful of in relation to ontology and epistemology. We provide these in Box 3.5.

Box 3.5

Important things to remember about epistemology and ontology

- The first thing to reflect on is what are the assumptions regarding reality, for you and for your study? For example, is it assumed that reality pre-exists human interaction with the world, or that our conscious interaction with our surroundings creates the reality we experience? This will inform your ontological position.
- Once you have considered what is being assumed about the nature of reality, this will directly relate to your understanding of how new knowledge about that reality can be generated. Your epistemological position as a researcher relates directly to the ontological presuppositions inherent to the project.
- Understanding the theory behind paradigms, ontology, and epistemology helps you to choose which theory to align yourself with as a researcher. Studying other authors will help you decide where to position your work theoretically (which may be different for different projects).

We have introduced you in this section to more information about various epistemologies within qualitative research. Before moving to the next section, we recommend you engage with the reflective activity in Box 3.6.

THEORY IN QUALITATIVE RESEARCH

> **Box 3.6**
>
> **Reflective activity on epistemology**
>
> Based on the brief introductions to each main epistemology, we invite you to start your decision-making regarding epistemology for your research project. In your research diary, write down your initial thoughts about the different epistemologies and make some decisions about where you need to direct your reading.

Methodology and method

We do not go into detail on methodology or methods at this point in the book, as we have chapters dedicated to these later. Rather, our purpose here is to introduce the conceptual issues so you can see how these are tied to axiology, ontology, and epistemology. During this conceptual discussion, we provide you with an overview of these in terms of what they mean for you and your project.

> **Key point!**
>
> Methods are different from methodologies, as methods provide a set of tools to do research, whereas methodology is a package comprised of theory, method, and other design elements.
>
> (Braun and Clarke, 2022)

Methodology is the connection between ontology and epistemology and determines your choice of methods. Simply, methodology is the study of methods (Stenbacka, 2001) and relates to how the researcher goes about finding out what they think can be known (Guba and Lincoln, 2004). That is, methodologies are procedural rules designed to guide researchers to explore social life and human behaviour (Hill, 1984).

> **Key point!**
>
> Methodologies are constrained by ontological and epistemological assumptions, and the choice of methods is informed by the given methodology.
>
> (Hesse-Biber and Leavy, 2004)

Your choice of methods can only make sense if they are anchored to a methodological and epistemological framework (Staller, 2013). So, the methodology you choose is the theoretical framework of your project. In qualitative approaches, these include phenomenological approaches, grounded theory, thematic design, discursive approaches, and others. Methods are those techniques, strategies, and tools that researchers use to complete their research inquiry. This includes data collection methods like interviews, focus groups, case studies, and so forth.

Author reflections and concluding remarks

In the spirit of reflexivity and transparency in our own research, our philosophical and theoretical position as researchers sits, broadly speaking, within a social constructionist epistemology (albeit we admit there are many variants of this). We advocate that language plays a powerful role in the construction of knowledge and that meaning is created through social interaction. Thus, we argue that methodological approaches and methods of data collection need to be used as tools to explore and investigate social and institutional interactions from the perspectives and voices of those participants pertinent to our research questions and aims (and we give you more guidance on this shortly in the book).

From Philip, Nikki, and Michelle

Predominantly, Philip tends to take a psychodynamically orientated, psycho-social position, favouring qualitative approaches to interviewing and analysis that draw heavily on concepts associated with psychoanalysis and psychoanalytic therapy (including ways they have been deployed in social theory). Nikki and Michelle favour discursive, language-based approaches, tending to use different forms of discourse analysis and conversation analysis. These are all detailed later in the book, so we do not provide explanations here, and only include this information to illustrate our own research positions. Providing this information demonstrates how our worldview shapes our research, which we use as examples to illustrate points in later chapters, and how our epistemology informs how we write and the way we work.

We close this chapter with the expert voice of Professor Nisha Dogra, a retired clinical academic who spent much of her career engaged in qualitative research in mental health and teaching about qualitative approaches. Professor Dogra was a former academic scholar at the University of Leicester and a Child and Adolescent Psychiatrist practising in the NHS. Her contribution can be found in Box 3.7.

Box 3.7

Practitioner perspective on the role of theory in qualitative research

Professor Nisha Dogra is an Emeritus Professor of Child Mental Health and a former practising psychiatrist. Here, she offers her reflections on the importance of theory in qualitative health research:

Before I offer my reflections on this chapter, I would like to reassure any readers who find themselves overwhelmed by the terminology and the volume of theories and approaches that they are not alone!

Given the complexity, there may be a tendency to dismiss the "theory" as irrelevant and a barrier to the research you want to do. To help highlight why an understanding of the theory is important, I would like to draw an analogy with clinical work and decision-making. Clinical practice follows a process of assessment before coming to a view about a potential disorder and the treatment options. It is unlikely that most clinicians would dismiss the idea that it is important to have a working knowledge of the theories behind the disorders and their potential treatments. The same would and should apply to any research we undertake.

The point that resonated most strongly with me and much of the research I have undertaken is that "Your values are embedded in your worldview, and this will influence all the decisions you make about your research project" (Hill, 1984).

I would go one step further and say that our worldview potentially impacts every decision we make, whether we are conscious of this or not. As researchers, we need to recognise our worldview and how it shapes the questions we ask and the methods we choose to answer them through the biases we carry. There may be a tendency to use the approaches with which we are comfortable with rather than those that properly address the research question we are posing. Our research will be better and more likely to have potentially usable outcomes if we ensure that we understand the approach we are using and why we are using it, as well as ensuring that the approach fits the research question. We can only ensure the approach we use is appropriate if we are aware of the alternative approaches and aware of why they are not suitable for the research question we have formulated.

References

Arneson, P. (2009). Axiology. In S. Littlejohn and K. Foss (Eds.), *Encyclopaedia of communication theory* (pp. 70–74). Thousand Oaks, CA: Sage.

Ashworth, P. (2003). The origins of qualitative psychology. In J. A. Smith (Ed.), *Qualitative psychology: A practical guide to research methods* (pp. 4–25). London: Sage.

Bendassolli, P. (2014). Reconsidering theoretical naïveté in psychological qualitative research. *Social Science Information*, 53(2), 163–179.

Bernard, H. (2011). *Research methods in anthropology: Qualitative and quantitative methods* (5th ed.). Plymouth: Alta Mira Press.

Blumer, H. (1969). *Symbolic interactionism; Perspective and method*. Englewood Cliffs, NJ: Prentice-Hall.

Borman, K., Lecompte, M., and Goetz, J. (1986). Ethnographic and qualitative research design and why it doesn't work. *American Behavioral Scientist*, 30(1), 42–57.

Braun, V., and Clarke, V. (2022). *Thematic analysis: A practical guide*. London: Sage.

Bryman, A. (2016). *Social research methods* (5th ed.). Oxford: Oxford University Press.

Chen, Y., Shek, D., and Bu, F. (2011). Applications of interpretive and constructionist research methods in adolescent research: Philosophy, principles and examples. *International Journal of Adolescent Medicine & Health*, 23(3), 129–139.

Creswell, J., and Creswell, D. (2018). *Research design: Qualitative, quantitative, and mixed methods approaches* (5th ed.). London: Sage.

Creswell, J., and Plano-Clark, V. (2011). *Designing and conducting mixed method research* (2nd ed.). Thousand Oaks, CA: Sage.

Cronenberg, S., and Headley, M. (2019). Dialectical dialogue: Reflections on adopting a dialectic stance. *International Journal of Research & Method in Education*, 42(3), 267-287.

Crotty, M. (2003). *The foundations of social research: Meaning and perspective in the research process*. London: Sage.

Crowell, S. (2010). Existentialism. In E. N. Zalta (Ed.), *The Stanford encyclopedia of philosophy* http://plato.stanford.edu/archives/win2010/entries/existentialism/

Diesing, P. (1965). Objectivism vs. subjectivism in the social sciences. *Philosophy of Science*, 33(1/2), 124–133.

Doucet, A., and Mauthner, N. (2006). Feminist methodologies and epistemology. In C. Bryant and D. Peck (Eds.), *Handbook of 21st century sociology* (pp. 36–45). Thousand Oaks, CA: Sage.

Edwards, D., Ashmore, M., and Potter, J. (2003). Death and furniture: Arguments against relativism. In M. Gergen and K. Gergen (Eds.), *Social construction: A reader* (pp. 231–236). London: Sage.

Fiss, O. (1994). What is feminism? *Faculty Scholarship Series, Paper 1331*, 413–428. Yale Law School Legal Scholarship Repository.

Florell, D. (2019). Idiographic versus nomothetic history: The first debate in school psychology. In M. Burns (Ed.), *Introduction to school psychology: Controversies and current practice* (pp. 217–241). Oxford: Oxford University Press.

Fraser, S., and Robinson, C. (2003). Paradigms and philosophy. In S. Fraser, V. Lewis, S. Ding, M. Kellett, and C. Robinson (Eds.), *Doing research with children and young people* (pp. 59–77). London: Sage.

Freshwater, D., and Cahill, J. (2013). International qualitative nursing research: State of the science in England, Wales and Scotland. In C. Beck (Ed.), *Routledge international handbook of qualitative nursing research*. London: Routledge.

Friedman, M., Metelerkamp, J., and Posel, R. (1987). What is feminism? And what kind of feminist am I? *Agenda: Empowering Women for Gender Equity, 1*, 3–24.

Glesne, C. (2015). *Becoming qualitative researchers: An introduction* (5th ed.). Boston, MA: Pearson.

Greene, J., and Hall, J. (2010). Dialectics and pragmatism: Being of consequence. In A. Tashakkori and C. Teddlie (Eds.), *Sage handbook of mixed methods in social and behavioral research* (2nd ed., pp. 119–143). Thousand Oaks, CA: Sage.

Guba, E., and Lincoln, Y. (2004). Competing paradigms in qualitative research: Theories and issues. In S. N. Hesse-Biber and P. Leavy (Eds.), *Approaches to qualitative research: A reader on theory and practice* (pp. 17–38). Oxford: Oxford University Press.

Gubrium, J., and Holstein, J. (2008). The constructionist mosaic. In J. Holstein and J. Gubrium (Eds.), *Handbook of constructionist research* (pp. 3–12). New York, NY: Guildford.

Harcourt, B. (2007). *An answer to the question: 'What is poststructuralism?' Public Law & Legal Theory Working Papers No. 156*. Chicago, IL: University of Chicago Law School.

Harding, S. (1987). Introduction: Is there a feminist method? In S. Harding (Ed.), *Feminism and methodology: Social science issues* (pp. 1–14). Bloomington, IN: Indiana University Press.

Harris, M. (1976). History and significance of the emic/etic distinction. *Annual Review of Anthropology, 5*, 329–350.

Hart, S. (1971). Axiology- theory of values. *Philosophy and Phenomenological Research, 32*(1), 29–41.

Hesse-Biber, S. (2017). *The practice of qualitative research* (3rd ed.). London: Sage.

Hesse-Biber, S., and Leavy, P. (2004). Distinguishing qualitative research. In S. Hesse-Biber and P. Leavy (Eds.), *Approaches to qualitative research: A reader on theory and practice* (pp. 1–17). Oxford: Oxford University Press.

Hill, M. (1984). Epistemology, axiology, and ideology in sociology. *Mid-American Review of Sociology, 9*(2), 59–77.

Hjørland, B. (2005). Empiricism, rationalism and positivism in library and information science. *Journal of Documentation, 61*(1), 130–155.

Hollis, M. (1994). *The philosophy of social science: An introduction* (Revised and updated). Cambridge: Cambridge University Press.

Hussey, J., and Hussey, R. (1997). *Business research*. Basingstoke: Palgrave.

Jaworski, W. (2016). Why materialism is false and why it has nothing to do with the mind. *Philosophy, 91*(2), 183–213.

Johnson, R. (2017). Dialectical pluralism: A metaparadigm whose time has come. *Mixed Methods Research, 11*(2), 156–173.

Kaufmann, W. (1975). *Existentialism: From Dostoevsky to Sartre*. New York, NY: Plume (Penguin).

Kelly, M., Ellaway, R., Reid, H., Ganshorn, H., Yardley, S., Bennett, D., and Dornan, T. (2018). Considering axiological integrity: A methodological analysis of qualitative evidence syntheses, and its implications for health professions education. *Advanced Health Science Education*, 23(4), 833–851.

Killam, L. (2013). *Research terminology simplified: Paradigms, axiology, ontology, epistemology, and methodology*. Sudbury, ON: Author.

King, N., and Brook, J. (2017). *Template analysis for business and management students*. London: Sage.

Kuhn, T. (1970). *The structure of scientific revolutions*. Chicago, IL: University of Chicago Press.

Law, S. (2007). *The great philosophers: The lives and ideas of history's greatest thinkers*. London: Quercus.

Lett, J. (1990). Emics and etics: Notes on the epistemology of anthropology. In T. Headland, K. Pike, and M. Harris (Eds.), *Emics and etics: The insider/outsider debate*. (pp. 127–142). Newbury Park, CA: Sage.

Lucy, N., and Mickler, S. (2008). The war on English: An answer to the question, what is postmodernism? *Transformations*, 16(1). http://transformationsjournal.org/journal/issue_16/article_01.shtml

Macquarrie, J. (1972). *Existentialism*. Philadelphia, PA: Westminster.

Madill, A., Jordan, A., and Shirley, C. (2000). Objectivity and reliability in qualitative analysis: Realist, contextualist and radical constructionist epistemologies. *British Journal of Psychology*, 91(1), 1–20.

Moreira, V. (2012). From person-centered to humanistic-phenomenological psychotherapy: The contribution of Merleau-Ponty to Carl Rogers's thought. *Experiential Psychotherapies*, 11(1), 48–63.

Moss, D. (2001). The roots and genealogy of humanistic psychology. In K. Schneider, J. Bugental, and J. Pierson (Eds.), *Handbook of humanistic psychology* (pp. 5–20). Thousand Oaks, CA: Sage.

Nguyen, T., Whitehead, L., Demody, G., and Saunders, R. (2022). The use of theory in qualitative research: Challenges, development of a framework and exemplar. *Journal of Advanced Nursing*, 78, e21–e28.

Onwuegbuzie, A., and Leech, N. (2005). Taking the "Q" out of research: Teaching research methodology courses without the divide between quantitative and qualitative paradigms. *Quantity & Quality*, 39, 267–229.

O'Reilly, M., and Kiyimba, N. (2015). *Advanced qualitative research: A guide to contemporary theoretical debates*. London: Sage.

O'Reilly, M., and Lester, J (2017). *Examining mental health through social constructionism: The language of mental health*. Basingstoke: Palgrave.

Ormston, R., Spencer, L., Barnard, M., and Snape, D. (2014). The foundations of qualitative research. In J. Ritchie, J. Lewis, C. McNaughton-Nicholls, and R. Ormston (Eds.), *Qualitative research practice: A guide for social science students and researchers* (pp. 1–26). London: Sage.

Padgett, D. (2008). *Qualitative methods in social work* (2nd ed.). Thousand Oaks, CA: Sage.

Paul, R., and Elder, L. (2020). *Critical thinking: Tools for taking charge of your professional and personal life* (2nd ed.). Oxford: Prentice Hall.

Peters, M. (2001). *Poststructuralism, marxism, and neo-liberalism: Between theory and politics*. Lanham, MD: Rowman and Littlefield.

Ponterotto, J. (2005). Qualitative research in counseling psychology: A primer on research paradigms and the philosophy of science. *Journal of Counseling Psychology*, 52(2), 126–136.

Pope, C., and Mays, N. (2020). The role of theory in qualitative research. In C. Pope and N. Mays (Eds.), *Qualitative research in healthcare* (4th ed.). Hoboken, NJ: John Wiley and Sons.

Ratner, C. (2002). Subjectivity and objectivity in qualitative methodology. *Forum: Qualitative Social Research*, 3(3), Art. 16. http://www.qualitative-research.net/index.php/fqs/article/view/829/1800

Ravitch, S., and Riggan, M. (2012). *Reason & rigour: How conceptual frameworks guide research*. Thousand Oaks, CA: Sage.

Reeves, S., Albert, M., Kuper, A., and Hodges, D. (2008). Why use theories in qualitative research? *British Medical Journal*, 337, a949.

Rennie, D. (1999). *Using qualitative methods in psychology*. Thousand Oaks, CA: Sage.

Risjord, M. (2022). *Philosophy of social science: A contemporary introduction* (2nd ed.). London: Routledge.

Robinson, O. (2011). The ideographic/nomothetic dichotomy: Tracing historical origins of contemporary confusions. *History & Philosophy of Psychology*, 13(2), 32–39.

Rosenau, P. (2004). *Postmodernism and the social sciences: Insights, inroads and intrusions*. Princeton, NJ: Princeton University Press.

Rosenthal, S., and Thayar, H. (2024). Pragmatism. https://www.britannica.com/topic/pragmatism-philosophy

Shook, J. R. (2023). *Pragmatism*. Cambridge, MA: MIT Press.

Smith, J. (1983). Quantitative versus qualitative research: An attempt to clarify the issue. *Educational Researcher*, 12(3), 6–13.

Snape, D., and Spencer, L. (2003). The foundations of qualitative research. In J. Ritchie and J. Lewis (Eds.), *Qualitative research practice: A Guide for social science students and researchers* (pp. 2–10). London: Sage.

Soiferman, L. (2010). *Compare and contrast inductive and deductive research approaches*. University of Manitoba.

Soini, H., and Kronqvist, E. L. (2011). Epistemology- a tool or a stance? In H. Soini, E. L. Kronqvist, and G. Hüber (Eds.), *Epistemologies for qualitative research* (pp. 5–8). Center for Qualitative Psychology.

Stack, G. (1998). Materialism. In the *Routledge encyclopedia of philosophy online*. London: Routledge.

Staller, K. (2013). Epistemological boot camp: The politics of science and what every qualitative researcher needs to know to survive in the academy. *Qualitative Social Work*, 12(4), 395–413.

Starks, H., and Trinidad, S. (2007). Choose your method: A comparison of phenomenology, discourse analysis, and grounded theory. *Qualitative Health Research*, 17(10), 1372–1380.

Stenbacka, C. (2001). Qualitative research requires quality concepts of its own. *Management Decision*, 39(7), 551–555.

Willig, C. (2008). *Introducing qualitative research in psychology* (2nd ed.). Milton Keynes: Open University Press.

Young, R., and Collin, A. (2004). Introduction: Constructivism and social constructionism in the career field. *Journal of Vocational Behavior*, 64, 373–388.

Zaidi, Z., and Larsen, D. (2019). Commentary: Paradigms, axiology, and praxeology in medical education research. *Academic Medicine*, 93(11s), S1–S7.

CHAPTER 4

Evidence-based practice and practice-based evidence

Learning objectives

This chapter enables the reader to:

- Identify what constitutes evidence.
- Appreciate the history of evidence-based medicine.
- Recognise what evidence-based practice is.
- Critically assess the value of qualitative evidence.
- Understand principles involved in the appraisal of research evidence.

Introduction

There has been a gradual growth in the development of qualitative methods in the field of health and an increasing acceptance of these as valuable across disciplines. Qualitative research approaches are now on many university research methods course curricula and there are entire journals that exclusively publish qualitative research papers. This growing devotion to qualitative research has implications for healthcare professionals as they engage with this field and undertake their own qualitative research projects. More specifically, this growth in popularity and developments in the field has implications for the value and translation of evidence generated from qualitative research into clinical practice.

The idea of "evidence" in healthcare was one founded predominantly in medicine, and now stretches across many areas of practice, including social care, education, and business. For the field of healthcare, evidence has become embedded in the ways practitioners go about their daily business and is a central tenet for benefiting patients and their families. The underpinning ideology is that health research should be transferable into the real-world work of clinical practitioners. As the goal of research in clinical settings is to maximise the effectiveness of practice, practitioners can see the necessity of generating and applying evidence through rigorous inquiry (Portney, 2020). In this chapter, our focus is on evidence-based practice. We introduce you to some of the core concepts associated with evidence and provide a critical narrative for how evidence generated through qualitative methods has been viewed and informed practice and care delivery in healthcare. Before we begin, we invite you first to reflect on your own thoughts about evidence-based practice by engaging in the activity in Box 4.1.

> **Box 4.1**
>
> **Reflecting on evidence-based practice**
>
> As part of our own research, we often discuss evidence-based practice with the clinical practitioners we work alongside. They have many ideas about what this means for their work and varying degrees of knowledge. We encourage you to take a moment to reflect on your knowledge and beliefs about the value of evidence in health and care settings and the benefits of evidence-based practice. Ask yourself these questions:
>
> 1. On a scale of 1–10 where would you rate your knowledge of evidence-based practice?
> 2. Where would you like it to be?
> 3. To what extent do you feel your own practice is informed by evidence?
>
> In your research diary, write a few sentences about your beliefs regarding the extent to which evidence-based practice is valuable, and how you view evidence generated through qualitative research methods.

What is evidence?

Let us start by asking what constitutes evidence. To be able to think about evidence-based practice, we must first think about the nature of evidence itself. In simple terms, evidence can be described as a cluster of facts that are conceived of as true (Melnyk and Fineout-Overholt, 2023). Researchers generate knowledge or "evidence" via a range of research methods, and this knowledge can be translated into clinical practice (Melnyk and Fineout-Overholt, 2023).

> **Key point!**
>
> In healthcare, it is widely advocated by organisations that patients should be provided with care that is based on the best research evidence available.

Thus, the directive for practitioners that their work ought to be guided by evidence is recognised in many countries and is established in a range of guidelines, for example, those provided by:

- The National Institute for Health and Care Excellence (NICE, UK).
- The Agency for Health Care Research and Quality (USA).
- The National Institute for Clinical Studies (Australia).

(Rycroft-Malone, Seers, Titchen et al., 2004)

In the context of healthcare, using research evidence to inform practice requires scrutiny (Rycroft-Malone et al., 2004), which relies on an understanding of how knowledge is generated. One way to think about evidence is to consider it as the accumulation of knowledge from different sources. In other words, practitioners require multiple sources of knowledge to inform a base of evidence (Rycroft-Malone et al., 2004). For Rycroft-Malone et al. (2004), this knowledge comes from four primary types of evidence:

- Research evidence.
- Clinical experience.
- Patient and family perspectives.
- Local context and environment.

We provide a brief overview of each type of evidence before we go into more detail about evidence-based practice.

Research evidence

If you are planning to do your own research project, then this is probably the type of evidence you are most interested in learning more about. Much evidence in healthcare is generated through research, and this kind of evidence usually (although not exclusively) involves academic researchers. For this to be more meaningful, we argue that academic research teams could work closely alongside clinical practitioners to promote making research findings applicable to the field of practice.

> **Key point!**
>
> Evidence from research can be generated using quantitative approaches, qualitative approaches, or a combination of the two.

We point out, however, that the scientific method is thought to be the most rigorous way of acquiring knowledge (Portney, 2020), although there are differences of opinion about what constitutes a scientific method. Mostly, randomised controlled trials (RCTs) have been considered the "gold standard", but other forms of evidence are also valuable, and the most appropriate method is the one that addresses the aims and objectives of a project and answers the research question (Cartwright, 2007; Gerstman, 2023).

Clinical experience

Much of the available literature about evidence-based practice refers to that generated using research methods. However, you should also recognise the value of clinical knowledge and experience as relevant sources of knowledge. Clinical knowledge is built via experience and training, and expertise develops over time.

> **Key point!**
>
> Experiential knowledge and expertise can only be thought of as evidence when it is shared and discussed and widely disseminated to others to learn from.
>
> (Rycroft-Malone et al., 2004)

Patient/service-user and family experiences

When developing evidence-based practice, those who use healthcare services also hold knowledge and information, as well as their families and carers. Service users and their families have a great deal of personal knowledge and experience that is central to understanding health. There are two types of service-user knowledge:

- Evidence that is available from the service-user's experiences of healthcare.
- Evidence that is available from service-users' knowledge of their own bodies and minds, as well as their personal and social contexts.

(Farrell and Gilbert, 1996)

Whilst service-user perspectives, and those of others, are often collected through research to generate research evidence, healthcare practitioners can also routinely gather helpful information from them to inform the care they provide, and more formally through quality improvement, audit, and service evaluations (as discussed in Chapter 2).

> **Key point!**
>
> Whilst there are commonalities, health, and illness are uniquely experienced, and service users have an individual lived perspective of their illnesses that may be best captured using qualitative methods.

Local context

The fourth type of evidence is that which arises from the context of care. This kind of evidence takes multiple formats, listed by Rycroft-Malone et al. (2004) as being:

- Audit or performance data.
- Cultural knowledge belonging to individuals and a healthcare organisation.
- Professional networks.
- Local and national policies.
- Information from all stakeholders.

It is helpful to be aware that this kind of knowledge and information is typically not considered the kind of evidence that would inform evidence-based practice. The challenge for this kind of evidence is that we need a better understanding of how it might be collected systematically, and the most appropriate ways to appraise it (Rycroft-Malone et al., 2004).

Evidence-based medicine
Now you have a more refined appreciation of evidence and the different ways it can be generated; we turn our attention to evidence-based practice. As the idea of evidence-based practice began in medicine, we first provide you with a brief overview of how this came about, starting with "evidence-based medicine". During the 1970s, David Eddy submitted a paper recognising that treatments and tests in medicine were typically not supported by good evidence or reasoning, and although the paper was retracted because of the negative reaction it received (Eddy, 2011), the idea gained traction as more critical voices joined the debate.

The evidence-based medicine movement was significantly influenced by Cochrane, a British epidemiologist who published a book critiquing the medical profession for failing to provide rigorous reviews of evidence that would help organisations deliver effective healthcare (Cochrane, 1972). Cochrane was hugely influential in the healthcare field, and there were calls for updates of systematic reviews and the synthesising of evidence to help inform decision-making (Melnyk and Fineout-Overholt, 2023). Alongside these calls for evidence, in 1991 the field of emergency medicine began to scrutinise resuscitation techniques, creating standards that others then began to follow (Timmermans and Berg, 2003). Evidence-based medicine thus entered the medical literature and was presented as an alternative to authority-based decision-making (Gambrill, 2019). Slowly evidence-based medicine began to gather momentum and was applied to practice.

The premise of evidence-based medicine, and subsequently evidence-based practice, was that decisions made in a healthcare context ought to be founded on the best available evidence and aligned with patient values and clinician judgement (Sackett, Rosenberg, Gray et al., 1996). Since Sackett and colleagues proposed their idea that evidence should inform treatment decisions, the definition of evidence-based practice has expanded. It now includes the systematic search for and critical appraisal of research and external evidence, the importance of clinical expertise aligned with evidence-based quality improvement work, and the inclusion of patient and family voices and values (Melnyk and Fineout-Overholt, 2023). In contemporary healthcare, evidence-based practice is seen as a cornerstone of service delivery.

The significance of evidence-based practice
The idea of evidence-based practice is founded a principle that quality care depends on the ability to make choices based on the best available evidence (Portney, 2020). The idea describes both a philosophy and a process (Gambrill, 2019). You may wonder how much evidence is needed and what the best type is to change practice, and it is helpful to recognise that the answer to this question depends on the questions being asked and the nature of the problem (Melnyk and Fineout-Overholt, 2023). Nonetheless, there has been significant investment in the healthcare infrastructure to incorporate the principles of evidence-based practice (Rycroft-Malone et al., 2004).

As a healthcare practitioner, you are likely to be encouraged or required by your organisation and related professional bodies to implement evidence-based practice in your work. Therefore, you probably take a problem-solving approach to your delivery of services which also integrates the best available evidence from a range of sources (Camargo, Iwamoto, Galvão et al., 2018). This means there are expectations from organisations that practitioners will have knowledge of the principles of evidence-based practice and develop essential competencies (Melnyk, Gallagher-Ford, and Fineout-Overholt, 2014). In healthcare, practitioner training typically develops "core competencies", and these provide a basis for a common language across health professions and clarity about expectations for optimal work (Albarqouni, Hoffmann, Straus et al., 2018). Yet, many healthcare practitioners are not able to define evidence-based practice, and there is often confusion about what it entails (Condon, McGrane, Mockler, and Stokes., 2016). As a result, some healthcare practitioners feel their competencies are insufficient for engaging in evidence-based practice in care delivery (Saunders, Gallagher-Ford, Kvist, and Vehviläinen-Julkunen, 2019). Furthermore, not only is it challenging to define core competencies of knowledge, skills, beliefs, and attitudes in terms of evidence-based practice (Melnyk et al., 2014), but the uptake of evidence-based practice core competencies in regular practice tends to be slow, and this can be a hindrance to organisations who aim to deliver evidence-based healthcare (Saunders et al., 2019).

As a clinician-researcher, although you may be engaging in your own research, it is also necessary to develop skills on how to appraise the research of others and how to translate the body of evidence into practice. This will also help with the development and quality of your own research. There are several steps offered by Melnyk, Fineout-Overholt, Stillwell, and Williamson (2010) to translate research into practice, and we outline these in Box 4.2.

Box 4.2

Steps for implementing evidence-based practice (Melnyk et al., 2010)

There are a series of steps for implementing evidence into your practice (from Melnyk et al., 2010):

1. Be reflective and frequently question your attitude toward evidence (and research more generally).
2. Elaborate on your clinical questions and consider what the best and most relevant evidence may be to answer them.
3. Engage in a search for evidence that might address the clinical problem you have identified.
4. Think critically about that evidence and assess the quality of the evidence you read.
5. Try to integrate the best evidence with your clinical expertise, whilst accounting for the preferences of those you are working with, including the client and their families, and carers.
6. Consider spending time evaluating your clinical decisions as aligned with the evidence you have critically assessed and reflect on the benefits and challenges.
7. Share your findings to promote change more widely and help others learn.

EVIDENCE-BASED PRACTICE/PRACTICE-BASED EVIDENCE

For evidence-based practice to be fully realised, the evidence needs to be available, the research published needs applicability to healthcare, and research needs to produce data that have utility for the setting in which those data are applied (Portney, 2020). Additionally, procedures and processes that are evidenced as effective need to be adopted in practice (Portney, 2020). This adoption into practice is central to improving healthcare quality and safety, improving patient outcomes, being cost-effective, and empowering practitioners and clients (Bodenheimer and Sinsky, 2014). We discuss this again later in the book in the context of knowledge exchange and impact.

Evidence hierarchies

Thus far, we have talked mostly about evidence and evidence-based practice in a general way and illustrated the development of its influence on contemporary health fields. We noted that definitions of evidence and considerations of evidence-based practice have relied heavily on ideas about "fact", "truth" and "science", and yet influential scholars also recognised the value of clinical judgement and the lived experiences of patients/clients.

In healthcare, different kinds of evidence have been hierarchically ranked in terms of value. An evidence hierarchy is, however, arguably problematic as it can perpetuate the view that qualitative evidence is somehow less robust or less useful than quantitative evidence. This misapprehends how different approaches and methods answer different kinds of questions and can even be used together to provide problem solutions.

> **Key point!**
>
> The evidence hierarchy has created a "politics of evidence" that influences how, when, and to whom qualitative methods are taught, funded, published, and implemented.
>
> (Morse, 2006)

Whilst qualitative researchers have fought hard to have the value of the approach recognised in health research (Morse, 2006), unfortunately, qualitative evidence is often positioned at the bottom of the evidence hierarchy, with randomised controlled trials (RCTs) at the top. RCTs are an important source of evidence. Nevertheless, in healthcare we also need a rich knowledge, and this requires a range of different approaches. Health research seeks to address a broad range of practical problems and raises many different types of questions. Decisions about whether to use quantitative or qualitative approaches to generate evidence are dependent on the research goals and questions. "If the goal is generalisability, then quantitative methods are accepted to be superior, but if the goal is a rich understanding of a particular phenomenon, then qualitative methods are indispensable" (McNeill, 2006, p. 151).

Arguably then, it makes little sense that qualitative research tends to be positioned at the bottom of the pyramid; rather, we need to generate evidence suitable for the problem and, where helpful, combine quantitative and qualitative evidence. Conceptualising evidence in a hierarchy and in a way that privileges "effectiveness", risks neglecting other applicable questions and other useful types of evidence that may inform a broader and more refined understanding (Evans, 2003). If the field of health fails to accept the full range of evidence types, then qualitative research will continue to be conceived as inferior, which risks reducing the emphasis on service user's voice (Lester and O'Reilly, 2015). Arguments about evidence and hierarchies have led to some criticisms about evidence-based practice and its place in healthcare. However, before we introduce you to those, we invite you to reflect on your own position by addressing the activity in Box 4.3.

Box 4.3

Reflecting on the evidence hierarchy

Your engagement with this book suggests to us that you are amenable to the idea that qualitative evidence is crucial in the field of healthcare. We also speculate that you can see how qualitative evidence might help to inform some areas of your practice. Now that you have been provided with some of the literature about evidence-based practice and the proposition that evidence can be ranked, we invite you to reflect on what you think about this.

In your research diary, write down where you think qualitative evidence should be in the hierarchy and whether there are more suitable ways of representing the value of different kinds of evidence in healthcare practice. How might you defend your qualitative research project to those who struggle to appreciate its value and who would argue that research resources might be better used for quantitative work?

The value of qualitative evidence

There are many reasons why qualitative evidence is important in healthcare practice. As researchers, we consider qualitative research to be immensely valuable to the field of health and believe its worth has been underestimated in some circles. We argue that qualitative evidence is crucial to explicate service user experiences and beliefs, as well as practitioner and service provider views (as well as others), in ways that quantitative evidence cannot capture (Lester and O'Reilly, 2015). These arguments notwithstanding, if you are going to identify yourself as a qualitative researcher and aim to contribute to the health evidence base in your area of practice, you need to be mindful of new ways of thinking about what is valued as evidence. Indeed, qualitative healthcare researchers must "take a much more nuanced and complex view of what constitutes evidence in health research" and challenge the idea that evidence is hierarchical (Xu and Storr, 2012, p. 1).

It is recognised that evidence that informs us about effective treatments, medication efficacy and safety, outcomes, and prevention in health conditions is crucial for improvements in the field. However, whilst outcomes research and quantitative evidence are vital for healthcare improvement, it is important to also attend to the findings of process research whereby qualitative evidence provides answers to different kinds of healthcare problems. There are numerous benefits to qualitative evidence, which we have detailed elsewhere (Kiyimba, Lester, and O'Reilly, 2019) and summarise in Box 4.4.

> **Box 4.4**
>
> **The value of qualitative evidence (Kiyimba et al., 2019)**
>
> Kiyimba et al. (2019) proposed a range of benefits of qualitative evidence, and we list these below:
>
> - The implementation of qualitative evidence can be empowering for service users, those whose voices contribute to the evidence, and those in receipt of improved practice.
> - Qualitative methods can illuminate communication practices that are effective and ineffective.
> - Evidence from qualitative research can explain the subjective experiences of health conditions as experienced by service users.
> - Evidence from qualitative research can illuminate the meaning that health and illness have for service users and other stakeholders.
> - Qualitative approaches can personalise evidence that reflects real-world experiences and knowledge.
> - Qualitative evidence provides new understandings of health and illness that can inform policies at the service, local, and national levels.
> - Listening to and hearing service-user voices and other stakeholders is essential for change in practice.
> - Using qualitative evidence helps generate new theories and ideas.
> - Implementing qualitative evidence provides opportunities for new discoveries and space to generate and identify new research problems and questions.
> - Qualitative evidence can provide a foundation for questions that can be addressed by quantitative investigations.

The strengthening of the evidence-based practice movement has, however, increased conversations about the value of different kinds of evidence for informing practice. This growth in emphasis on evidence has created tensions about the legitimacy of qualitative research and, consequently, some scholars have pushed for qualitative research to be "more scientific" to conform to the boundaries expected (Lather, 2013). This has led some in the qualitative community to orient more to post-positivist approaches (St Pierre, 2016), and yet whilst this may have value, it is not always appropriate or theoretically congruent. Further, qualitative scholars are acutely aware of how evidence is often ranked in the politics of health research, and in a competitive funding environment, need to find ways to ensure qualitative research is taken seriously. Indeed, when research environments are under financial pressure, this tends to be more challenging for qualitative researchers, who face more difficulties in getting their approaches taught, pedagogies about those approaches published, and implemented (Morse, 2006).

To complement your own reflections on the value of qualitative research and its position in the evidence hierarchy, we asked Dr Tina Adkins for her expert opinion on this matter. We present her thoughts in Box 4.5.

> **Box 4.5**
>
> **The views of Dr Tina Adkins on the value of qualitative evidence**
>
> Dr Tina Adkins is a Research Assistant Professor and Director of The Sue Fairbanks Psychoanalytic Academy for the Texas Institute for Child & Family Wellbeing at the University of Texas at Austin.
>
> During my years working with foster and adoptive families, I realised these caregivers were not receiving the kind of training and information they both needed and craved to handle not only the emotional needs of traumatised children in their care but the stress of therapeutic parenting in a complicated and often unhelpful system. I started collecting qualitative data around their struggles, successes, expectations, and hopes. Qualitative methods allowed me to explore in detail their caregiving experiences. As a result of the deeper knowledge and nuanced understanding I gleaned, I was able to develop an intervention for these caregivers to meet their specific needs.
>
> This qualitative data guided the development of this intervention, helping me create something truly unique and a type of intervention that was not being offered to these caregivers but could be quite useful and meet a real need. First, it helped me develop a training that was psychoeducational in nature but based on a clinical intervention … one that went deeper than just sharing information. "Family Minds" is a brief mentalising intervention that helps caregivers both connect around their shared experiences and reflect deeper about themselves and the children in their care.
>
> Piloting this intervention, I collected even more qualitative data to really tailor this intervention for the caregivers in my community. For an intervention to have an impact quantitatively, it must be designed to both target what you are trying to impact/change, but also in a way that meets the needs of the population it is designed for. By gathering feedback via evaluations and interviews, I was able to roll out an intervention that had a much higher chance of producing quantitative evidence of efficacy. An experimental study on this intervention was very positive and showed a statistically significant impact of this intervention for caregivers and the children in their care. I am confident that my qualitative data was vital for the development of this intervention and significantly contributed to the fact that it is now an "evidenced-based practice". Instead of thinking of these two different research methods as either/or, we need to remember that mental health research is made stronger when qualitative and quantitative methods are used together.

Criticisms of evidence-based practice

The idea of an evidence hierarchy has not been fully accepted by academics or by practitioners. The literature holds several critiques against the conceptualisation of evidence-based practice, but also about the organisation of evidence and its value to inform decision-making in practice.

> **Key point!**
>
> Practitioners do not generally disagree with the principle that healthcare should be delivered based on what works well, rather the disagreement tends to be about what evidence is and how practitioners should use that evidence to inform their decisions in a clinical environment.
>
> (Rycroft-Malone et al., 2004)

A central criticism of an evidence hierarchy is that in the real world of healthcare practice, practitioners tend to base their decisions and reasoning on a range of sources, including research evidence, but also on case reports, training, experience and expertise, personal knowledge, and their knowledge of the person in front of them (Miller and Miller, 2011). In the evidence-based practice movement, it has been argued that the rhetoric of evidence and focus simply on "standards" have led to a "watered-down" competition, reduced autonomy, limited innovation and creativity, and an unhelpful focus on politics (Timmermans and Berg, 2003). Thus, if research evidence does not translate effectively into the typical everyday work of practitioners, then its value is questionable. The problem with evidence-based practice is that much of the evidence generated to inform practice is produced from artificially controlled research, which may not correspond to the complexities of real-world work with service users (Green, 2006). This issue of knowledge mobilisation and impact, we return to toward the end of the book.

Clearly, a significant criticism of evidence-based practice relates to its implementation in the real world of healthcare. There are several individual barriers identified to implementation reported by Alatawi, Aljuhani, Alsufiany et al. (2020), which are:

- Lack of awareness, knowledge, and skills.
- Practitioner attitudes and experiences.
- Disciplinary terminology.

As well as organisational barriers, which are:

- Lack of resources.
- Lack of support and supervision.
- Insufficient time.
- Lack of training and education.

Thinking critically about evidence

Whilst there have been broad criticisms of the evidence-based practice movement, it nonetheless retains a huge appeal across healthcare and remains a central endeavour for organisations and politics. We recognise that you are likely to be expected to work this way in your daily practice and therefore it is important that you can take a critical position on the evidence that you engage with.

When you are making decisions in practice, you are likely to be using a range of clinical skills, strategies learnt in your training, and implementing recent evidence. Decisions you make will be informed by theories and methods, recommended interventions, and the extent to which you involve the service user (Gambrill, 2019). In so doing, you need to be reflective and think critically to consider what can be done to improve things and draw upon your relevant skills and knowledge to question your assumptions (Paul and Elder, 2020). Thus, critical thinking skills are integral to the process and implementation of evidence-based practice (Gambrill, 2019), as practices and policies based on evidence need to be evaluated and assessed by those implementing them.

There is a skill in reading evidence in a critical way to determine its quality before you use it in your practice. A procedure to do this was developed by Bashir and Dziemidowicz (2021), which we reproduce in Box 4.6.

Box 4.6

Appraising research evidence (Bashir and Dziemidowicz, 2021)

To critically appraise a specific piece of evidence, there are several steps for you to follow:

- Determine whether the study has addressed a clearly focused issue. This can be considered by examining the aim and nature of the study and ascertaining if the design was appropriate for the aim.
- Identify who the population being studied were. This means examining the inclusion and exclusion criteria of the study, deciding if that sample was an accurate representation of the population, and determining whether any participants withdrew from the research.
- Interpret the findings by matching them to the goals of the study and seeing if these are appropriate for the methodology.
- Assess for bias to see if any confounders were identified and if bias was minimised, appreciating that the idea of bias is not always appropriate for qualitative evidence as the subjectivity of the researcher is acknowledged (sometimes foregrounded) and managed through reflexivity.
- Determine if the study is applicable to your practice and think about how that might be achieved.

In determining whether the evidence you have appraised is applicable to your practice, you will need to think about implementation. This is a multistep process, and Umesh, Karippacheril, and Magazine (2016) provided some practical steps to do this, which we reproduce in Box 4.7. We consider the issue of translating research findings into implications for practice, that is, of implementation, in more detail in the final chapter.

Box 4.7

Implementing evidence in practice (Umesh et al., 2016)

To critically appraise health evidence, there are several steps:

- Formulate a question you believe is pertinent for improving the lives of those you work with and/or their families.

- Undertake a thorough search of the literature to identify what might be the best, i.e. the most appropriate, evidence to address your question.
- Assess that evidence critically, evaluating its quality against the appropriate quality markers for the approach utilised by the authors, and consider the applicability of that evidence to the question you developed.
- Take steps to apply that evidence in your practice.
- Monitor the application of the evidence and assess whether the outcomes or processes have improved.

Practice-based evidence

Potentially, the solution to some of the criticisms of evidence-based practice is practice-based evidence. Practice-based evidence emphasises participatory approaches and the promotion of sharing experiences and expertise. Arguably, this has the advantage of meaningfully involving practitioners in the generation of evidence, particularly when research is designed with practical applicability in mind (Fox, 2003). The key factor in understanding practice-based evidence is that it involves collecting information about the efficacy of treatment in "routine practice". In other words, a specific research protocol to collect data from matched samples is not attempted, as might be the case where evidence is being collected that will become the "evidence base" for evidence-based practice. The point of practice-based evidence is to find *meaningful* ways to collect information about the benefits of the treatment.

Key point!

There is some overlap between evidence-based practice and practice-based evidence; thus, the distinction between the two is not clear-cut.

Practice-based evidence has been considered valuable because of differences in the conceptualisation and language of academically orientated empirical research. Led by practitioners at a grassroots level, gathering evidence is for the purpose of informing and improving practice and tends to be less formal than data gathered specifically for research purposes (Margison, Barkham, Evans et al., 2000). Practice-based-evidence is thus seen to have more real-world authority for practitioners (Fox, 2003). Practice-based evidence places greater emphasis on the realities of practitioners' work. Thus, practice-based evidence is an approach that retains high quality but is developed in real-world settings to be implemented in those settings (Portney, 2020). The goal driving practice-based evidence is to better understand the healthcare environment and use those insights to inform the research environment, rather than the other way around (Gabbay and Le May, 2011).

Although individual practitioners may be involved in gathering practice-based evidence, another popular and beneficial approach is the formation of practice research networks (PRNs). These are defined as a "network of clinicians that collaborate to conduct research to inform their day-to-day practice" (Audin, Mellor-Clark, Barkham et al., 2001, p. 241). One area of practice that is notoriously difficult to gather evidence about its efficacy through highly formalised research methods such as randomised controlled trials is counselling and psychotherapy. In this field of work, clinician-researchers are likely to gather data that will constitute practice-based evidence and may form practice research networks for this purpose. Audin et al. (2001) identified that within this context there have emerged several different types of PRNs (also known as practice-based research networks or PbRNs), and we provide a reference source for each type for you to explore examples:

- **Grassroots**: These are characteristically organic in that there is a natural evolution of a group or network of practitioners (e.g. Huet, Springham, and Evans, 2014).
- **Developmental**: This is a more systematic or phased approach whereby a network of practitioners collaborating will gradually build up a resource of clinical tools (e.g. Sales, Farrández-Berrueco, Sanahuja, and Moliner, 2024).
- **Central or single site**: This is where research expertise tends to be centralised at a single centre and a natural hierarchy of data emerges (e.g. McAleavey, Castonguay, and Xiao, 2014).
- **Star or multiple sites**: This approach looks more like a network of nested data that emerges naturally. An example by Cooper, McGinnis, and Carrick (2014) demonstrates this multilevel evidence approach within a network of primary or secondary schools.

Author reflections and concluding remarks
From Nikki
As a Clinical Psychologist it makes total sense to me that commissioners of services and health insurance companies would like reassurances that the interventions they are funding will be effective in reducing the distress of the people the service is provided for. In terms of quality assurance and ethicality, I agree that service providers should be accountable for providing services that are beneficial to those who engage with their services. An obvious way to achieve this is to look to the pool of published research to examine which therapies or interventions have evidence that they work. The logic is that only those interventions that have some concrete empirical evidence of their effectiveness would be listed as approved interventions by the commissioners of those services. However, the flaw in this approach, as we have discussed in this chapter, is twofold. First, some interventions are notoriously tricky to measure because of the qualitative nature of what "success" looks like for those service users and service providers. Second, there is still a preference in the literature for conducting trials about treatment efficacy using quantitative approaches.

When these two factors are combined, the result is that those interventions best assessed via qualitative approaches have less published research evidence available than interventions that lend themselves better to quantitative investigation. This means there may be more treatment modalities that do work in practice, but do not have as many research studies examining their effectiveness, and the ones that do are qualitative, and therefore excluded from the meta-analyses used to inform decisions about the types of approaches that constitute evidence-based practice. What I have observed is that there are therefore very few "mainstream" treatments in the field of mental health that are "approved" by commissioners of services as having a sufficiently robust evidence base to warrant their endorsement. In practice, several things happen as a result: i) only a limited range of psychological interventions are offered to clients, ii) a wider range of interventions are actually offered, but are adapted so that they can claim to be within the designated range, and iii) those who wish to practice outside of this limited range operate in private practice where there is less regulation.

Obviously quality assurance is essential, and thankfully most clinical practitioners are affiliated with a professional body that requires ongoing professional development and adherence to protocols of ethical practice. This offers some security to the public, who may be, to a greater or lesser degree, informed about what interventions they are accessing and what evidence there may be for their effectiveness. Additionally, service users very often "vote with their feet"; quite pragmatically, a individual is at liberty to simply stop attending sessions which they are not finding beneficial and perhaps look elsewhere. From my perspective, the burgeoning of collaborative networks of clinician-researchers involved in developing practice-based evidence is an excellent way to navigate some of the practical challenges of this debate. As someone who has worked with a wide range of very experienced and skilled practitioners, I appreciate the fact that they are often best placed to make intelligent decisions about what to evaluate and how. Most practitioners choose to work in the field they do because they genuinely want to help people; they want to make a difference. This means they are motivated to figure out "what works". This might not look as organised and formal as large randomised controlled trials, but it is arguably more targeted to the specific service need and the specific interventions provided. I would encourage all practitioners to find meaningful ways to measure the efficacy of the work that they are involved in.

References

Alatawi, M., Aljuhani, E., Alsufiany, F., Aleid, K., Rawah, R., Aljanabi, S., and Banakhar, M. (2020). Barriers of implementing evidence-based practice in nursing profession: A literature review. *American Journal of Nursing Science, 9*(1), 35–42.

Albarqouni, L., Hoffmann, T., Straus, S., Olsen, N. R., Young, T., Ilic, D., Shaneyfelt, T., Hanes, R., Guyatt, G., and Glasziou, P. (2018). Core competencies in evidence-based practice for health professionals. Consensus statement based on a systematic review and Delphi survey. *JAMA Network Open, 2*(1), e190281.

Audin, K., Mellor-Clark, J., Barkham, M., Margison, F., McGrath, G., Lewis, S., Cann, L., Duffy, J., and Parry, G. (2001). Practice research networks for effective psychological therapies. *Journal of Mental Health, 10,* 241–251.

Bashir, S., and Dziemidowicz, K. (2021). Critical appraisal: How to evaluate research for use in clinical practice. *The Pharmaceutical Journal, 306*(7950), 1–15.

Bodenheimer, T., and Sinsky, C. (2014). From triple to quadruple aim: Care of the patient requires care of the provider. *Annals of Family Medicine, 12*(6), 573–576.

Camargo, F. C., Iwamoto, H. H., Galvão, C. M., Pereira, G. A., Andrade, R. B., and Masso, G. C. (2018). Competences and barriers for the evidence-based practice in nursing: An integrative review. *Revista Brasileira de Enfermagem, 71*(4), 2030–2038.

Cartwright N. (2007). Are RCTs the gold standard? *BioSocieties, 2*(1), 11–20.

Cochrane, A. (1972). *Effectiveness and efficiency. Random reflections on health services.* London: Nuffield Provincial Hospitals Trust.

Condon, C., McGrane, N., Mockler, D., and Stokes, E. (2016). Ability of physiotherapists to undertake evidence-based practice steps: A scoping review. *Physiotherapy*, *102*, 10–19.

Cooper, M., Mcginnis, S., and Carrick, L. (2014). School-based humanistic counselling for psychological distress in young people: A practice research network to address the attrition problem. *Counselling & Psychotherapy Research*, *14*(3), 201–211.

Eddy, D. M. (2011). The origins of evidence-based medicine: A personal perspective. *American Medical Association Journal of Ethics*, *13*(1), 55–60.

Evans, D. (2003). Hierarchy of evidence: A framework for ranking evidence evaluating healthcare interventions. *Journal of Clinical Nursing*, *12*, 77–84.

Farrell, C., and Gilbert, H. (1996). *Health care partnerships*. London: Kings Fund.

Fox, N. (2003). Practice-based evidence: Towards collaborative and transgressive research. *Sociology*, *37*(1), 81–102.

Gabbay, J., and Le May, A. (2011). *Practice-based evidence for healthcare: Clinical mindlines*. London: Routledge.

Gambrill, E. (2019). *Critical thinking and the process of evidence-based practice*. Oxford: Oxford University Press.

Gerstman, B. B. (2023). There is no single gold standard study design (RCTs are not *the* gold standard). *Expert Opinion on Drug Safety*, *22*(4), 267–270.

Green, L. (2006). Public health asks of systems science: To advance our evidence-based practice, can you help us get more practice-based evidence? *American Journal of Public Health*, *96*(3), 406–409.

Huet, V., Springham, N., and Evans, C. (2014). The art therapy practice research network: Hurdles, pitfalls and achievements. *Counselling & Psychotherapy Research*, *14*(3), 174–180.

Kiyimba, N., Lester, J., and O'Reilly, M. (2019). *Using naturally occurring data in health research: A practical guide*. Cham, Switzerland: Springer.

Lather, P. (2013). Methodology-21: What do we do in the afterward? *International Journal of Qualitative Studies in Education*, *26*(6), 634–645.

Lester, J., and O'Reilly, M. (2015). Is evidence-based practice a threat to the progress of the qualitative community? Arguments from the bottom of the pyramid [Special issue; 20th Anniversary edition]. *Qualitative Inquiry*, *21*(7), 628–632.

Margison, F. R., Barkham, M., Evans, C., McGrath, G., Clark, J. M., Audin, K., and Connell, J. (2000). Measurement and psychotherapy. Evidence-based practice and practice-based evidence. *British Journal of Psychiatry*, *177*, 123–130.

Mcaleavey, A., Castonguay, L., and Xiao, H. (2014). Therapist orientation, supervisor match, and therapeutic interventions: Implications for session quality in a psychotherapy training PRN. *Counselling & Psychotherapy Research*, *14*(3), 192–200.

McNeill, T. (2006). Evidence-based practice in an age of relativism: Toward a model for practice. *Social Work*, *51*(2), 147–156.

Melnyk, B., and Fineout-Overholt, E. (2023). *Evidence-based practice in nursing & healthcare: A guide to best practice* (3rd ed.). Philadelphia, PA: Wolters Kluwer.

Melnyk, B., Fineout-Overholt, E., Stillwell, S., and Williamson, K. (2010). The seven steps of evidence-based practice. *American Journal of Nursing*, *110*(1), 51–53.

Melnyk, B., Gallagher-Ford, L., and Fineout-Overholt, E. (2014). The establishment of evidence-based practice competencies for practicing registered nurses and advanced practice nurses in real-world settings: Proficiencies to improve healthcare quality, reliability, patient outcomes, and costs. *Worldviews on Evidence-Based Nursing*, *1*(1), 5–15.

Miller, C., and Miller, D. (2011). The real-world failure of evidence-based medicine. *The International Journal of Person Centered Medicine*, *1*(2), 295–300.

Morse, J. (2006). The politics of evidence. *Qualitative Health Research*, *16*(3), 395–404..

Paul, R., and Elder, L. (2020). *Critical thinking: Tools for taking charge of your professional and personal life* (2nd ed.). Oxford: Prentice Hall.

Portney, L. (2020). *Foundations of clinical research: Applications to evidence-based practice*. Philadelphia, PA: F.A Davis Company.

Rycroft-Malone J., Seers K., Titchen A., Harvey, G., Kitson, A., and McCormack, B. (2004). What counts as evidence in evidence-based practice? *Journal of Advanced Nursing, 47*(1), 81–90.

Sackett, D., Rosenberg, W., Gray, J. A., Haynes, R. B., and Richardson, W. S. (1996). Evidence-based medicine: what it is and what it isn't. *British Medical Journal, 312,* 71–72.

Sales, A., Farrández-Berrueco, R., Sanahuja, A., and Moliner, O. (2024). Knowledge mobilisation strategies for responsible and inclusive academic research. *European Journal of Higher Education, 14*(1), 20–39.

Saunders, H., Gallagher-Ford, Kvist, T., and Vehviläinen-Julkunen, K. (2019). Practicing healthcare professionals' evidence-based practice competencies: An overview of systematic reviews. *Worldviews on Evidence-Based Nursing, 16*(3), 176–185.

St. Pierre, E. (2016). Practices for the "new" in the new empiricisms, the new materialism, and post qualitative inquiry. In N. Denzin and M. Giardina (Eds.), *Qualitative inquiry and the politics of research.* Walnut Creek, CA: Left Coast Press.

Timmermans, S., and Berg, M. (2003). *The gold standard: The challenge of evidence-based medicine and standardization in health care.* Philadelphia, PA: Temple University Press.

Umesh, G., Karippacheril, J., and Magazine, R. (2016). Critical appraisal of published literature. *Indian Journal of Anaesthesia, 60,* 670–673.

Xu, M., and Storr, G. (2012). Learning the concept of researcher as instrument in qualitative research. *The Qualitative Report, 17*(21), 1–18.

CHAPTER 5

Planning a project

> **Learning objectives**
>
> This chapter helps the reader to:
>
> - Develop a research question.
> - Differentiate project aims, objectives, outputs, and outcomes.
> - Write a research proposal.
> - Develop ideas and a plan for a literature review.
> - Critically assess the literature.
> - Assess the importance of a pilot study.

Introduction

If you are undertaking a research project in health, then planning your project is crucial. Before you start the research process, you need to plan and map out the process and design. This means you need to undertake a literature search, design your research question, anchor it to your methodology and theoretical foundation, and create a strong research proposal. The process of planning any type of qualitative research project is iterative, which means it is not linear, but that you cycle back through different stages as you go along. While you are likely to start with an initial research topic you read more about, the formal development of a research question and a structured literature review are preceded by multiple layers of thinking, reading, engaging, and creating. Also, the methodological approach you ultimately decide to use will require slightly different processes in relation to this. In this chapter, we guide you through some of these early steps in planning your research project.

Designing a research question

> **Key point!**
> The research question is fundamental to your research project and is something you need to consider from the very early stages of your work.

When undertaking qualitative research, you need a strong underpinning research question. The prospect of having to develop a "good" or robust research question can create some anxiety for those less familiar with the research process. Your research question will inform your methodology and associated methods and is underpinned by your theoretical and epistemological position. It is therefore advisable to start with your question, rather than the methods, and think about how it links to your theories and positionality. This is because research questions guide the choice of methodology, methods, recruitment choices, data collection methods, and data analysis.

> **Key point!**
> A poorly defined research question will likely result in you losing focus and direction and may create challenges for you later in the process of the research project.

It takes time to develop a research question and involves dialogue with your supervisor, mentor, or team members, so we encourage you to keep this in mind and avoid rushing to formulate a question (White, 2017). It is often underestimated by new researchers how the research question will shape and direct their study. Although good questions do not guarantee good research, it is the case that questions that are poorly thought through will create problems at various stages of the project (Agee, 2009). Talking to stakeholders who will be affected by your research is a good place to start. You need to ask yourself, who is the research for, and who will benefit? A research question that is guided by the needs and priorities of your participant population is likely to have real-world currency but may need to be shaped to work effectively within an academic landscape.

These considerations notwithstanding, it is helpful to remember that your research question is not static. Your research focus can change, be adapted, and refined as you work through the various research processes (Agee, 2009; Hennink, Kaiser, and Weber, 2017). In other words, your question will evolve as it is iteratively derived, with first iterations being tentative and exploratory, before becoming more specific and refined (Creswell and Poth, 2018). Consequently, the process of developing the question is a reflective process, which underscores the strength of the qualitative approach (Agee,

2009). In finalising your research question, the associated methodological approach will influence how the question is worded, and we acknowledge there are different types of research question (Doody and Bailey, 2016; Ritchie, Lewis, McNaughton, and Nicholls, 2014; White, 2017):

- **Explanatory questions** – seek to explain phenomena and examine the reasons for or the associations between what exists.
- **Generative questions** – seek out new ideas or aid in the development of theories or actions.
- **Contextual questions** – are designed to describe the nature of what exists.
- **Evaluative questions** – critically assess the effectiveness or value of something.
- **Exploratory questions** – investigate and enrich our understanding of phenomena where there is little or limited available information.
- **Ideological questions** – have a goal of building the ideology of a position.
- **Descriptive questions** – have the goal of describing phenomena.
- **Emancipatory questions** – research that addresses these kinds of questions is based on a liberatory ethos and seeks to engage in social actions related to specific phenomena.

Writing your research question

In developing your research question, you need to articulate what you want to achieve (Agee, 2009). Agee emphasised that by doing this, you will be making an inquiry about a specific topic and seeking to identify the perspectives of a specific sample of the population. In developing your research question, we also encourage you to be mindful of the ethics of the research and the ethical implications of seeking to answer the research question. Often, ethical considerations in developing research questions are not reflected upon carefully enough by researchers, but this is a central issue in health research when studying the lives of people, especially if it involves vulnerable or marginalised groups and examining sensitive topics (Agee, 2009). Thus, we argue that the research question you decide upon ultimately needs to be taken from an ethically considered position (O'Reilly and Parker, 2014). This is because research questions can inadvertently contribute to the stigma of certain health conditions, may fail to reflect the priorities of populations, may be motivated by profit, or may be poorly constructed and fail to generate useful knowledge or ultimately reinforce assumptions upon which they are based (Dubois, 2008). Another aspect of the ethics of the research question is to understand your motives for engaging in the planned research project, and to consider who will benefit. When participants are generous enough to sacrifice their time and share their knowledge, experience, and views, we need to respect and honour that and ensure our research adds to the pool of knowledge which may serve (in some way) to improve the circumstances of the population that the research sample represents. We outline a list of things to remember in writing your question in Box 5.1.

Box 5.1
Things to remember when writing your research question

As you write your research question, remember these points:

- A broad question is a useful starting point and can help you develop your sub-questions. By creating an overarching question, you can capture the main goals of your study (Agee, 2009).
- Remember that your positionality, epistemology, ontology, and explanatory theories will be connected to your research question and that the theoretical framing of a research study may inspire additional questions or sub-questions (Agee, 2009).
- Utilise the research evidence and wider literature to help shape your initial thinking as you develop your research question (Doody and Bailey, 2016).
- Keep your research question focused and related to your research aims (Doody and Bailey, 2016).
- Think critically about any taken-for-granted assumptions, as this can support the articulation of transformative viewpoints (Mattick, Johnston, and de la Croix, 2018).
- A good research question will guide the researcher to collect data that provides new insights and produces original and helpful knowledge to influence practice (Mattick et al., 2018).

While the points to remember are valuable, we also offer some practical guidance for developing your own question in Box 5.2.

Box 5.2
Practical steps to write a research question

It can be a tricky process to produce a good research question. There are, all the same, practical steps you can take to navigate this process effectively:

- As you read, think, reflect, and do research, you will generate ideas and have moments of inspiration, so it is useful to keep a specific file on the computer or a section of your research diary to note these down, so they are not lost (Agee, 2009).
- Have one or more brainstorming sessions on your own or with others to create idea clouds, lists, or messy idea boards. While this will need to become more organised as you progress, these more imaginative sessions can help in generating questions (O'Reilly and Parker, 2014).
- Make sure your question aligns with your topic of interest, which will help keep it focused, and think about who will benefit from answering it (Mattick et al., 2018).
- Explore the literature to see what questions have already been addressed in the area and how those have been framed to help you think about the type of question you want to ask and how it can be clearly articulated and relevant to previous research concerned with the same topic (Mattick et al., 2018).

- Your research question will need to have relevance to the clinical area you are working in or undertaking research in. The generation of knowledge by answering the question should help inform practice (Riva, Malik, Burnie et al., 2012).
- Although your question may begin as a broad concern, it will need to become more specific over time so that it has direction and impact (Mattick et al., 2018).
- Work with other people, contemplating and playing with different ideas. Engage a supervisor, mentor, manager, or other person with more research experience to help critically appraise your question.
- Keep a record of different iterations of your question, as you may find you return to an older version of it and redevelop that if you are not satisfied with the way your question changes.

Consistent with this practical guidance, there are different models in the literature designed to facilitate the process of iterative question development. We highlight two of these below – the STEPS model and the PICOT model.

The STEPS model was devised in our earlier work (O'Reilly and Parker, 2014) and was created for qualitative researchers. This model proposed that a research question needs to contain five core characteristics, and we have updated these to now be:

- Specific – the field of study should be narrow and defined.
- Timed – the question should frame the project within an achievable timeline.
- Enquiry – this refers to the nature of the question and is part of what the question is addressing.
- Participants – this refers to the population being studied.
- Subject – this refers to the topic of interest being studied.

STEPS is not a prescriptive model for articulating a research question but rather is designed to provide a guide for novice researchers. In this model, we proposed there is a "what" aspect of a question and a "how" aspect. The "what" part refers to the fact that the question should show the nature of the inquiry, the type of participants, and the specific nature of the subject being studied. The participants should be mentioned in the question to indicate the focus of the inquiry, and the subject gives a sense of what health topic is being studied. In terms of the "how" aspect, the question needs to be specific and within a timeframe that is realistic.

An example question could be:

> What experiences do autistic children in primary school have of engaging with sporting events?

In this question, we see the *enquiry*, "what", the *participants*, "autistic children", and the *subject*, "engaging in sporting events". The question is *specific* to a certain condition, a certain population, and a certain area of their lives, and it is achievable to address, that is, in a reasonable *time frame*.

The PICOT model has been widely utilised for generating research questions that inform randomised controlled trials (RCTs) (Guyatt, Drummond, Meade, and Cook, 2008), but arguably the format is still useful if adapted for designing a qualitative research question.

P = Population – the sample for your project.
I = Intervention – the intervention the participants will receive (not all qualitative work has an intervention).
C = Comparison – who you will be comparing your population with, the comparison group. In an RCT, this would be a control group, but in qualitative research you will not have one.
O = Outcome – how you plan to measure the effectiveness of the intervention, but qualitative work has different kinds of outcomes.
T = Time – the duration of the data collection period.

Developing a question using the PICOT model affords a basis to understand a clinical area of investigation and its relevance to current literature (Riva et al., 2012). The PICOT format involves a comparison and an intervention, which qualitative health research is less likely to involve. While some qualitative health research may have an element of comparison and may examine the perceived impact of an intervention, it will not measure phenomena in the same way as quantitative research. Therefore, if you use the PICOT model, you will have to adapt it to suit your approach. One way in which PICOT has been adapted is for qualitative research evidence synthesis in the form of the SPIDER model; that is, S - Sample, PI - Phenomenon of Interest, D - Design, E - Evaluation and outcome, and R- Research approach (Cooke et al., 2012).

Differentiating aims, objectives, outputs, and outcomes

Central to developing a good research question and informing the research process is being clear about the aims and objectives of your study and having some sense of what the desired outputs and outcomes will be. However, it requires reflection and consideration to develop a robust aim and set of objectives, and this will take time to consider. Thus, we provide some guidance on how to develop these.

Aims

In determining the aims of your project, you need to describe the overall purpose of what you are hoping to accomplish in a general sense (Doody and Bailey, 2016). By developing a clear statement of project aims, the readers of your work will be able to make a judgement about whether you have achieved your purpose (Tully, 2014).

> **Key point!**
>
> Aims are usually general and thus normally positioned at the beginning of the project, as they are broad and introductory.
>
> (Thomas and Hodges, 2010)

There are different types of aim statements, and these were described by Newman, Andrews, Magwood et al. (2011) as utilised to:

- Make a prediction.
- Add to the knowledge base.
- Have a personal, social, institutional, or organisational impact.
- Test a new idea.
- Understand complex phenomena.
- Measure change.
- Generate new ideas.
- Examine the past.

As you develop your aims statement, describe what it is you are trying to achieve. You might use phrases like "to map", "to critically assess", "to build", "to synthesise", "to examine", "to investigate", "to explore", or "to design".

Objectives

Developing your aims statement provides a basis for determining your objectives. Objectives are more specific than an aim and map more directly against your research question (Grove, Gray, and Burns, 2014). Five of the more common objectives (as described by Johnson and Christensen, 2014, and by Onwuegbuzie and Leech, 2006) are:

- **Exploration** – using mostly inductive methods to explore a concept, construct, situation, event, or phenomenon to advance understanding.
- **Description** – identification and description of the antecedents, nature, and cause of the phenomenon.
- **Explanation** – the development of theory for the purpose of explaining relationships between concepts.
- **Prediction** – the use of pre-existing knowledge or theory to predict future outcomes.
- **Influence** – manipulating a setting or variables to produce an anticipated outcome.

The research objectives need to be specific and build on the aims statement. Usually, researchers have two or three objectives, and it is considered good practice to number these, so they are clearly identifiable (Thomas and Hodges, 2010). Your objectives need to be practical and achievable and tend to use words like "collect", "recruit", "measure", "produce" "analyse", or "create". For example, Farrugia, Petrisor, Farrokhyar, and Bhandari (2010, p. 281) provided a hypothetical example in intra-operative fluoroscopy where an objective could be: "to determine the effect of treatment A as compared to treatment B on patient functional outcome at 1 year". Thus, the objective was "to measure" the effectiveness of a specific treatment. We note that this was in relation to quantitative research rather than qualitative, but it should help you to see how an objective is formulated.

When developing a set of objectives, there is some agreement that these should be SMART, as described by Ogbeiwi (2017) and outlined in Box 5.3.

> **Box 5.3**
>
> **SMART objectives (Ogbeiwi, 2017)**
>
> SMART objectives refer to the following characteristics:
>
> - **S**pecific – exact, clearly identifying what you intend to accomplish.
> - **M**easurable – quantifiable.
> - **A**ppropriate – aligning with the needs of the target audience.
> - **R**ealistic – achievable with the resources available.
> - **T**ime-specific – within a certain timeframe.

Aims and objectives (summarised)

It is crucial that your research aims and objectives are connected and help ensure you meet the goals of your project. We provide a set of practical tips for developing your aims and objectives, as proposed by Thomas and Hodges (2010) in Box 5.4.

> **Box 5.4**
>
> **Developing aims and objectives guidance from Thomas and Hodges**
>
> Often aims and objectives are developed together:
>
> - Make sure you give yourself enough time to think through the aims and objectives and do not rush in developing them.
> - Undertake a lot of reading in the area and see what other researchers have achieved.
> - Consider what your technical terms and concepts are.
> - As part of your literature review, link your objectives to the conclusions of your review to strengthen how your objectives are anchored to the current evidence.
> - Draft your aims statement and your objectives, and keep revising these until you are happy with the final version.
> - Share these with your colleagues, supervisors, peers, and other experts.
> - Ensure your aims and objectives are feasible.
> - Make sure your aims are distinguishable from your objectives and put them in separate sentences. Ideally, objectives should be numbered.
> - Your aims and objectives should not be vague or ambiguous.

Outputs

Your project is going to produce various outputs, and it is helpful to think about what these might be and what you hope to accomplish. These tend to be more tangible outcomes arising from the project. For example, you might want to produce an information leaflet for a group of patients, a toolkit for oncologists to use in practice, or a communication tool for speech and language therapists. Thus, the outputs of your project are the products resulting from it. More formally, your outputs can be academic outputs produced to meet the expectations of academic work.

We encourage you to recognise that if your research is funded, there will likely be a strong emphasis on anticipated outputs from funders. For example, the UK funding body, Wellcome Trust, states the following: "we expect the researchers we fund to manage their research outputs in a way that will achieve the greatest health benefit" (Wellcome Trust, n.d., n.p). Your research may produce new insights, institutional models, technical innovations, products, services, or training (Belcher and Halliwell, 2021). Outputs can also take the form of data sets, discoveries, theories, policies, recommendations, or even processes like dialogue and networking, and in that sense, outputs are the knowledge, innovations, and services produced by the research (Belcher and Halliwell, 2021).

Outcomes

Your outcomes will be connected to your outputs, but these are broader and less specific. Outcomes are connected to your aims in terms of what you hoped to accomplish, that is, the changes that you wanted to achieve from the project. For example, this may be increased awareness of something for a professional group, such as particular consideration in clinical decision making, increased medication adherence, or improved confidence in carers.

> **Key point!**
>
> It is helpful to develop a set of outcome indicators so you have some way of knowing whether you have achieved your outcomes and to what extent.

Notably, outcomes relate to the benefits of the research. These are the changes that can be identified, like changes in knowledge, confidence, attitudes, skills, or relationships that manifest as a change in behaviour, which may be at an individual, group, or organisational level (Belcher and Halliwell, 2021). Belcher and Halliwell argued that there are different kinds of outcomes: academic and societal. As a clinician-researcher, there can be tension related to the balance of these when considering that the primary focus of research ought to be the improvement of an aspect of health or social well-being.

Outputs and outcomes (summarised)

Your outputs and outcomes will be very important for the dissemination, translation, and impact of your research, and these are matters we will return to toward the end of the book. Often outputs and outcomes are conflated, but it will be helpful to bear in mind that these are different. For example, Magowan (2019) distinguished between outcomes as denoting what you want or need to achieve and outputs as the items or actions that allow you to achieve those outcomes.

For instance: You may have an *output* of producing 50 information leaflets about medication adherence for people with diabetes. The intended *outcome* of providing the information leaflets may be an increased adherence to prescribed medication by 50 individuals diagnosed with diabetes per region involved in the study within a six-month timeframe.

Alternately: You may have an *output* of a toolkit for 200 secondary school teachers to use with children and young people in educating them about searching for credible mental health information online. The intended *outcome* may be an increase in children's use of credible health web sources of mental health information in school and at home.

Or: You may have an *output* of an evidence-based training programme to deliver to 100 trainee nurses. From this, you may intend to have an *outcome* of increased confidence in delivering care within two weeks of delivery.

Notably, then, outcomes tend to result from outputs. They are also a precursor to impact (Belcher and Halliwell, 2021).

Writing a research proposal

In planning your research project, it is common to write a research proposal that accounts for your main decisions, plans, and what you anticipate will happen as a result of undertaking the project. The research proposal outlines the practical and theoretical components of your planned project and is something you develop in detail over time. In our earlier work, we explained the different audiences who might engage with your research proposal (O'Reilly and Parker, 2014):

- **You** – you are a relevant audience for your proposal, as this document will help you track your decisions and plans for the work.
- **Ethics committees/governance panels** – your research will need ethical governance and oversight, and part of the proposal will demonstrate the scientific and ethical credibility of your plans.
- **Educational institutions** – it may be the case that you are undertaking a qualification, and your project is to be assessed as part of the programme of study. The proposal will serve as a basis for discussions with supervisors.
- **Peers/team members** – if you are working with others, the proposal can be a co-created document where you share your ideas, plans, and decisions.
- **Funding bodies** – you may be seeking funding for your research, and a formal proposal will be part of the process.

How to write a proposal

Although there is no universal template for a proposal, you will benefit from following any guidance provided by the institution you are writing it for, as there can be standard forms associated with certain organisations. However, there are some general features that a proposal usually contains, and we guide you through these.

> **Key point!**
>
> The audience(s) you are writing for will likely have different expectations, so consider those as you write and remember to check word lengths and required headings.
>
> (O'Reilly and Parker, 2014)

Title page: Your proposal should have a title page with an original, memorable, but informative title and other useful details, like your name, email address, and date.

Background and literature review: The proposal needs a short summary review of the key literature in the field, with an introduction section that illustrates what the research problem is, why it is important to address, and briefly what research evidence currently exists in the area. The literature review should provide a brief critical appraisal of the evidence and guide the reader toward the relevance and need for your work.

Aims, objectives, and research questions: Here it is necessary to provide the reader with a rationale for your work, illuminating the aims and objectives, your research questions, and potential outputs and outcomes. You can also illustrate how you will address any gaps in knowledge and how you will contribute to knowledge and evidence.

Approach and methods: This section outlines your decisions on methodology, methods, and theory. It provides your reader with information about the project design and a rationale as to why a qualitative design and specific methodological approach are appropriate to meet your aims and address your questions. This section of the proposal addresses practical considerations and contains details about recruitment, sampling, methods of data collection, and so forth.

Ethics: In this section, you need to demonstrate a commitment to ethical governance, processes, and principles. Any sensitivities, vulnerabilities, and possible risks, safety, and safeguarding concerns should be noted in this section, as should any formal governance procedures you will adhere to.

Contribution and impact: Most health research has the goal of making a contribution to practice and having value to a population. This is your opportunity within the proposal to illustrate the longer-term goals and possible impacts your research will have.

Timescale: It is useful to provide an anticipated timescale for your project, including any planning and recruitment, ethics processes, and reviewing that might be included. The time indicators need to be realistic, achievable, and sensible, with contingencies for delays built in.

Budget: Depending on the nature of the project and the audience, you might also need to include a breakdown of the costs involved in your project.

Logic models

Logic models are primarily associated with evaluation research but can be a helpful visualisation and planning tool in qualitative research too. Visually representing the process of research evaluation is growing in popularity (Jones, Azzam, Wanzer et al., 2020), with the logic model being widely used (Chen, 2014). Logic models tend to be used in evaluative research as they can represent the causal processes where interventions produce outcomes (Mills, Lawton, and Sheard., 2019). Although largely associated with quantitative health research, Mills and colleagues noted that logic models can be used by qualitative researchers as some qualitative research is conducted in the form of process evaluations with a goal to produce theories about how interventions work, which is referred to as a theory of change (Moore, Audrey, Barker et al., 2015).

In process evaluations, the diagrammatical form of a logic model helps visualise the process of knowledge generation and knowledge transfer (Stone and Lane, 2012).

> **Key point!**
>
> It can be useful to create a logic model to visualise core components of your research, especially if there is an evaluation part of your work.

The logic model visually represents the main activities in your research programme and illustrates how those activities lead to the outputs and outcomes (Knowlton and Phillips, 2012). In other words, the logic model is an organisational tool for designing an evaluation and highlighting the relevant elements of the programme (McLaughlin and Jordan, 2004). McLaughlin and Jordan outlined the central features of logic models, which are outlined in Table 5.1.

Developing your logic model should follow a series of steps, and we would encourage you to seek out visual examples from others to help you. McLaughlin and Jordan (2004) argued there are five steps to producing your logic model, which we outline in Box 5.5.

> **Box 5.5**
>
> **Practical steps to produce a logic model (McLaughlin and Jordan, 2004)**
>
> 1. **Collect the relevant information** – this should be a team effort and draw on expertise regarding the programme or intervention, including from partners, stakeholders, and service users/customers.
> 2. **Describe the problem and its context** – define the need for the programme, while identifying who is involved in the programme.
> 3. **Define the elements of the model** – when building your logic model, you need to categorise the information you have collected, and identify the activities, resources, short-term and long-term outcomes.
> 4. **Draw out your model** – this should capture the logical flow and links that exist across the process. This enables you to organise the information and show how aspects of the model are connected.
> 5. **Verify your model** – as you iteratively build your logic model, it needs continuous evaluation regarding the goals of representing the programme logic, how the programme works, and the conditions that support this. This process should involve engaging appropriate stakeholders.

Mills et al. (2019) argued that part of the challenge with using logic models for qualitative research is that there are different kinds of logic models, and researchers need to be mindful of this. Indeed, they created a typology of four types of logic models. These are described in Table 5.2.

Table 5.1 Features of a logic model (McLaughlin and Jordan, 2004)

Feature	Description
Resources	The human and financial resources needed.
Activities	The actions needed to produce outputs.
Outputs	The products, services, or good produced.
Consumers/audience	People are needed to engage with the programme to enable actions that lead to results. Staff and stakeholders need to consider the population groups the programme will serve.
Outcomes	The changes or benefits of the activities and outputs.

Table 5.2 Typology of logic models (Mills et al., 2019)

Logic model	Description
Type one	Feature a list of intervention components and outcomes and can be useful in the planning of an intervention.
Type two	Focus on the central aims of the evaluation to understand the contextual factors that enable or limit delivery. This type has a linear structure and moves from inputs to outputs to outcomes.
Type three	Entails connections being drawn between model factors. This type fully represents the respective logics of interventions by displaying exactly how they work to produce various outcomes. It is typically illustrated using a flow chart indicating how an input leads to an outcome. Usually these are used to develop and test hypotheses about the relationship between intervention components and outcomes. The focus resides with the intervention rather than the intervention setting.
Type four	While not technically a logic model, this type falls under the broad rubric of Promoting Action on Research Implementation in Health Services (PARIHS). This type is context-sensitive and can include aspects of the traditional PARIHS model structure. A type four logic model shows that a researcher can qualitatively model the specifics of complex interventions.

Developing a grant application

One possible purpose of your research proposal is to acquire funding for your research project. The challenge is that acquiring research funding is competitive, and it can be difficult to convince the funder that your research is worthy of investment. When you write a research proposal for a funder, it needs to demonstrate the gaps in current knowledge, a focused way in which the research question will address the identified gap, and the skills and competencies of the research team (Brownson, Colditz, Dobbins et al., 2015). Arthurs (2014) argued it is necessary to:

- Demonstrate why the project is important and how it is different.
- Identify the resources needed.
- Identify the type of grant needed.

- Explore which funders are appropriate.
- Provide reasons why the project deserves funding.

You need to be realistic in your application process. If you have not applied for funding before then you might start by considering a small grant, possibly provided via a local funder or charity group (Arthurs, 2014). Whichever funding stream you apply to, you need to be well-informed about the process, the funder's aims, mission and priorities, its review process, and map your proposal using these (Gitlin, Kolanowski, and Lyons, 2021). In measuring the value of your research proposal, a funding body is likely to focus on the three Ps (Arthurs, 2014):

1. **The person** – your skills, competencies, experience, qualifications, and aspirations.
2. **The project** – this needs to be novel, have potential scientific merit, clear aims and objectives, and a realistic timeframe and budget.
3. **The place** – the institution you represent needs a strong track record, appropriate expertise, facilities, mentors, and research environment.

When writing your research proposal for funding, show how your interests are mapped against funder expectations (Gitlin et al., 2021). Despite this complexity and challenge, there are many benefits of seeking and obtaining research funding. Gitlin et al. (2021) argued that these are:

- Providing a basis to initiate a programme of research.
- Advancing knowledge in your field.
- Supporting pedagogical initiatives.
- Supporting institutional activities.
- Building a career profile.
- Expanding opportunities for education.
- Building a reputation in research and that of your organisation.
- Legitimising your research programme.

> **Key point!**
>
> Many funding bodies publish their acceptance rates which can often be as low as 5–10% with little feedback. It is helpful to learn from the process and important not to be deterred despite it seeming very challenging.
>
> (Arthurs, 2014)

While we have provided you with some guidance on how to write a research proposal, there are some useful tips to think about if this proposal is for the purpose of acquiring funding. Brownson et al. (2015) offered some ideas about what to include in a funding proposal and we outline these in Table 5.3.

In closing this section, we offer some tips for successful grant writing from Sathian, Simkhada, van Teijlingen et al. (2016) in Box 5.6.

Table 5.3 Writing a proposal for funding (Brownson et al., 2015)

Section	Tips
Abstract	This is the first impression you give to your reviewers. The abstract should include: a brief background of the project, the questions and aims, the objectives, the significance of the project and its relevance to practice, innovation in the work, the methods, and potential implications of the work.
Aims	This is critical for setting up the study and should include 2–4 realistic aims and not overpromise on what will be delivered. The aims should frame the proposal, and each aim should have a rationale and a sentence on how it will be accomplished.
Significance	It is necessary to define the scope of the problem, the gap in knowledge, and the importance of addressing that issue. Some reference to relevant research literature is needed, and you should comment on how addressing this gap can serve the purpose of improving health.
Innovation	Try to show the originality of your work and the contribution it will make, and show how this issue has not been adequately addressed to date. Highlight what is innovative about your proposed approach, methods, or methods or theory.
Approach	This is likely to be the longest section of your proposal and has the most bearing on whether you are successful. This shows how you will meet your aims and convince the reviewers of the potential impact.

Box 5.6

Writing a grant proposal (Sathian et al., 2016)

Sathian et al. provided their top ten tips for writing a grant application proposal, and we offer them here to help you in your process:

1. Check your eligibility to apply and look at previous examples of successful projects.
2. The application needs to start from a good idea, and this needs to fit with the main goal of the funder. You can find this information on funders' websites.
3. Spend time ensuring you understand the key elements of the application and address them. These will be used by reviewers and assessors to evaluate the proposal, including the proposed project's scientific merit, relevance to funding priorities, potential impact for wider society, strengths of the team, the plan for implementing the research process, outputs and outcomes, and dissemination plan.
4. Think like a reviewer. Remember that reviewers will be experienced scholars and will evaluate your proposal in relation to its strengths and weaknesses, as well as in terms of the experience and skills of the research team.
5. Ensure your summary or abstract is clear, logical, well-articulated, and concise. Organise your proposal according to the funder's guidance. Make sure your aims and objectives are clear and your approach robust. Do not neglect to proofread and check spelling and grammar, as well as references.

6. Be clear about how your goals and expected results relate to the priority of the funding programme.
7. Write your proposal clearly and provide sufficient information about your approach and methods.
8. Provide a clear rationale for the budget.
9. Share your proposal and gain advice and feedback from experienced experts.
10. Make sure the application form is complete and correct and submitted on time.

The literature review

Writing a literature review is a central part of the research process. There are different kinds of literature reviews, including scoping reviews, systematic reviews, and narrative reviews. In essence, a literature review is a systematic method for identifying, evaluating, and synthesising evidence (Fink, 2005). When you start searching and looking at the literature, you may feel overwhelmed by the amount written about any topic or issue. There are some things you can do to help you manage this, including:

- Clarifying the purpose of your project – the more defined your project is, the more focused your search will be.
- Utilising the expertise of your research team, supervisor, colleagues, or other experts to help identify relevant sources.
- Starting with a general search engine, like Google Scholar, to get a sense of the literature in and around your topic.
- Using the electronic databases associated with your discipline and topic.
- Considering what else you might need to read – remember that academic journal articles are not your only source for a literature review. Books and chapters, as well as news articles, credible web sources, and personal accounts, can also be useful sources of information.

It can be helpful to start broad, as reading widely can help with your understanding of the issues pertinent to your project. It might be that you do not find anything specific to your project. However, try to also recognise that while there may be very little that is specific to what you are looking for, there will be literature addressing wider, related topics. Your search should be methodical and follow the procedure of the type of review you are going to do. Broadly, there are six steps, as outlined by Templier and Paré (2015):

1. Formulate the research question and objective.
2. Search the literature.
3. Screen for inclusion.
4. Assess the quality of included studies.
5. Extract data.
6. Analyse data.

Before we provide information about different types of literature reviews, we offer some general practical guidance in Box 5.7.

> **Box 5.7**
>
> **Guidance on doing a literature review**
>
> There are some useful things to consider when searching the literature and writing your review:
>
> - Ensure your literature review has direction and provides a clear, logical argument.
> - Bring in core disciplinary concepts and theories as you shape your review.
> - The literature review provides background and context regarding the need for research evidence, and your review should be organised around your research question, aims, and objectives.
> - Your argument should not just describe the evidence but should critically assess its value – this is why it is called a literature review; it is a critical appraisal of the literature and not simply a report on it (or an annotated bibliography). The argument can be built around themes and pertinent issues.
> - One purpose of the literature review (for some approaches) is to summarise and synthesise what we know about the topic and identify gaps in knowledge.
> - Identify and critique the theories, concepts, and methods that relate to the evidence.
> - Your review needs a clear introduction that sets out the aims of the review and the central features of the argument to come. Use the introductory section to define the topic, set the context, provide a rationale for the review's importance, and set out the overall organisation of the review.
> - The conclusion of your review should summarise the core features of the argument you have presented, identify the gaps in knowledge, make suggestions for future directions, and have a clear concluding sentence that leads to the need for your research.

There are lots of different types of literature review and we do not provide details on all of them. We introduce you to a typology here and then provide further information on some of the most common kinds. Grant and Booth (2009) created a typology of literature reviews, which is:

1. **Critical review** – provides an extensive overview of the literature and critique of the quality of the evidence. This is not simply a description of the evidence in the field but includes analysis and conceptual considerations. The critical review presents, analyses, and synthesises material from a range of different sources.
2. **Narrative review** – examines published material over a wide range of subject matter, which are at various levels of completeness. This is generally a broad overview of the evidence, which can make it difficult to generalise from. There are common characteristics in a literature review in the sense that it focusses on published evidence and involves a process for identifying materials for inclusion, selecting materials for inclusion, synthesising them in textual, tabular, or graphical format, and analysing the contribution or value of that evidence.
3. **Mapping review** – this kind of literature review was developed by the Evidence for Policy and Practice Information and Co-ordinating Centre (EPPI-Centre) and is designed to categorise the existing evidence base on a given topic area. The goal is

to identify gaps in knowledge as a means of identifying avenues for future reviews or research.
4. **Meta-analysis** – this is a type of review that combines the results of quantitative studies in a statistical way. A meta-analysis needs all included studies to be sufficiently similar. This includes characteristics of the population, the intervention, and the comparison made.
5. **Mixed-studies or mixed-methods review** – any combination of methods where one component is a literature review.
6. **Overview literature review** – is a general term used for summarising the literature. This type of review surveys the literature and describes its characteristics.
7. **Qualitative systematic review or qualitative evidence synthesis** – this is a method that compares findings from qualitative research. The goal of this may be to develop new theory or a new narrative on an issue or an "interpretative translation". The focus of this kind of review is to identify themes or constructs from the included qualitative studies.
8. **Rapid review** – this type of review is based on a recognition of the time constraints in synthesising evidence to inform research, policy, and practice. This method uses systematic review methods to search and critically assess evidence in a rapid way.
9. **Scoping review** – is a type of review that provides a preliminary assessment of the scope and size of the existing evidence base. The aim of this type of review is to identify the nature and extent of research evidence on a topic.
10. **State-of-the-art review** – this is a subtype of the general "literature/narrative review" that tends to focus on more current matters and literature. A state-of-the-art review provides a new perspective on an issue or highlights areas that need further research.
11. **Systematic review** – this is the best-known kind of review which seeks to systematically search and synthesise a body of evidence. It has a transparent method of reporting.
12. **Systematic search and review** – this kind of review combines the strengths of a critical review with a comprehensive search strategy. This kind of review addresses broad questions.
13. **Systematised review** – this kind of review attempts to take one or more elements of a systematic review process while not claiming the output of a systematic review.
14. **Umbrella review** – is a mechanism for aggregating the findings of several reviews, thus compiling evidence from multiple reviews. Each review drawn upon focuses on a broad problem or health condition where there are two or more interventions, and thus the umbrella review pulls together results.

Developing a systematic review

In the field of health, there are many systematic reviews conducted for various reasons across diverse fields and to address different questions (Munn, Peters, Stern et al., 2018). During the 1990s, the Cochrane group was developed (Jordan, Munn, Aromataris, and Lockwood, 2015) and the Cochrane procedure is a commonly used framework for systematic reviews, with researchers registering their review or review protocol on the Cochrane database.

Broadly defined, a systematic review is a research synthesis conducted by a group of researchers with specialist skills with a goal of identifying the international evidence pertinent to a specific issue, usually to inform practice or identify future research need (Pearson, 2004). A systematic review requires the use of a structured and pre-defined process using rigorous methods, and as such, these reviews are considered central in evidence-based healthcare (Munn, Porritt, Lockwood et al., 2014). Munn et al. noted there are five main purposes for conducting a systematic review:

1. To identify and explore the international research evidence.
2. To confirm current practices and identify new ones.
3. To identify and inform areas for future research.
4. To investigate where there is conflict in results.
5. To produce statements that might guide decision-making.

The systematic review was a product of the evidence-based practice movement and represented a significant change from the position of expert consensus to a need for evidence-led guidance for the evolution of clinical knowledge (Burgers, Grol, Klazinga et al., 2003). For a review to be considered systematic, it requires a clearly formulated question, should identify studies that are relevant, critically appraise the quality of that research, and summarise the evidence using an explicit methodology (Cook and West, 2012). Cook and West observed that when done well, a systematic review should contribute to the wider literature and add to the body of knowledge to meaningfully inform research, policy, and practice.

There are a set of procedures to follow in doing a systematic review, and these are identified by Sharma, Gordon, Dharamsi et al. (2015) and outlined in Box 5.8. If it is something you are interested in using, we also recommend you attend a training course on undertaking systematic reviews, as this is a specialist task requiring specific skills.

Box 5.8

Doing a systematic review (Sharma et al., 2015)

There are a series of steps to follow in doing a systematic review:

1. **Inception of the review** – where the problem needs to be identified to guide the method, scope, and focus of the review.
2. **Scoping searches are useful** – check the Cochrane database of systematic reviews. This is useful to identify any existing evidence synthesis work and consider the depth and breadth of the evidence.
3. **Assemble a review team** – with appropriate expertise.
4. **Create a work plan** – this should be in the form of a protocol to delineate the actions for the review, the rationale for it, the methodology, and scope.
5. **Formulate the review question** – refine and focus this question.
6. **Plan the search** – the efficacy of the question should be considered, and operational definitions clarified. Make decisions about what to include and what not to include. You

will need to refine inclusion and exclusion criteria and think about language and the time period of published literature.
7. **Perform the search** – use appropriate literature search databases for the field and topic (e.g. SCOPUS, MEDLINE, ERIC, PsycINFO). Select studies using the inclusion and exclusion criteria. At least two reviewers are needed to reduce random error or bias. Start with the title, keywords, and abstract and if ineligible, exclude the article. If there is disagreement, then the full article should be read. If disagreement cannot be resolved, a third reviewer can be consulted.
8. **Extract the data from the studies** – it is necessary to extract the descriptive data, the methodological data, and information on the intervention. You also need to make a quality assessment of the study.
9. **Synthesise and analyse the data** – do this by making a statement about the evidence and gaps in knowledge.
10. **Discuss** – conclude the review.
11. **Report** the review.

> **Key point!**
>
> It is possible to streamline or accelerate the systematic review process by using rapid review methodologies.
>
> (Ganann, Ciliska, and Thomas, 2010)

Developing a scoping review

You may choose to do a scoping review rather than a full systematic review. A scoping review is a study aiming to rapidly map the core concepts in a research area and identify the core sources and types of evidence (Arksey and O'Malley, 2005). Arksey and O'Malley argued that a scoping review is useful when areas of research are early in development to map the current state of knowledge, and rather than conducting a quality assessment like a systematic review, a scoping review instead seeks to identify the breadth of the literature.

The scoping review is becoming an increasingly popular way of synthesising research evidence (Pham, Raji, Greig et al., 2014) to examine the extent, range, and nature of research on a topic and to determine the value and possible scope of doing a full systematic review (Levac et al., 2010). A scoping review aims to map the literature on a topic (Arksey and O'Malley, 2005), but a systematic review should summarise the best available evidence and assess the quality of it (Campbell Collaboration, 2013).

In determining whether you want to do a systematic review or a scoping review, it is worth thinking about when a scoping review is most useful. Munn et al (2018) argued that a scoping review can be especially helpful when:

- You want to determine the scope or coverage of the literature on a specific topic.
- You need a clear indication regarding the volume of literature and studies available.

- You want to explain the emerging evidence when it is unclear and determine more specific questions to ask for a systematic review (see Armstrong, Hall, Doyle, and Waters 2011).
- You want to report on evidence that addresses and informs practice in the field and seek information about how research has been conducted.

Arksey and O'Malley (2005) represent the scoping review as involving five distinct stages:

1. Identify the research question.
2. Identify relevant studies.
3. Select studies.
4. Chart the data.
5. Collate, summarise, and report the results.

Developing a thematic or narrative review

It is worth noting that some qualitative researchers conduct their literature review much later in the research process, as they do not take an *a priori* approach to the topic or phenomenon, and they do not set out to fill a gap in knowledge. Rather, they take a much more iterative approach to engagement with evidence, their literature searching being informed by the analytic process rather than a systematic approach to keywords and researcher knowledge. In these cases, researchers tend to undertake a general literature review, a narrative review, or a thematic review, which are all typically similar in ambition and process. A narrative review or general literature review tends to cover a broad range of evidence for inclusion and synthesises that evidence in the form of a narrative and demonstrates the value of that knowledge (Grant and Booth, 2009).

Some qualitative researchers organise the material into themes to provide the argument with a structure that maps against the issues that were yielded through analysis of participants' contributions. By providing a thematic review of the evidence, the writer can provide a rich and contextualised exploration of the topic and demonstrate a collective understanding across time, space, and place to make an argument and provide a theoretically informed assessment of the state of knowledge in a particular area (Braun and Clarke, 2022).

Reading research articles critically

To be able to do any kind of review, you need to read each article you might include in it critically. When including articles that have used qualitative methods in your review, you will need to assess whether it describes an important problem, whether the methodology is appropriate to address the problem and utilised in a rigorous and cogent way, and whether the perspective of the researcher is included (Greenhalgh and Taylor, 1997).

> **Key point!**
> It is helpful to read the article through fully first to get a general sense of what was found. Reading the article for a second time is then useful, but this time make critical notes as you do so.

As you make your notes about a research article or other piece of literature, it is necessary to provide a clear assessment of the argument presented and the conclusions drawn by the authors, and identify any limitations of the work. This will require you to weigh up the strength of the argument compared to those made by other authors. When reading the article, you should have a sense of what type of study was conducted, and this will enable you to evaluate whether the design adopted was appropriate or not (Greenhalgh, 1997). We have previously identified a series of steps that can be useful to help you critically assess an article (O'Reilly and Parker, 2014), and these are outlined in Box 5.9.

> **Box 5.9**
>
> **Critiquing a research article (O'Reilly and Parker, 2014)**
>
> There are a series of steps you can follow to critique an article:
>
> 1. Make sure you write down the reference for the paper in full or import the citation using appropriate software so that you have all the details of the article you are critiquing.
> 2. Read through the abstract and create a memo of the key points contained in it. You might want to copy the abstract into your notes, but make sure you do not plagiarise it in your own writing.
> 3. Read through the introduction or background section of the article. This will be where the authors set out and comment on the evidence in the field and note the gap in knowledge they identify. You might also use this to note other references to follow up in the field.
> 4. Identify the aims of the study and make a note of them. Be clear on what these are when you start assessing whether the author/s met their aims and objectives. Consider how this contributes to the healthcare field.
> 5. Read the methods of the study and note any apparent limitations. You can write these in list form. Consider how the methodological decisions were rationalised.
> 6. Explore the recruitment strategy and sampling, and consider how this was or was not appropriate for the design.
> 7. The ethics section will add transparency, and you can make a judgement about the ethicality of the processes.
> 8. Assess the results or findings of the article. Think about how well these are reported, if they are understandable, and if they are clearly presented; you can summarise these in a simple format for your notes.
> 9. Identify the conclusions drawn and judge whether these are consistent with the stated aims and objectives. Think about what the contribution is.
> 10. Summarise your critique and identify the core strengths and limitations of the work.

Critically assessing the literature will require some familiarity with the quality indicators associated with qualitative research. It can be difficult to make these assessments because of the heterogeneity in the paradigm, meaning that different approaches require different kinds of appraisals (Kuper, Reeves, and Levinson, 2008). To make these assessments, we recommend you read further about the quality indicators of certain methodologies.

Conducting a pilot study

A necessary aspect of your research project can be to pilot your idea and methods before you undertake the substantive project. The pilot study is typically associated with quantitative research, especially RCTs, as a way of checking the feasibility of the main project, to prevent any significant flaws that may be costly further down the line if left unchecked (Polit and Beck, 2017). A pilot study is, in this way, a "mini version" of the main study and provides a mechanism to test aspects of the project (like the data collection methods) (van Teijlingen and Hundley, 2002).

Pilot phases can also be supportive for a qualitative health research project. By completing a pilot study, you will be able to gain feedback from the population you are working with as well as other relevant stakeholders. Thus, when you plan your project, build in time to undertake your pilot study and be mindful that they often take longer than anticipated to conduct properly. Pilot studies can vary in how long they take to complete and in their depth and intensity, depending on the purpose of the pilot work.

There are a range of benefits to undertaking a pilot study, as we have outlined in our earlier work (O'Reilly and Parker, 2014):

- Undertaking your pilot study will enable you to identify any issues of access. You can utilise this to build rapport with gatekeepers and to gain information that may benefit the main study. This provides you with an opportunity to test out your communication strategies and promote interest among organisations and/or potential participants.
- Exploring the process of implementing your ethical procedures is a considerable benefit to your research. The pilot study allows you can test your consent procedures and identify any barriers. It also provides a mechanism for checking that your participants understand the ethical principles and identify any issues related to potential harms.
- Data collection is fundamental to the research process, and evaluating your methodology via the pilot study allows you to explore the practical issues related. It affords you an opportunity to gain feedback on how to improve the process and test any participatory or additional techniques.
- The pilot study has the benefit of providing a space to check the viability of your ideas and processes. This provides information to inform the main project. As a researcher, you can anticipate possible barriers and use this information to demonstrate to others that the project is feasible.

Overall, the pilot study has the benefit to the researcher of identifying potential areas of weakness for the main study and enabling them to take steps to address them (van Teijlingen and Hundley, 2002). In closing this chapter, we invite you to think about how you might plan and implement your own pilot study for your research project by engaging with the reflective activity in Box 5.10.

Box 5.10

Reflective activity on the pilot study

One very useful aspect of planning a research project includes the pilot phase of your work. We invite you to think about the following questions and write down your reflections in your research diary:

1. What steps will you take to involve your stakeholders in planning and implementing a pilot study?
2. What are the specific issues you want to test out through the pilot study, and how do you anticipate this will be helpful for your main project?

Author reflections and concluding remarks

From Philip

The process of planning a research project can be laborious. A great deal of work goes into formulating a research question, project aims, objectives, outputs, and outcomes, as well as writing a proposal, seeking funding, and reviewing relevant literature. There is a temptation to view the planning stage for a study simply as a stepping stone one must navigate to get to the doing of *real* research, i.e. of gathering and analysing data and finding things out. Yet, the planning stage is very much part of the substance of research inquiry. A poorly conceived project is unlikely to produce serviceable knowledge, i.e. insights or findings that can meaningfully inform the development of care delivery or contribute to wider debates or an evidence base.

For me, this lesson reinforces how, for busy healthcare practitioners, working as part of a team can be highly advantageous in sharing the burden of a research project and the value added by the diverse expertise that team members can bring to the endeavour. Some projects are, of course, driven primarily by a single individual (notably, the clinician-researcher completing PhD research), but, even in this scenario, the knowledge and support of supervisors and others (e.g. library staff) can be invaluable.

Further, having been involved in a range of different research projects in the fields of health and social care, of varying scope, I have increasingly become aware of how the process of planning a project gets easier with experience. Over time, one does (gradually) become more acquainted with the different components this planning entails and learns lessons about navigating this terrain, which can be reflected upon and used, for instance, in successfully obtaining research funding for a small study.

References

Agee, J. (2009). Developing qualitative research questions: A reflective process. *International Journal of Qualitative Studies in Education*, 22(4), 431–447.

Armstrong, R., Hall, B., Doyle, J., and Waters, E. (2011). "Scoping the scope" of a Cochrane review. *Journal of Public Health*, 33(1), 147–150.

Arskey, H., and O'Malley, L. (2005). Scoping studies: Towards a methodological framework. *International Journal of Social Research Methodology*, 8, 19–32.

Arthurs, O. (2014). Think it through first: Questions to consider in writing a successful grant application. *Pediatric Radiology*, 44, 1507–1511.

Belcher, B., and Halliwell, J. (2021). Conceptualizing the elements of research impact: Towards semantic standards. *Humanities & Social Sciences Communications*, 8(183).

Braun, V., and Clarke, V. (2022). *Thematic analysis: A practical guide*. London: Sage.

Brownson, R., Colditz, G., Dobbins, M., Emmons, K., Kerner, J., Padek, M., Proctor, E., and Stange, K. (2015). Concocting that magic elixir: Successful grant application writing in dissemination and implementation research. *Clinical & Translational Science*, 8(6), 710–716.

Burgers, J., Grol, R., Klazinga, N., MAkela, M., and Zaat, J. (2003). Toward evidence-based clinical practice: An international survey of 18 clinical guideline programs. *International Journal of Qualitative Health*, 15(1), 31–45.

Campbell Collaboration. (2013). What is a systematic review? http://www.campbellcollaboration.org/what_is_a_systematic_review/

Chen, H. (2014). *Practical program evaluation*. Thousand Oaks, CA: Sage.

Cook, D., and West, C. (2012). Conducting systematic reviews in medical education: A stepwise approach. *Medical Education*, 46(10), 943–952.

Cooke, A., Smith, D., and Booth, A. (2012). Beyond PICO: The SPIDER tool for qualitative evidence synthesis. *Qualitative Health Research*, 22(10), 1435–1443.

Creswell, J., and Poth, C. (2018). *Qualitative inquiry and research design* (5th ed.). Thousand Oaks, CA: Sage.

Doody, O., and Bailey, M. (2016). Setting a research question, aim and objective. *Nurse Researcher*, 23(4), 19–23.

DuBois, J. (2008). *Ethics in mental health research: Principles, guidance, and cases*. Oxford: Oxford University Press.

Farrugia, P., Petrisor, B., Farrokhyar, F., and Bhandari, M. (2010). Research questions, hypotheses and objectives. *Canadian Journal of Surgery*, 53(4), 278–281.

Fink, A. (2005). *Conducting research literature reviews: From the internet to paper* (2nd ed.). London: Sage.

Ganann, R., Ciliska, D., and Thomas, H. (2010). Expediting systematic reviews: Methods and implications of rapid reviews. *Implementation Science*, 5, 56–66.

Gitlin, L., Kolanowski, A., and Lyons, K. (2021). *Successful grant writing: Strategies for health and human service professionals*. New York, NY: Springer.

Grant, M., and Booth, A. (2009). A typology of reviews: An analysis of 14 review types and associated methodologies. *Health Information & Libraries Journal*, 26, 91–108.

Greenhalgh, T. (1997). How to read a paper: The Medline database. *British Medical Journal*, 315, 180–185.

Greenhalgh, T., and Taylor, R. (1997). How to read a paper: Papers that go beyond numbers (qualitative research). *British Medical Journal*, 315, 740–743.

Grove, S., Gray, J., and Burns, N. (2014). *Understanding nursing research: Building an evidence-based practice* (6th ed.). St Louis, MO: Elsevier Saunders.

Guyatt, G., Drummond, R., Meade, M., and Cook, D. (2008). *Users' guides to the medical literature: Essentials of evidence-based clinical practice* (2nd ed.). Chicago, IL: McGraw Hill.

Hennink, M., Kaiser, B., and Weber, M. (2017). Code saturation versus meaning saturation: how many interviews are enough? *Qualitative Health Research*, 27(4), 591–608.

Johnson, R., and Christensen, L. (2014). *Educational research: Quantitative, qualitative, and mixed approaches* (5th ed.). Thousand Oaks, CA: Sage.

Jones, N., Azzam, T., Wanzer, D., and Skousen, D., Knight, C., and Sabarre, N. (2020). Enhancing the effectiveness of logic models. *American Journal of Evaluation*, 41(3), 452–470.

Jordan, Z., Munn, Z., Aromataris, E., and Lockwood, C. (2015). Now that we're here, where are we? The JBI approach to evidence-based healthcare 20 years on. *International Journal of Evidence-Based Healthcare*, 13(3), 117–120.

Knowlton, L., and Phillips, C. (2012). *The logic model guidebook: Better strategies for great results*. Thousand Oaks, CA: Sage.

Kuper, A., Reeves, S., and Levinson, W. (2008). An introduction to reading and appraising qualitative research. *British Medical Journal*, 337, 404–407.

Levac, D., Colquhoun, H., and O'Brien, K. (2010). Scoping studies: Advancing the methodology. *Implementation Science*, 5(1), 69.

Magowan, K. (2019). Outcomes versus outputs: What's the difference. BMC blogs. https://www.bmc.com/blogs/outcomes-vs-outputs/

Mattick, K., Johnston, J., and de la Croix, A (2018). How to... write a good research question. *The Clinical Teacher*, 15(2), 104–108.

McLaughlin, J., and Jordan, G. (2004). Using logic models. In J. Wholey, H. Hatry, and K. Newcomer (Eds.), *Handbook of practical program evaluation* (2nd ed., pp. 7–32). San Francisco, CA: Jossey-Bass.

Mills, T., Lawton, R., and Sheard, L. (2019). Advancing complexity science in healthcare research: The logic of logic models. *BMC Medical Research Methodology, 19*, 55.

Moore, G. F., Audrey, S., Barker, M., Bond, L., Bonell, C., Hardeman, W., Moore, L., O'Cathain, A., Tinati, T., Wight, D., and Baird, J. (2015). Process evaluation of complex interventions: Medical research council guidance. *British Medical Journal, 350*, 1258.

Munn, Z., Peters, M. D. J., Stern, C., Tufanaru, C., McArthur, A., and Aromataris, E. (2018). Systematic review or scoping review? Guidance for authors when choosing between a systematic or scoping review approach. *BMC Medical Research Methodology, 18*, 143.

Munn, Z., Porritt, K., Lockwood, C., Aromataris, E., and Pearson, A. (2014). Establishing confidence in the output of qualitative research synthesis: The ConQual approach. *BMC Medical Research Methodology, 14*, 108.

Newman, S., Andrews, J., Magwood, G., Jenkins, C., Cox, M., and Williamson, D. (2011). Community advisory boards in community-based participatory research: A synthesis of best processes. *Preventing Chronic Disease, 8*(3), A70.

Ogbeiwi, O. (2017). Why written objectives need to be really SMART. *British Journal of Healthcare Management, 23*(7), 324–336.

Onwuegbuzie A., and Leech, N. (2006). Linking research questions to mixed methods data analysis procedures. *Qualitative Report, 11*(3), 474–498.

O'Reilly, M., and Parker, N. (2014). *Doing mental health research with children and adolescents: A guide to qualitative methods*. London: Sage.

Pearson, A. (2004). Balancing the evidence: Incorporating the synthesis of qualitative data into systematic reviews. *JBI Reports, 2*, 45–64.

Pham, T., Raji, A., Greig, J., Sargeant, J., Papadopoulos, A., and McEwen, S. (2014). A scoping review of scoping reviews: Advancing the approach and enhancing the consistency. *Research Synthesis Methods, 5*, 371–385.

Polit, D., and Beck, C. (2017). *Nursing research: Generating and assessing evidence for nursing practice* (10th ed.). Philadelphia, PA: Wolters Kluwer.

Ritchie, J., Lewis, J., McNaughton, C., and Nicholls, C. (2014). *Qualitative research practice: A guide for social science students and researchers* (2nd ed.). Thousand Oaks, CA: Sage.

Riva, J., Malik, K., Burnie, S., Endicott, A., and Busse, J. (2012). What is your research question? An introduction to the PICOT format for clinicians. *Journal of the Canadian Chiropractic Association, 56*(3), 167–171.

Sathian, B., Simkhada P., van Teijlingen, E., Roy, B., and Banerjee, I. (2016). Grant writing for innovative medical research: Time to rethink. *Medical Science, 4*(3), 332–333.

Sharma, R., Gordon, M., Dharamsi, S., and Gibbs, T. (2015). Systematic reviews in medical education: AMEE Guide 94. *Medical Teacher, 37*(2), 108–124.

Stone, V., and Lane, J. (2012). Modeling technology innovation: How science, engineering, and industry methods can combine to generate beneficial socioeconomic impacts. *Implementation Science, 7*, 44.

Templier, M., and Paré, G. (2015). A framework for guiding and evaluating literature reviews. *Communication of the Association for Information Systems, 37*(6), 112–137.

Thomas, D., and Hodges, I. (2010). *Designing and planning your research project: Core skills for social and health researchers*. London: Sage.

Tully, M. (2014). Research: Articulating questions, generating hypotheses, and choosing study designs. *Canadian Journal of Hospital Pharmacy, 67*(1), 31–34.

Van Teijlingen, E., and Hundley, V. (2002). The importance of pilot studies. *Nursing Standard, 16*(40), 33–36.

Wellcome Trust. (n.d.). How to complete an outputs management plan. https://wellcome.org/grant-funding/guidance/how-complete-outputs-management-plan

White, P. (2017). *Developing research questions* (2nd ed.). London: Bloomsbury.

CHAPTER 6

Types of qualitative research

Learning objectives

This chapter enables the reader to:

- Identify different approaches to qualitative research.
- Critically assess the value of those approaches.
- Differentiate the approaches at a conceptual level.
- Recognise the relevance and importance of quality in approaches.
- Identify debates about mixing qualitative methodologies.
- Identify debates about mixing qualitative methods.

Introduction
Clinician-researchers need to make decisions regarding the most appropriate methodology and methods to address the area of research interest they are investigating. These decisions need to be theoretically informed, with a clear and congruent rationale. The clinician-researcher benefits from an awareness the different kinds of approaches, and the associated underpinning frameworks. The goal of this chapter is to introduce you to the most common qualitative approaches. Choosing your approach needs to be congruent with your theoretical and epistemological position, and will guide your ethical decisions, planning decisions, method choices and processes. This chapter provides an overview of the core premises of several, and later in the book, where we consider the associated methods of analysis, we provide some guidance on how to use those methods in practice. Aligned with these issues, we also address areas of quality, and how to assure quality within qualitative research. We consider the different arguments proposed in the field., and conclude with some consideration of multi-method studies, in the sense of using more than one qualitative method or methodology.

Thematic approaches

Thematic approaches to qualitative research are probably the most commonly used. Because of that, we devote a chapter to undertaking a thematic analysis later in the book. At this stage, we introduce you to this set of qualitative approaches to give you the foundational knowledge needed to help you understand the approach and determine whether this is the most suitable one for your project.

The thematic approaches have been arguably strengthened and clarified by the work of Braun and Clarke, who have provided a range of materials for those seeking to practice this analytic approach. The thematic approaches are as a set of methods of analysis that can be used to identify, analyse, and report general patterns across a data corpus (Braun and Clarke, 2006). In this way, the thematic approaches allow for the descriptive organisation of data, that facilitates interpretation of various aspects related to a research topic (Boyatzis, 1998). Whilst mostly descriptive in their approach, there is some interpretation of data.

> **Key point!**
>
> The thematic approaches provide accessible and robust methodologies for those new to qualitative research.
>
> (Braun and Clarke, 2022)

Theory is important for the thematic approaches, and you can re-visit Chapter 3 to remind yourself of the details. Whilst thematic approaches are theoretically flexible, they are not theory free, and so it is essential if you use one of these approaches that you acknowledge your ontological and epistemological assumptions (Braun and Clarke, 2022).

The thematic approaches utilise thematic analysis to describe and interpret data to understand the issues at stake in relation to the research focus/foci. In so doing, these approaches offer a method for developing, analysing, and interpreting patterns across the data, and this requires a systematic process of data coding so that themes can be developed (Braun and Clarke, 2022).

> **Key point!**
>
> Thematic approaches are more of a method for analysis than an overarching methodology.
>
> (Braun and Clarke, 2022)

The thematic approaches offer a set of tools, concepts, techniques, practices, and guidelines that help the researcher to organise, interrogate and interpret their data (Braun and Clarke, 2022). In this sense, Braun and Clarke see thematic analysis (TA) as a method of data analysis but note that this is not a single approach as there are different types of TA, which differ in their approach and procedures. This is important for clinician-researchers, as there has been confusion in the literature with many authors claiming to be undertaking one type of TA, associated with an influential article on TA by Braun and Clarke published in 2006, when, in fact, they were doing a different kind, which Braun and Clarke themselves critique (see Braun and Clarke, 2022). Thus, the thematic approaches have been conceptualised by Braun and Clarke (2022) into three clusters

- Coding reliability.
- Codebook.
- Reflexive.

Coding reliability thematic approaches

The coding reliability thematic approaches are united by their commitment to post-positivism, and this epistemological position shapes the way in which the approach is used due to the belief of seeking an unbiased truth from the data (Braun and Clarke, 2022). The goal is to create a coding frame either deductively from pre-existing theory or inductively by familiarisation with data. This kind of approach to TA follows the "scientific method – a researcher starts with theory, develops hypotheses (themes) and conducts an experiment (coding) to test (find evidence for) the hypotheses (themes)" (Braun and Clarke, 2022, p. 238).

A coding reliability approach uses a structured coding practice and requires reliability across coders to agree code accuracy (Braun and Clarke, 2019). It necessitates the involvement of multiple coders to code the data and to determine whether the codes have been organised at a sufficiently high level that the coding is reliable (Braun and Clarke, 2022). Thus, the underpinning post-positivist theory and the goal of reliability mean that this approach leans towards quantitative ideas. Some scholars have argued that coding reliability thematic approaches serve as a bridge between the quantitative and qualitative paradigms (e.g. Boyatzis, 1998; Guest, MacQueen, and Namey, 2012). Conversely, other scholars have argued that this notion of bridging the divide is insufficient, as it relies on a limited definition of qualitative research as a set of tools rather than as a combination of both philosophy and techniques (Braun and Clarke, 2022) and fails to account for the broad range of qualitative approaches and more critical orientations (Willig, 2008).

Codebook thematic approaches

A more moderate thematic approach that combines the principles of qualitative research and a structured coding developmental process is the codebook thematic approach (Braun and Clarke, 2019). In this thematic approach, a codebook is developed in a structured way, but coding reliability is not encouraged (Braun and Clarke, 2022). There are various codebook approaches to thematic analysis, including matrix analysis, framework analysis, network analysis, and template analysis,

Like other thematic approaches, template analysis provides a framework for organising and analysing data to produce a set of codes, which can either be descriptive or interpretive (King, 2004). The codebook can be developed deductively, before analysis begins, or inductively following some familiarisation with the data (Braun and Clarke, 2022). Either way, the focus for template analysis is to build a template which is applied to subsequent transcripts (King, 2012). Therefore, the blend of inductive and deductive processes, with some a priori codes identified before engaging with data, facilitate the development of the template. In this way, codebook thematic approaches are considered advantageous for researchers new to qualitative enquiry because of the flexibility and structure and are commonly used in applied research (Braun and Clarke, 2022).

Reflexive thematic approaches

Reflexive thematic analysis was developed and advocated by Braun and Clarke (2006), although at that time it did not carry this label. This thematic approach has the advantage of being flexible and can be undertaken from a range of different theoretical positions (Braun and Clarke, 2022). It is labelled reflexive because of the importance of the subjective, situated, and questioning role of the reflexive researcher (Braun and Clarke, 2019). This means that the researcher takes an active role in the selection and categorisation of data into themes (Braun and Clarke, 2006). In other words, "reflexive research treats knowledge as situated, and as inevitably and inescapably shaped by the processes and practices of knowledge production, including the practices of the researcher" (Braun and Clarke, 2022, p. 12).

There are different forms of reflexive thematic analysis so reflexive thematic analysis cannot be considered a single method (Braun and Clarke, 2022). Braun and Clarke argue that reflexive thematic approach provides analytic and interpretive tools. It involves a process of meaning-making and meaning-telling, and thus the focus for this thematic approach is on the different layers of meaning (Braun and Clarke, 2022). Here, in Box 6.1, we remind you of some key things about the thematic approach.

Box 6.1

Thematic approaches: things to remember

There are several things to remember if you select a thematic approach for your research. We list these below:

- Thematic approaches are a useful place to start a learning journey in qualitative research for novice researchers.
- Thematic analysis, as a method of analysis, is not a singular method. There are multiple thematic approaches.
- Some thematic approaches lean toward a quantitative theoretical basis whilst others are much more strongly qualitative in their orientation.
- The process of coding, labelling, thematising, organising, interpreting, and writing is different across the thematic approaches.
- The aims and goals of the thematic approaches are also different.

Phenomenological approaches

Phenomenology is a type of qualitative research that involves exploring lived experiences (Neubauer, Witkop, and Varpio, 2019). Thus, phenomenological approaches seek to describe the "essence of a phenomenon" by investigating it from the perspective of those with experience of it (Teherani, Martimianakis, Stenfors-Hayes et al., 2015). There are different types of phenomenology, and these are founded in different schools of philosophy. Thus, any choice you make about a phenomenological approach will reflect a guiding philosophy (Neubauer et al., 2019). Some approaches are more descriptive, others are more interpretive (Davidsen, 2013). The goal of phenomenology in qualitative research is to explore the experience and meanings of individuals, to capture the way in which the phenomenon is experienced (Giorgi and Giorgi, 2003).

> **Key point!**
>
> Phenomenology can be characterised as a "movement" as it is a dynamic philosophy comprised of different currents that are related but not homogenous.
>
> (Davidsen, 2013)

The difference across phenomenological approaches is reflected in the writings of key scholars who have contributed to this area. Whilst there are many scholars contributing to this approach, three pertinent contributors were highlighted by Davidsen (2013). We outline these in Table 6.1.

Table 6.1 Influential scholars in phenomenology (as described by Davidsen, 2013)

Scholar	Influence
Husserl	In his early writing, Husserl studied how phenomena in the world are constituted by human consciousness. Psychologists adopted Husserl's methods and created a phenomenological psychology, although Husserl himself raised some objections. Husserl argued it is possible for researchers to seek to "bracket off" their presuppositions.
Heidegger	Heidegger prompted an existential turn for phenomenology with a goal of understanding existence. Heidegger proposed that phenomenology relies on description, but that all description inevitably involves interpretation and thus phenomenology has a hermeneutic direction. Time and temporality were pertinent, with experience understood in a temporal context between past, present, and future.
Gadamer	Gadamer aligned with Heidegger's argument that phenomenology has a hermeneutic direction. Gadamer emphasised the idea that the human existence is hermeneutic. In his work *Truth and Method* (Gadamer, 1989), he argued that humans are influenced by prejudices and our openness to the world is biased. Thus, any interpretation is necessarily selective and a form of perspectivism. Gadamer claimed all understanding is linguistic, and language is our basis for understanding.

Amongst the various phenomenological approaches in qualitative research, two commonly drawn upon are transcendental (descriptive) and hermeneutic (interpretive) (Neubauer et al., 2019).

Husserl is the key figure associated with transcendental phenomenology, also known as the descriptive approach, where the goal is to achieve "transcendental subjectivity", where the researcher's influence over the research is frequently inspected and any preconceptions are neutralised, so they do not impact the study (Lopez and Willis, 2004). In this type of phenomenology, the researcher must not allow their subjectivity to inform the descriptions offered, and the lived experience is best approached by a researcher who can shift from the participants' descriptions of their lived experiences to universal essences of the phenomenon (Davidsen, 2013). For transcendental phenomenology, the researcher brings no definitions, expectations, assumptions, or hypotheses to the research, and assumes a position of a *tabula rasa* (the blank slate), using participants' accounts of their own experiences to develop an understanding of the essence of a phenomenon (Neubauer et al., 2019).

Heidegger is the key figure associated with hermeneutic phenomenology, also known an interpretative approach. Whereas Husserl's epistemological focus was on the nature of knowledge, Heidegger's ontological focus was on the nature of being and temporality (Reiners, 2012). For hermeneutic phenomenology, humans are actors in the world and research following this approach focuses on the relationship between the individual and their lifeworld; a concept which refers to how individuals' realities are influenced by the world they live in (Lopez and Willis, 2004). From this perspective, individuals are considered to always understand themselves within their worlds, even if they are not always consciously aware (Staiti, 2012) where consciousness is conceptualised as the formation of historically lived experiences (Lopez and Willis, 2004). Arguably, no individual can step outside their lifeworld and cannot experience a phenomenon without referring to their own background (Neubauer et al., 2019). For hermeneutic phenomenology, there is no expectation to bracket off the researcher's perspective as this approach recognises the researcher is not independent of their own lifeworld. A person's past experiences and knowledge are considered valuable assets, rather than being a hindrance to the inquiry (Neubauer et al., 2019).

Interpretative phenomenological analysis (IPA)

Interpretative phenomenological analysis was pioneered by Jonathan Smith and is influenced by both Husserl and Heidegger (Smith, Flowers, and Larkin., 2009). The goal of IPA is to explore the personal lived experiences of participants in depth, and how they make sense of those experiences, through an approach which is idiographic, inductive, and interrogative (Smith, 2004). Smith explained that IPA is phenomenological in that its core concern resides with the individual's perceptions of objects or events, and it is hermeneutic in that it focuses on how participants make sense of their personal and social world. As indicated by its name, IPA advocates a strong interpretive position (Sandberg, 2005).

Using IPA is a useful approach to delve deeply into the lives and experiences of participants. Tala Noweisser, a registered psychologist in Lebanon, explained how she applied this methodology to her work on political instability and children's wellbeing in Box 6.2.

> **Box 6.2**
>
> **Practitioner view of IPA – Tala Noweisser**
>
> Tala Noweisser is a psychologist working in Lebanon and is currently completing her PhD. Tala's research is focused on children and their parents and explores their insights and perspectives on political instability and children's wellbeing. To accomplish her research, she used IPA as an approach and method of analysis. The following are her own words:
>
> I am a Registered Psychologist in Lebanon and for the past six years, I have been supporting university level students through their personal and academic journeys. I found it fascinating to be utilising some of the most humanistic, non-judgemental, and empathic approaches through IPA interviews, like those employed in a therapeutic session, to elicit and capture the meaning of the emotions associated with the participants' lived experiences whilst staying mindful to not slip back to my counselling role.
>
> The IPA interviews instilled a comfortable and a natural atmosphere for participants to articulate their experience of the instability in Lebanon in real-time manner. Because some of the experiences that participants shared in interviews were of high value to them, and because IPA offered the space for a conversational-like interview, they provided a thorough account to the meaning they hold to what they have gone through whilst expanding on the repercussions echoed in other aspects of their life. Using IPA as a methodology granted participants the freedom to elaborate on what mattered to them the most. IPA appeared to be most fitting within a collectivist culture that relies heavily on dialogue and language to share their experience with others.

We now invite you to try the reflective activity in Box 6.3.

> **Box 6.3**
>
> **Reflective activity on phenomenology**
>
> Consider the value of phenomenology for the topic you are interested in. Consider the implications of different phenomenological approaches for your project and develop an account of these in your research diary.

Discursive approaches

There are a range of discursive methodologies under the rubric of language-based approaches. These include discourse analysis, ethnomethodology, socio-linguistics, and conversation analysis. These approaches have been used widely in healthcare research, and are useful in exploring health, communication, and social interaction in health settings. Language-based approaches are a distinctive way to explore human behaviour in both organisational and everyday settings, as well as how members conduct their institutional business in organisational settings through language (Potter and Hepburn, 2012). Thus, language-based approaches attend primarily to interactional practices that constitute social life, and it is these that are the central tenet of investigation (Lester, O'Reilly, and Steele, 2023). Whilst there are many different discursive approaches, we outline the four most common here.

Discourse analysis

Discourse analysis is an umbrella concept covering discursive approaches, with an interest in how social processes inform the ways knowledge claims can be constructed as objective and factual representations of the world (Wooffitt, 2005). There are many types of discourse analysis, including critical, Foucauldian, Bhaktian, and discursive psychology. Despite differences between these types, they all share a view that language is performative of social actions. Thus, discourse analysis focuses on the study of language and language use (Wetherell, 2001), and these approaches are united in their focus on the study of talk and text as used in social practice (Potter, 1997).

Some discourse approaches have a more critical lens and take a socio-political position; a concern for the way language is shaped by (and shapes) social and political context. These include critical and Foucauldian discourse analysis (Arribas-Ayloon and Walkerdine, 2008; van Dijk, 1993). Other discourse and language-based approaches take a more micro-focus, like discursive psychology (DP) and conversation analysis (CA) (Edwards and Potter, 1992; Sacks, 1992). The more micro-focused discursive approaches do not presume social inequalities or power differentials, but rather examine how speakers interact and if and how they elect to make inequality or asymmetry relevant (Lester, O'Reilly, Kiyimba, and Wong, 2018).

Discursive psychology

Discursive psychology was developed during the 1980s and 1990s, primarily by the UK-based scholars Derek Edwards and Jonathan Potter (Edwards and Potter, 1992). This language-based approach orients to psychological matters, like memory or cognition, as made visible through discourse (Edwards, 1997). Thus, their foundational text introduced an approach that challenged the orthodox, cognitivist ways of making sense of psychological phenomena (Edwards and Potter, 1992). The interest is not on people's intentions, mental states, or motives, but instead how those mental states are treated as a concern for members of the interaction (Te Molder, 2015). Discursive psychologists see talk as performative of social action (Edwards and Potter, 1992) and study psychological constructs including memory, identity, and agency from the perspective of social actors engaged in an interaction are managed and navigated by those involved (Te Molder, 2015). Three main aims of discursive psychology are outlined by Wetherell (2007) and we summarise these in Table 6.2.

It is notable that the different strands of discursive psychology are united by core premises but have different approaches to research and analysis. We set out these three strands in Table 6.3.

Critical discourse analysis

Critical discourse analysis is sometimes referred to as critical discourse studies to distinguish the approach as an applied critical practice (van Dijk, 2008). Researchers using

Table 6.2 Three aims of discursive psychology (Wetherell, 2007)

Aim	Description
To focus on language as a way of examining psychological topics	Discursive psychology examines psychological topics with a focus on language, including social categories, emotions, attribution, representations, memory, identity, and gender. Thus, role identities are treated as flexible constructs created by organisations and individuals to perform social actions within settings.
To attend to theorising	Discursive psychology attends to different ways of theorising and studying psychological constructs through talk.
To advance methods	Discursive psychologists seek to advance qualitative methods across fields where language is a central focus, not just in psychology. This is accomplished by moving away from what people think they do, to investigate research problems that are driven by exploring language as occurring naturally in organisational practices. In doing so, understandings of mental states are reconfigured as discursively and socially constructed phenomena.

Table 6.3 The three strands of discursive psychology

Type	Description
The first strand	This was the earliest form of discursive psychology which emerged from the work of Potter and Wetherell (1987). They brought a focus on interpretive repertoires, the building blocks used by speakers when constructing their version of the world. This strand tends to have a broader interest in cultural identity and power.
The second strand	This approach grew in popularity during the 1990s, with the seminal text of Edwards and Potter (1992). This strand saw the shift toward studying everyday conversations and natural institutional settings (Lester et al., 2023). This strand focused on psychological constructs as being produced in and through interaction (Edwards and Potter, 1992).
The third strand	This approach developed later in the 1990s, as discursive psychology became heavily influenced by conversation analysis and ethnomethodology (Lester et al., 2018). This form of discursive psychology became increasingly interested in the sequential organisation of talk, as well as attending to the detail of the talk (e.g. Edwards and Potter, 2017). Thus, the engagement with conversation analysis moved researchers to attend more specifically to the micro-features of interaction (Potter, 2012).

a critical discourse approach seek to investigate the role of language in the production and maintenance of power dynamics within social structures, and analysts examine how discourse manages to sustain and legitimise inequalities (Wooffitt, 2005). In this way, those practising critical discourse analysis take an explicit socio-political position and focus on the role of language in the (re)production of the dominance of elite groups, institutions, and forms of knowledge (van Dijk, 2008). Researchers using critical discourse analysis typically have assumptions (based on empirical and anecdotal evidence) that there are pre-existing power inequalities in society (as opposed to some other kinds of discourse analysis which argue these are created and made relevant through interaction). However, often these inequalities are difficult to "pin down" in terms of exactly how they occur and are perpetuated.

By drawing on the micro tools of discourse analysis, researchers of this group use transcripts of institutional and everyday conversations or scrutinise publicly available texts to try to identity where these inequalities happen in concrete terms in people's interactions. Examples of subtle dominance in verbal conversations might be that one person talks more than the other person, interrupts the other person, or disagrees with them frequently. Analysis of transcripts can allow for tangible, even measurable, evidence. Similarly, analysis of texts such as newspapers or magazines might involve examining language used to describe or portray a particular social group. Where a large corpus of data examples is collected, trends in language use may highlight a weighting towards pejorative or undermining language used about specific groups of people. Where media may be saturated with certain types of descriptors, this can provide evidence for hypothesising about why certain groups in society continue to be marginalised or subjugated through processes of systemic oppression.

Conversation analysis
Conversation analysis (CA) was pioneered by Harvey Sacks during the 1970s. Conversation analysis is a methodology that advocates the study of social interaction, paying special attention to the details of "talk-in-interaction" as well as the sequential order of talk (Sacks, 1992). The goals of conversation analysis are to provide explanations of how social members of an interaction make sense of and respond to one another through talk, and to examine ways in which people perform social actions through language in context (Hutchby and Wooffitt, 2008). It is argued by conversation analysts that through the design of conversational turns, people make visible the "happenings" of social life, and the sequential nature of interactions show that an individual's turn in talk sets up a normative expectation of what comes next (Sacks, 1992). Examination of sequence organisation shows that talk is responsive to the conversational turn immediately prior to it (Heritage, 2011), and through turn design, a speaker constructs their subsequent turn, which is understood as performing a social action (Drew, 2013).

> **Key point!**
>
> In conversation analysis, there is a distinction between two foci, mundane, everyday talk, and that characteristic of institutional settings.
>
> (Antaki, 2011)

A distinction between different conversation analysis types has been referred to as that between traditional or pure conversation analysis and applied conversation analysis (Lester and O'Reilly, 2019). Whilst Sacks' early work focused on institutional data from a Suicide Prevention Centre, his attention was caught by the sequential order of the turns of talk, which became more of a focus to him than its institutional basis. We note that the distinction between pure and applied CA is somewhat blurred, and there is some overlap between traditional and applied conversation analysis (Lester and O'Reilly, 2019). Notably, institutional interactions have features that distinguish them from everyday talk, and in institutional settings, professional identities become relevant to the work-based activities people are engaged in (Drew and Heritage, 1992).

To draw this section on the language-based approaches to a close, we provide you with the view of Dr Alison Drewett, a speech and language therapist who has experience of these approaches in her research exploring talk in inpatient mental health care. In Box 6.4, Alison shows her perspective on the value of these qualitative approaches for research addressing health topics in healthcare settings.

Box 6.4

Practitioner view of language-based approaches – Dr Alison Drewett

Dr Alison Drewett is a Specialist Speech and Language Therapist with experience of working in Adult Learning Disability, Autism and Mental Health services. She is also a Research Associate at Loughborough University on the DECODE project which aims to find meaningful ways to produce health information for people with learning disabilities and their carers. She was recently awarded her PhD with the University of Leicester. Here she writes about her discursive research.

My research investigated staff communication with autistic adults in mental health hospitals about their care. It uses a mixed-methodologies qualitative design to examine "work as done" via video-recordings of ward rounds, and "work as imagined" using reflexive interviews with staff and clients. The research uses critical discursive psychology as a methodology to analyse the video-recordings of ward rounds. This approach provided a framework to examine the natural data of the real conversations using the concepts of interpretive repertoires, ideological dilemmas, and subject positions. These foundational concepts shone a light on how clients were represented in talk, e.g. as mental health or autistic and illuminated the common-sense ideas that pertained to these identities that were occasioned in the talk.

The concept of ideological dilemmas helped to provide an account of how and why client narratives differed inter- and intra-staff and how these conceptualisations performed different actions. Significantly, the critical component allowed for an acknowledgement of power as central to available discourses, the epistemic claims of staff, and category entitlements of professionals. Language-based approaches are critical to deconstruct how work is done in healthcare, and to recognise the importance of social interactions as maintaining and reproducing inequalities in health outcomes for individual clients.

Narrative approaches

Narrative approaches are those that recognise the extent to which the stories that people tell can provide a range of insights into their lived experiences, and into how people make sense of their lives and worlds (Thorne, 2000). As individuals live their lives, they have continuous experiences and interact with the world around them through dialogic interactions (Moen, 2006). Moen (2006) pointed out that a natural way of recounting one's experiences is through storytelling, as this provides a way of creating order out of experience. For some scholars, there has been a focus on the narrative approaches as a method of research inquiry (e.g. Connelly and Clandinin, 1990), whereas others have suggested narrative approaches are not a method but a frame of reference where narratives are the producers and transmitters of reality (e.g. Heikkinen, 2002).

According to Moen (2006), there are three commonalities across the narrative approaches to qualitative research:

- First – people tend to organise their experiences of the world into narratives.
- Second – the stories people tell are dependent on past and present experiences, as well as the person's values. These stories also depend on the audience, and when and where they are told.
- Third – there is a multi-voicedness occurring within narratives, whereby other people's perspectives become articulated within the story.

Theory is important to the narrative approaches, and these approaches tend to be united by an underlying philosophy that one can access real people in real settings through the "painting" of their stories (Wang and Geale, 2015). Narrative approaches are underpinned by narrative theory which promotes the idea that people are born into a storied world (Murray, 2003). In this way, narrative approaches support researchers gaining insights into the participant's world from their point of view (Thorne, 2000). Researchers utilising narrative approaches can hold different ontological and epistemological positions, including symbolic interactionism, social constructivism, and different forms of realism (Riessman, 2008). For example, in health research, participants may articulate their health and illness experiences through the narrative process, with their experiences being variously constructed as the person negotiates shifting meanings (Wang and Geale, 2015). There are different types of narrative approach for research and Riessman (2008) described four types which we outline in Table 6.4.

Table 6.4 Four types of narrative approach (Riessman, 2008)

Type of approach	Description
Thematic narrative approach	Focuses on what is said, that is, the content of the narrative. This approach identifies common thematic elements.
Structural narrative approach	The focus of this approach is on how a narrative is spoken and looks at the narrative form, including the organisation of units into discourse and the other structural features.
Dialogic narrative approach	This is a more interpretative approach focusing on the contexts that shape the person's narrative, including how it is "multi-voiced" in the present conversation.
Visual narrative approach	Focuses on visual artefacts and explores why and how these are produced, how they can be made and how they are interpreted with the participants.

There are arguably several benefits of using the narrative approach in qualitative research. First, this approach assumes humans are natural storytellers and there is a simplicity in encouraging people to tell stories (Butina, 2015). Second, depth of meaning is made possible through the narrative approach, as people reveal great amounts of information about themselves through stories (Savin-Baden and van Niekerk, 2013). Third, gathering depth is simple to acquire as stories generally include thick descriptions which in narrative language refer to detail (Butina, 2015).

Ethnographic approaches
It was during the late 19th century that ethnography grew in popularity across a range of disciplines, although it is thought to have originated in anthropology (Fetterman, 2010). There is no singular definition of ethnography as it denotes a set of approaches but is typically used to explore how people make sense of their everyday lives, particularly through observing them (Hammersley and Atkinson, 2007). Ethnography is an approach to research requiring immersion when investigating people's cultures and social worlds and involves observing and being part of those worlds (Thorne, 2000). Ethnographic approaches are therefore considered both a method and a product, giving rise to the phrase "an ethnography" (Fetterman, 2010).

Like with the other qualitative approaches, there are different types of ethnographic approach, including classical and critical ethnography and autoethnography (Grbich, 2013) as well as video reflexive ethnography (Iedema, Forsyth, Georgiou et al., 2007). Whichever form of ethnography you choose, it is essential to clarify the epistemological position as they vary across approaches. For example, Staller (2013) argued that the epistemologies are typically as follows:

- Classical ethnography, which is usually underpinned by objectivism.
- Critical ethnography, which is commonly underpinned by social constructionism (but is congruent with other epistemologies).
- Autoethnography, which is usually underpinned by subjectivism.

Notwithstanding these general distinctions, ethnographers have been influenced by a wide range of epistemological positions including functionalism, pragmatism, symbolic interactionism, hermeneutics, post-structuralism, feminism, post-modernism, and Marxism (Hammersley and Atkinson, 2007).

Video reflexive ethnography
Video reflexive ethnography (referred to as VRE) investigates how interactional work is accomplished, and is guided by the four key principles as described by Iedema, Carroll, Collier et al. (2019):

- **Exnovation** – illumination of practice from practitioner level, bottom up, looking closely for the opportunity for change.
- **Reflexivity** – active process of reflection on research in a shared capacity rather than individual.

- **Collaboration** – professionals, patients/clients and other stakeholders are viewed as experts.
- **Care** – participants should feel safe and cared for.

The fundamental principle of VRE is to collect data from multiple sources, typically video or audio recordings of real-world interactions as well as reflection on those data and conversations with those participants, usually through interviews. As such, video data are prioritised as this captures the complexity of *work as done* (WAD) as opposed to *word as imagined* (WAI) (Hollnagel, Wears, and Braithwaite, 2015). The reflexive aspect of this ethnographic approach connects with the idea of the idea of the researcher-as-insider as they utilise the video data to encourage reflection and encourage greater depth in dialogue.

Like other forms of ethnography, epistemology and theory are aligned. VRE is not anchored to a specific epistemology or methodology, and thus the researcher needs to be mindful to provide a clear rationale for their decision-making (Carroll and Mesman, 2018). The VRE approach does not place theoretical constraints on the researcher as the conversations with participants are viewed as opportunities to share ideas and develop new collaborative ways of thinking about a research topic (Iedema and Carroll, 2010).

Autoethnography

Autoethnography is a method focused on the researcher's personal experience in describing and interpreting experiences, practices and beliefs (Adams, Ellis, and Holman-Jones, 2017). Adams et al. argued that those practicing autoethnography hold the idea that personal experiences are imbued with cultural and political norms and expectations and so rigorous and constant self-reflection is crucial to the research. This reflexive aspect of autoethnography highlights how people give meaning to their lives and their struggles (Bochner and Ellis, 2002). Scholars using this approach focus therefore on personal experiences and offer accounts of those experiences in ways that complement or address gaps in existing social science research (Adams et al., 2017). Adams et al. further noted that autoethnography has a goal of articulating insider knowledge of cultural experiences where those who have experienced cultural problems like racism, loss or illness can talk about them in ways that are different from outsiders.

Psychoanalytically informed approaches

Psychoanalytic approaches, often referred to as psychoanalytically informed or psychosocial approaches, share with clinical psychoanalysis a concern for role of the unconscious in human experience and action. In the UK, over the past 20 years or so, there has been increasing interest in how ideas from psychoanalytic therapy can be applied in the "extra-clinical" context of qualitative social research (Frosh, 2010; Holmes, 2013; Lapping, 2011). This interest has, in part, been driven by the concerns of psychodynamically orientated practitioner researchers in psychotherapy and health and social care, and a desire for research which gets close to the social and emotional complexity of practice and service user experience (see, for example, Cooper, 2009).

Various frameworks and methods can be deemed "psychoanalytically informed" in nature when psychoanalytic ideas are used by the researcher. These include a range of qualitative approaches, such as those that are interview-based, include participant observation, and discourse analysis, as well as forms of action research which directly benefit the participants or organisations involved, for instance, by facilitating group-based reflection on professional practice.

One influential example of a psychoanalytically based approach is Hollway and Jefferson's (2013) "free association narrative interview method (FANIM)". This method draws heavily on the psychoanalytic concept and technique of free association, as well as psychoanalytic ideas around unconscious mental functioning, transference and countertransference. With the approach, borrowing from the theory and practice of psychoanalytic therapy, the research interviewer acts like a therapist in different ways as a quiet, empathic listener, following the concerns of the participant as they speak and narrate their experience. As well as audio-recording, the researcher records detailed "process" notes after the interview, detailing aspects the audio-recording would not pick up, i.e. of body language, notable "moments" in the interview and their own experience as interviewer. These data are then used to consider the affective dimensions of the interview and how emotions may have been passed between the participant and interviewer by unconscious processes of projection and identification. In initial interviews at least, questions are phrased in an open way or as requests, for example, "tell me about your experience of …" This is viewed as eliciting richer, more nuanced and experience-rich responses, which involve storytelling rather than "well-worn", more predictable responses. When analysing the interview material, the researcher is as (if not more) interested in the form as they are the content of what is related, i.e. how things are told as much as what is told. The "associative" ordering of what is said as well as other phenomena the therapist would usually be attuned to, such as repetition, slips of the tongue, and pauses, are all considered valuable to attend to in considering matters of personal or unconscious significance.

Like other psychoanalytically informed methods, Hollway and Jefferson's approach has informed several studies in healthcare research, not limited to topics related to psychotherapy (see Archard, 2020, 2021). However, the application of ideas from psychoanalytic therapy in the extra-clinical context of qualitative research is complicated terrain (Archard and O'Reilly, 2022; Frosh, 2010), and there are risks of it involving an expert-driven application of psychoanalytic understanding, where the researcher is positioned to make speculative judgements about unconscious experience (Frosh and Baraitser, 2008).

We have also previously noted that the way in which psychoanalytically informed methods are used does not map straightforwardly onto certain conventions associated with the practice and writing up of research (Archard and O'Reilly, 2022). Notably, if an analysis is concerned with unconscious processes, it may not be appropriate to return findings and preliminary analyses of data to participants. Research and therapy diverge in different ways in theory and practice and whilst participating in qualitative research may have quasi-therapeutic qualities, participants may not wish to be exposed to certain "insights" and the researcher not able to share them in a safe and ethical way. In this way, careful thought needs to be given to how this type of method can be used in practice. In particular, as a researcher using this type of method, you will a need to reflect on whether certain analytic and practical strategies may be used to offset the excesses of an expert-driven use of psychoanalysis, for example, by using multiple theoretical lenses to examine data (Frosh and Emerson, 2005), and completing a greater number of interviews when sharing analyses with participants over time (Hoggett, Beedell, Jimenez et al., 2010).

Nevertheless, psychoanalytically informed methods can be highly beneficial in developing rich conceptualisations of researcher and participant subjectivity and can enrich researcher reflexivity by introducing a concern for aspects of research relationship that would not usually be acknowledged, i.e. for the psychodynamics of the research encounter. We invite you to reflect on what you have learned about this approach in Box 6.5.

Box 6.5

Reflective activity on psychoanalytic approaches

We have noted that there are range of issues to reflect on when using a psychoanalytic approach in qualitative research, but that it can also enrich one's understanding of the researcher endeavour by way of a close concern for intersubjective and unconscious processes.

Consider how this type of research approach may or may not be relevant for your research project and what it might add in terms of understanding the phenomena you are seeking to investigate. Consider also what some of the risks involved might be in the using this type of approach. We suggest you make an entry in your research diary so you can thoughtfully address these issues.

Grounded theory approaches

Grounded theory approaches are another set of approaches that can be undertaken in different ways, under an umbrella concept and methodology. The term "grounded theory" refers to both the method of inquiry and the product of inquiry (Charmaz, 2005). The grounded theory approach emerged originally from the collaboration between Glaser and Strauss (1967), who pioneered an approach to transcend the boundaries between data collection and analysis that pervaded research at that time (Willig, 2008). During the early development of the approach, the aims were to develop an inductive way to conceptualise data collected with a goal to develop an explanatory theory of psychological and social processes within those environments where they took place (Glaser and Strauss, 1967). As the grounded theory approach has developed and evolved, and different iterations of it emerged, so too have the aims. The aim of modern grounded theory approaches is to explore basic social processes, but to also gain an understanding of the multiplicity of interactions that produce variations within those processes (Heath and Cowley, 2004).

Over time, grounded theory has diversified, and Glaser and Strauss themselves also went on to develop slightly different approaches from one another. Glaser stayed with the original grounded theory approach (Heath and Cowley, 2004), and Strauss, along with colleague Corbin, reformulated the classic version (Annels, 1996). Whilst these two approaches share theoretical and methodological similarities, there are some epistemological differences. Ontologically, Glaser and Strauss offered a compromise between extreme empiricism and relativism and argued that knowledge claims made by analysts should be based on how individuals interpret reality (Suddaby, 2006). Other approaches to grounded theory however take a different epistemological position, being informed by symbolic interactionism (Starks and Trinidad, 2007), social constructionism (Burck, 2005), or constructivism (Charmaz, 2005).

> **Key point!**
>
> The objective of grounded theory is to generate an overarching, encompassing theory of social or psychological processes.
>
> (Biggerstaff, 2012)

Grounded theory approaches aim to identify and integrate categories within the data (Willig, 2008) using a constant comparative method of analysis (Charmaz, 2006). In that way grounded theory is a systematic way to undertake research that makes explicit its strategies for the analysis of data, so that an explanatory theory can be generated to offer an abstract understanding of one or more concerns being studied (Charmaz and Thornberg, 2021). Taking a grounded theory approach to data, means the researcher is open to learning about their participants' lives and experiences, and means there is a transparency about that learning process (Charmaz and Thornberg, 2021).

Action research

Action research does not represent a single approach, but instead refers to a family of approaches that have been used within a range of areas (Brydon-Miller, Greenwood, and Maguire, 2003). The action research approaches are those that are concerned with practice (Avison, Lau, Myers, and Nielsen, 1999) and are participatory in nature (Koshy, Koshy, and Waterman., 2010), which have made them popular in health research. Action research is sometimes described as a cooperative enquiry, with aims for utility for healthcare researchers as it is designed to improve conditions and practices within organisations (Lingard, Albert, and Levinson, 2008). It can be a catalyst to needed organisational change.

> **Key point!**
>
> There is not a universally agreed definition of action research, but there is agreement that these are research approaches that seek to inform and influence practice, and thus action research is an orientation and purpose of enquiry, rather than research methodology.
>
> (Reason and Bradbury, 2001)

A central benefit of action research approaches is the focus on generating solutions to practical problems, as well as the inclusion and empowerment of those who are working in practice-based environments (Meyer, 2000). This strength is recognised because of the commitment to knowledge sharing, promotion of change and focus on problem-solving (Reason and Bradbury, 2001).

Types of action research

Whilst there are similarities across action research approaches, Avison et al. (1999) distinguish four main types:

1. Action research that focuses on change and reflecting on practice.
2. Action science that aims to resolve conflict between espoused and applied theory.
3. Participatory action research which involves collaboration with participants as co-researchers.
4. Action learning that is designed to also be pedagogical and support experiential learning.

Despite the differences across the approaches, there are principles anchoring them together. According to Cordeiro and Soares (2018), the four main principles of action research are:

1. Action research approaches are committed to participation and collaboration.
2. They all entail a cycle of planning, action, observation, and reflection.
3. Knowledge building through action research requires a focus on participants' realities.
4. All action research approaches are committed to social change and problem-solving (see also Cordeiro and Soares, 2018).

Thus, whilst action research approaches have different goals and assumptions, a focus on learning by doing remains central to the activities of the researcher (Jacobs, 2018).

Action research is particularly useful in the field of health. This is because this approach takes the position that practice informs research and research informs practice synergistically (Avison et al., 1999; Brydon-Miller et al., 2003). This is accomplished by combining theory and practice, where researchers and practitioners promote reflection and change by moving through an iterative cycle of activities and reflective learning (Avison et al., 1999). Aligned with this, action research works to address traditional power hierarchies by bridging gaps between research and action (Gray, Wong-Wylie, Rempel et al., 2020).

> **Key point!**
>
> Action research relies on researchers working with stakeholders to accomplish change that benefits them.
>
> (Huang, 2010)

To address power hierarchies, action researchers emphasise the democratic and participatory process of researcher, combining reflection with action, and practice and theory, so that practical solutions are pursued within the communities (Reason and Bradbury, 2001).

Participatory research refers to approaches that are committed to inclusivity, as well as social or environmental justice (Cargo and Mercer, 2008), through collaboration and empowering participants to be included in the decisions about the research processes (Liegghio, Nelson, and Evans., 2010). Liegghio et al. noted that participatory action research focuses on knowledge production and action through the meaningful participation of vulnerable populations in a collaborative way to address asymmetrical relations.

Participatory action research requires flexibility from the researcher to attend to issues arising among members in situ, and to be mindful of the social conditions that may produce or reproduce oppression (Liegghio et al., 2010). By attending to oppression, power and vulnerability, participatory action research creates possibilities to transform power relations (Haarmans, Nazroo, Kapadia et al., 2022).

Quality in qualitative research
When undertaking any qualitative study, due consideration needs to be given to how the work conforms to appropriate quality standards. Establishing what these standards are, however, is debated among researchers. For quantitative research, there are clear checklists available to measure quality. However, in qualitative research, universalised checklists have been subject to criticism (Barbour, 1998; Lester and O'Reilly, 2021). Although this criticism does not mean qualitative research cannot have defensible rigour, it is important to be aware of the differences in measuring quality between qualitative and quantitative approaches. We therefore discuss these universal ideas first, and then provide the counter argument that the heterogeneity in the approach requires more specificity in terms of quality.

Homogeneity arguments
A central challenge for qualitative research relates to the degree of ambiguity about which quality criteria to apply to the work because of the diversity across methodologies, and we have noted that this can be especially difficult when synthesising qualitative inquiry for review or funding purposes (O'Reilly and Kiyimba, 2015). To address some of the early criticisms targeted toward qualitative evidence, scholars began to create specific quality markers to produce universal criteria checklists constructed to be appropriate across the paradigm. For some of these checklists, there was merely an adaptation of language associated with quantitative research, i.e. with reference to concepts like validity, reliability, and generalisability. However, as time progressed, more philosophically congruent frameworks were developed. In 2003, Spencer, Ritchie, Lewis et al. identified 29 different qualitative quality frameworks, and two decades later, there are inevitably many more. The challenge inherent to these frameworks is that they treat qualitative methodologies as homogenous, in the sense that they propose the same set of criteria should be applied to any of the different ways of doing qualitative research.

There are various checklists with overlapping indicators (albeit using slightly different terms), and two of those that are frequently cited are a general checklist proposed by Tracy (2010), and the 32-item COREQ (COnsolidated criteria for REporting Qualitative research) checklist that Tong, Sainsbury, and Craig (2007) designed for research involving interviews and focus groups (*note, however, that this treats interviews as if they are a straightforward homogenous method, and as we note in Chapter 14 there is diversity within interviewing*). For your information, and critical reflection, we provide an overview of the core eight universal markers offered by Tracy (2010) in Table 6.5, and a summary of Tong et al.'s COREQ checklist which they grouped under three domains in Table 6.6.

Collectively there are many individual indicators contained within these homogenous universal checklists around the different processes of completing a qualitative research project. The significance of these is that they are designed to promote methodological integrity, often referred to by those with a more positivist leaning as validity.

Table 6.5 Eight universal indicators of quality in qualitative research (Tracy, 2010)

Indicator	*Description*
Worthy topic	Research conducted should be timely and significant.
Rich rigour	There should be sufficient data to support the claims being made and findings should be rich in detail.
Sincerity	The end goal should be achieved through transparency and honesty, with a clear audit trail.
Credibility	The reporting should be trustworthy, and findings should be plausible and achieved via in depth description.
Resonance	There should be a goal to meaningfully translate the research findings for audiences in a way that resonates with the reader.
Significant contribution	The study should aim to extend knowledge and/or improve practice.
Ethics	There are protocols that attend to the iterative process of research ethics.
Meaningful coherence	The study should accomplish its stated purpose and use methods that relate to relevant theory and the body of research in which the enquiry is situated.

Table 6.6 COREQ quality indicators (Tong et al., 2007)

Domain	*Broad issues*
Research team and reflexivity	There is clear reference to the identities and personal characteristics of the researchers, and the nature of their relationship with participants.
Study design	The study has a sound theoretical framework, with appropriate participant selection. The study design considers the setting of the study and attends to the quality of the data collection.
Data analysis and reporting	There is appropriate data coding and analytic process. The process of reporting the findings is clear and relevant to the aims and questions of the project.

With respect to qualitative research, validity relates to whether knowledge claims are an accurate representation of reality (Spencer et al., 2003). However, this relies on a philosophical ideal that there is an objective reality to represent. Hence, the concept of validity is more often repositioned in qualitative work as trustworthiness of the interpretations and conclusions drawn (Stiles, 1993). In relation to trustworthiness of interpretations, the way in which findings are framed should clearly connect back to the ontological and epistemological foundation of the work (O'Reilly and Kiyimba, 2015), and there needs to be transparency about how the findings are linked to the relationship between the researcher and the participants (Stenbacka, 2001).

The interpretations of the researcher need to be verified in some way by the audience, and thus researchers must present sufficient evidence in disseminating their findings of their processes and interpretations for the audience to be able to make such judgement (Lester and O'Reilly, 2021). Thus, for those using universal criteria to judge quality, you will find a range of concepts used. We provide a brief overview of some of these given the relevance arguments made regarding heterogeneity:

- **Credibility** – a demonstration of transparent and honest reporting of how researcher influences were identified and addressed. These may include the researcher's training and experience, how the participants were recruited, and the funding source or personal connections (Johnson, Adkins, and Chauvin, 2020).
- **Transferability** – the extent to which the findings may be likely to be similar in other population groups. To ascertain this, it is helpful to provide the reader with information about numbers of participants, how they were sampled, their geographical location, characteristics of participants, and the timeframe of data collection and analysis (Shenton, 2004).
- **Reflexivity** – requires the researcher to reflect and report on their role and identity during the process to consider how they have shaped and influenced the project and its findings (Finlay, 2003).
- **Transparency** – refers to the need to provide a full an honest account of the project by giving rich and detailed description with a clear rationale (Spencer et al., 2003).
- **Auditability** – the degree of clarity provided so that the decisions and choices made during the study can be systematically reviewed (Nair, 2021).
- **Trustworthiness** – the extent to which the findings represent reality (Guba and Lincoln, 1994).
- **Sampling adequacy** – the adequacy of the sample size, sample composition, and sample representativeness to be able to make claims from the data (O'Reilly and Parker, 2013).
- **Ethicality** – an iterative and meaningful approach to ethics is needed, not only in terms of formal governance, but also in terms of evidence of a responsive navigation of ethical considerations as part of the process of research.

Whilst universal checklists can be useful to appraise qualitative research, they are limited in their reach if the person evaluating the work is not able to extrapolate to the specific methodological variations of the research they are engaging with. Some universal markers may be translated differently or mean slightly different things in relation to some methodological approaches or may be applied in a different way, and some markers are simply not relevant for certain qualitative approaches.

We therefore tend to favour those approaches to ensuring quality that more directly engage with the heterogeneity of qualitative research, and more explicitly recognise how any universal markers are applied in context. As Barbour put it in 2001, "if we succumb to the lure of 'one size fits all' solutions, we risk being in a situation where the tail (the checklist) is wagging the dog (the qualitative research)" (2001, p. 1115). Indeed, as acknowledged by Rolfe (2006, p. 308) "the continued failure to agree on universal criteria for judging quality in qualitative research is symptomatic of an inability to identify a coherent 'qualitative' research paradigm" as the concept of homogeneity does not exist outside of generic texts. As such, we invite you to consider your own position on the value or lack of value of universal quality checklists and engage with the reflective activity in Box 6.5.

Box 6.5

Reflective activity on universal quality checklists

Based on the two universal checklists provided here, consider how you might use one when designing your qualitative health research project. Make a note in your research diary or discuss with a colleague:

- Considering your project, how many of these criteria have you already planned for?
- Which quality measures have you not yet considered?
- How will you ensure that you demonstrate each aspect of quality to your audience?
- Are there any problems with trying to utilise a universal criteria checklist to your chosen methodological approach and research design?

Heterogeneity arguments

Our argument in this chapter is that whilst the quality criteria that have been developed to assure robustness in qualitative research may be suitable across a spectrum of methodologies, the way those criteria are applied will likely vary. Thus, when research is appraised by reviewers, funders or other audiences, the framework, theory, goals and objectives, and standards in relation to methods need to be aligned with the methodological approach (Lester and O'Reilly, 2021). Consequently, although universal criteria can be helpful in giving an overview of the issues of quality, it is necessary to have an understanding of what quality means specifically within each methodology or approach so that researchers can be confident they are not being judged against inappropriate standards. In fact, it has been strongly argued that there is great within-group diversity across the qualitative paradigm, and any assessment of quality must account for that diversity (Meyrick, 2006; Sandelowski and Borroso, 2002).

Because of the criticisms levied toward universal checklists and a potential overreliance on these to appraise qualitative research, it has been argued instead that a different approach is needed, one that accounts for the heterogeneity in approaches (Barbour, 1998; O'Reilly and Kiyimba, 2015; Lester and O'Reilly, 2021). By taking a more nuanced approach to quality, it is possible to emphasise and celebrate the diverse nature of different forms of qualitative research, whilst still accepting the need for formal quality criteria for each of those approaches. In recognising diversity, it is generally accepted that there are differences in the epistemological, ontological, ethical, and political assumptions of those different types of qualitative research (Moccia, 1988).

> **Key point!**
>
> There is a broad range of epistemological positions in qualitative research, and this means the qualitative paradigm is simply too broad for any scholar to produce a single set of universal quality criteria.
>
> (Sandelowski and Borroso, 2002)

We now invite you to consider your own position on the value of specific quality checklists in the reflective activity in Box 6.6.

> **Box 6.6**
> **Reflective activity on specific quality checklists**
>
> Based on your reading in this chapter, please write in your diary the extent to which you think universal checklists are useful for qualitative health research. Make a note of your reasons and as you complete the chapter, see if you change your mind.

Given we are advocating there should be a more specific approach to quality in qualitative research that accounts for the heterogeneity within the paradigm, we encourage you to engage with further reading. As you engage with more literature on this subject, it is helpful to recognise that academic discussion about the relevance of quality criteria has evolved over time. This is not a peripheral issue in theorising and practicing research, rather practising researchers need to contribute to the methodological literature to help novice researchers ensure that when they are employing a specific qualitative approach, they can also assure its quality (see Lester and O'Reilly, 2021). Indeed, we recommend you refer to the articles in the special issue to see how each of the common qualitative methodologies are considered in terms of their quality indicators. The editorial for the issue is this:

- Lester, J.N., and O'Reilly, M. (2021). Introduction to special issue quality in qualitative approaches: Celebrating heterogeneity. *Qualitative Research in Psychology*, *18*(3), 295–304.

Mixing qualitative approaches – mixing qualitative methods

We recognise that as a qualitative health researcher you may be engaged with a bigger-scale project that mixes methods or approaches. The very concept of a "mixed-methods" research study usually refers to a project having both a quantitative strand and a qualitative strand, and this can be conceived of as inter-paradigm research. This kind of mixing has become increasingly popular in recent years, especially in health research as it is seen as a holistic way to address research problems. Whilst this kind of mixing approaches is quite common in modern research and it may be the type of project you are doing, it is not what we are concerned with in this chapter. Instead of reiterating the vast literature on mixing quantitative with qualitative research, we turn our attention to the much smaller work that has been concerned with researchers mixing their methods within the qualitative paradigm – that is, what we have termed intra-paradigm research (O'Reilly and Kiyimba, 2015).

When researchers mix quantitative and qualitative approaches in one study, the rationale for this is to improve the robustness of the project and extend the scope of the findings (Bazeley, 2018), and to overcome any weaknesses in a single research design (Bryman, 2016) by capitalising on the strength of each approach (O'Cathain and Thomas, 2006). On this basis, one might assume that combining two or more qualitative approaches, or two or more qualitative methods could have similar benefits. Problematically, however, there is less written about the benefits and challenges of doing so, and even the concepts used are different for such activity. For example, if you consult the literature, you will find terms like "qualitative mixed-methods design", "multiple-method design" (Morse, 2009), "multi-methods" (Anguera, Blanco-Villaseñor, Losada et al., 2018), and "pluralism" (Barker and Pistrang, 2005).

We argue that there is a difference between research that combines two or more qualitative methodologies and research that mixes two or more qualitative methods. As we noted earlier in the book, there is a difference between methodology and method and therefore the tensions or challenges that can arise from "mixing" these also change. We have noted that our preference is for the concept of a "synthesised methodologies study", referring to the mixing of methodologies, and a "mixed qualitative methods study", where it is the methods that are mixed under the rubric of a single approach (O'Reilly and Kiyimba, 2015). We clarified that in a synthesised methodologies study, the mixing does not occur until both single parts are completed, and the integration of findings and application of research messages occurs as the final stage. In a mixed qualitative methods study, the integration occurs from the beginning and the two or more datasets are analysed together. This is possible because of the overarching single design, methodology, epistemology, and ontology.

Mixing intra-paradigmatic research is not straightforward, as qualitative research is heterogenous, with many different approaches, different epistemologies, and different ontologies, thus creating philosophical tensions that need to be addressed and resolved before mixing (O'Reilly et al., 2020). It has often been thought that intra-paradigmatic research is less problematic than inter-paradigmatic research because of the misconception that qualitative research is a united approach (Barbour, 1998). But as Barbour has observed, that is inaccurate, as whilst qualitative research has some uniting characteristics, there are different methodologies, theories, and methods meaning that this paradigm is complex with many differences at a range of levels that need to be reconciled. Researchers need to be wary that there are difficulties in mixing potentially epistemologically incompatible qualitative methodologies (Wimpenny and Gass, 2000), and often when combining those methodologies, researchers do not always anchor their work with an identifiable epistemological perspective (Caelli, Ray, and Mill., 2003). It is further important to consider the ontological foundation of the research, as there is a greater likelihood of epistemological congruence when the two methodologies are underpinned by the same ontology (Annells, 1996).

> **Key point!**
>
> The difference between an overarching methodology and the different methods of data collection and analysis are essential to consider when trying to reconcile epistemological and ontological issues with intra-paradigmatic research.
>
> (O'Reilly et al., 2020)

Triangulation, integration, and crystallisation of data
Triangulation

The concept of *triangulation* was originally developed in the context of surveying and navigation as a technique to identify a location via multiple points of reference. However, in the context of research, the concept has been modified to refer to the inclusion of multiple methods, types of data, theories or perspectives in a way that strengthens a research project (Denzin and Lincoln, 2011). Triangulation then, is often associated with studies using multi-methods, especially in research involving a combination of quantitative and qualitative methods. In work that uses multiple qualitative methods, triangulation can also be a helpful concept, referred to as data triangulation, when multiple data collection methods are drawn upon, methodological triangulation, when combining methodologies, investigator triangulation, for the involvement of multiple researchers, and theoretical triangulation, when combining theories (Denzin, 1978). Indeed, for qualitative research, triangulation requires the researcher to explore the data collected via different methods (Shih, 1998) or triangulate through multiple coders whereby the data are coded independently and then compared (Patton, 1999).

> **Key point!**
>
> In the context of qualitative research, triangulation should not be understood as a means for validating findings, but instead is a way of providing different perspectives in relation to a specific phenomenon.
>
> (Flick, 2017)

There are some qualitative researchers who align their work with post-positivist thinking and deploy triangulation in seeking to enhance the credibility of the analysis and findings, whereas others, conversely, deploy the term to refer to capturing richness and diversity of perspectives on a phenomenon (Denzin and Lincoln, 2011). On this basis, in terms of quality in qualitative research, it is necessary for the researcher to describe exactly what they are triangulating, how they are doing it, and how they are incorporating the findings of this triangulation (Varpio, Ajjawi, Monrouxe et al., 2017). There has been some useful advice in the literature on how to achieve this in practice and we summarise guidance provided by Bazeley (2018) in Box 6.7.

> **Box 6.7**
>
> **Practical steps for triangulation (Bazeley, 2018)**
>
> There are various practical ways in which triangulation can be used to organise complementary data and Bazeley argued there are six steps:
>
> 1. The first step is for the researcher to create a list of themes or shared concepts that relate to the research questions and multiple data sets. These concepts need to be based on an understanding of the individual cases constituting the sample.
> 2. The second step necessitates the researcher juxtaposing sources by generating a matrix of quotes from the data and frequencies of occurrences to compare each concept and the frequency of each in the entire dataset.
> 3. The third step is to assess convergence, in other words the triangulation goal. The researcher identifies where the coded data has agreement, partial agreement, or when there are gaps when identified issues are covered in one set of findings but not another. As part of this step, it can be helpful to explore if the differences relate to the nature and/or focus of the data set, or to the conditions in which data were collected, or if they represent a legitimate difference in the findings.
> 4. The fourth step is to assess completeness which in practice necessitates the researcher comparing the nature and scope of the unique topic areas for each dataset and identify similarities and differences.
> 5. The fifth step is an important step in cases where multiple coders and researchers are involved in the research, as these analysts compare their assessments regarding the convergence and completeness of the data and consider any areas of disagreement.
> 6. The sixth step requires the researcher to develop a unified description and interpretation of each concept and merge the information together.

The principle of triangulation is not without its critics, and in qualitative research specifically, there are some controversies regarding its use. Triangulation requires the merging of two or more sets of data from different sources, and a main interpretation is provided to see if there are similarities across them (Morgan, 2018). Morgan argued that the triangulation of qualitative and quantitative data sets can be problematic for three reasons:

1. On theoretical and practical grounds. In relation to theory, two methodologies from quantitative and qualitative approaches will have competing epistemological foundations (albeit not necessarily in mixed qualitative approaches). In relation to practice, it can be difficult to take two sets of findings obtained through different methods and integrate them in a meaningful way.
2. It is arguable that quantitative and qualitative methods are too different to be able to study "the same thing".
3. The differences in data collection methods and analytic approaches between quantitative and qualitative mean the findings/results cannot be meaningfully compared.

Integration

Integration describes an intentional process of using quantitative and qualitative data interdependently so that a research goal can be achieved (Bazeley, 2018). For example, when health researchers undertake evaluative research such as a randomised controlled trial and subsequently seek to integrate the results with qualitative analysis of the process of the intervention (Richards, Bazeley, Borglin et al., 2019). Integration is when the researcher brings together core findings from different parts of the project, or different datasets. Put differently, integration denotes the extent to which the two sets of findings are coherent and represent the explanatory strength of the project (Fetters, Curry, and Creswell, 2013). Integration can also involve the production of visual aids to demonstrate the overlaps in findings, or a comparison (Richards et al., 2019). There is a case in the literature that there are benefits to the integration of two different data sets, particularly in the case of mixed methods. This is because qualitative data can be used to assess the validity of quantitative findings or quantitative data can be used to generate a sample for qualitative research or to explain qualitative findings (Fetters et al., 2013). In this section however, we consider ways to integrate findings from two or more qualitative methods or methodologies.

Ravitch and Carl (2016) proposed that an integrated approach to analysing qualitative data involves five elements:

1. Data analysis is considered an iterative and recursive process. In other words, the researcher recognises analysis as an active ongoing process and builds their analysis in such a way as to recognise the layers and complexities of the data. The analytic process needs to be transparent. How the researcher has managed the data should be clearly described.
2. The analysis should involve both formative and summative stages. It is necessary to closely attend to the ways in which questions are asked of participants, and how those questions shape participants' responses, and to examine how follow-up questions are asked.
3. The analytic process requires the triangulation of data and theory. Triangulation is an aspect of data integration, and theoretical triangulation enables the researcher to account for multiple theoretical perspectives, whilst data triangulation necessitates looking at different data sources for differences as well as the ways the data support emergent theory. Analytic data triangulation requires the researcher to organise analysis of data to consider the data from different analytic angles.
4. Power relations should be recognised, as well as ethical concerns relating to research analysis. The research holds a great deal of interpretive authority, that is power when interpreting participants' experiences and narratives. Other people's lives are represented by the researcher, and they should be mindful that interpretations of data into "findings" are not simply collected and claimed but co-constructed. Transparency is therefore essential in the interpretive process.
5. Analysing data requires a process of seeking and engaging with an alternative perspective, especially those that challenge those of the researcher. Collaboration is therefore useful to realise an authentic data analysis. As part of the process of

analysis, the researcher's assumptions and biases should be explicitly explored. This will be supported through critical conversations between team members or with research supervisors in an open-ended way and analytic memos could be shared whilst preliminary analytic ideas are interrogated.

There are different levels at which the data may be integrated. One way is to integrate at a *methods* level. This is where the integration occurs by linking the methods of data collection with analysis (Creswell and Piano-Clark, 2011), which can be achieved through connecting, building, merging, or embedding (Fetters et al., 2013). Fetters et al. conceptualised the process of integration through different domains. Integrating through connecting is when one type of data connects with another through the sampling frame, when participants are identified for one method through the other method. Integration through building is when the insights from analysis of one set of data inform the other, and thus the later method builds on the former. Integrating through merging is when the researcher brings the two datasets together for comparison, and integrating via embedding is when data collection and analysis are linked at multiple points and involves a combination of connecting, building, and merging.

It is also possible to integrate at an *interpretation* and *reporting* level. At the interpretation and reporting level, the integration can occur through narrative, data transformation or through joint displays (Fetters et al., 2013). For Fetters et al., to integrate through narrative, multiple findings are described in a single or series of related reports. This can take different forms: through data transformation means one type of data must be converted into the other type of data, and when transformed they are then integrated; and through joint displays, researchers integrate the data by bringing the multiple data together through visual means to generate new insights beyond the information gained from each independently.

Crystallisation
Crystallisation is an alternative concept to triangulation. Richardson and St Pierre (2005) noted that it is a more appropriate term than triangulation as it indicates a recognition there are more than three angles or positions from which to view social phenomena. In this respect, crystallisation can be considered something of a point of contrast to the, arguably, more two-dimensional, fixed idea of triangulation, capturing instead the multiple endeavours of researchers to embrace complexity in interpreting the experiences of multiple participants (Denzin and Lincoln, 2011).

As a concept, crystallisation is of value for researchers using qualitative methods. This is because when crystallisation occurs, projects incorporate a range of facets on the qualitative continuum to maximise the benefits of contrasting approaches to analysis and representation and are also self-referential of their partiality (Ellingson, 2017). Ellingson proposed that crystallisation manifests in qualitative work that offers nuanced interpretations about a phenomenon, represents ways of producing knowledge across multiple points of the qualitative spectrum, and uses more than one genre of writing. In this way, crystallisation typically prompts a degree of reflexivity of the researcher's sense of self and role in the process and serves as a critique to positivist claims to objectivity via an independent "view from nowhere".

Author reflections and concluding remarks
From Nikki, Philip, and Michelle

In our work, we have noticed that the relatively lower status of qualitative research compared to quantitative research that still exists in healthcare contexts can sometimes tempt qualitative researchers to add a quantitative component to their work to bolster its apparent credibility. Our argument is that if a piece of research is conducted rigorously in line with the quality criteria for that methodology, then it can stand as a valuable contribution to the knowledge base in its own right. A newer approach to combining methodologies as discussed in this chapter, is to subject the same data set to two different methodological analyses, or to combine two different qualitative data sets in the same study.

We emphasise here the difference between inter- and intra-paradigmatic mixed methods approaches. In our experience of qualitative research, there have been occasions when it has appeared profitable to us to engage in an intra-paradigm qualitative mixed methods study. For example, this might be to evaluate the data from different perspectives, perhaps at first taking a macro-qualitative approach such as thematic analysis to look for overarching themes in a naturally occurring data set to establish *what* the main practices are that are observable. Following this, it may be advantageous to reanalyse the same data set using the lens of a micro qualitative approach, such as a discourse analysis, to explore further how those practices are being co-constructed in the data. Presenting these two forms of analytic findings alongside one another can add depth as well as breadth to the way in which answering the research question is approached. However, we strongly caution those who may be keen to engage in intra-paradigm qualitative mixed methods research to think carefully about the congruence of the intended approaches to ensure compatibility.

The difference in qualitative research from quantitative is that it is has a much broader scope of variety in relation to epistemic possibilities and options. Qualitative research is a heterogenous paradigm in the sense that, due to this variability, some qualitative approaches simply do not fit well with others. Just because the two chosen approaches are both qualitative does not assure a successful and meaningful combining can be realised. At an epistemic level, the first consideration is to ensure that both chosen approaches sit within the same epistemic framework – a social-constructionist methodology for example would need to be paired with another social-constructionist methodology for there to be the required synergy to draw any meaningful conclusions from the combining of approaches. Similarly, there needs to be congruence with the data collection method and the analytic methodology. For example, we much prefer to collect naturally occurring rather than researcher generated data to explore the social actions occurring in a particular context. As a clinician-researcher, it is important to understand how participants operate in a real-life context, and how they engage in social actions in situ. For example, different learning will occur by watching a video of a doctor patient interaction than by interviewing one party or the other after the interaction. What we can observe occurring in a real-life exchange is particularly helpful for informing clinical practice and helps us to see exactly what is going on rather than relying on impressions and memories of events.

Our advice is that, before collecting any data, the whole research project is mapped out, with thought given to what data is being collected, how, and why. We also recommend that careful consideration is given to how best to answer the research question whilst holding a commitment to maintaining congruence throughout the research design process. Ultimately, a piece of research that has not been adequately thought through in this way, will possibly not meet the quality criteria required for publication, or for inclusion in a meta synthesis of research in the field. Taking time at the planning stage and asking for advice and support from an academic researcher with experience in qualitative approaches, and experience in combining them for mixed methods studies will help ensure your hard work is not in vain.

References

Adams, T., Ellis, C., and Holman-Jones, S. (2017). Autoethnography. In J. Matthes (Ed.), *The international encyclopedia of communication research methods* (pp. 1–11). John Wiley & Sons.

Anguera, M., Blanco-Villaseñor, A., Losada, J., Sánchez-Algarra, P., and Onwuegbuzie, A. (2018). Revisiting the difference between mixed methods and multimethods: Is it all in the name? *Quality & Quantity, 52*(6), 2757–277.

Annells, M. (1996). Grounded theory method: Philosophical perspectives, paradigm of research, and postmodernism. *Qualitative Health Research, 6*(3), 379–393.

Antaki, C. (2011). Six kinds of applied conversation analysis. In C. Antaki (Ed.), *Applied conversation analysis: Intervention and change in institutional talk* (pp. 1–4). Basingstoke, Hampshire: Palgrave MacMillan.

Archard, P. J. (2020). Psychoanalytically informed research interviewing: Notes on the free association narrative interview method. *Nurse Researcher, 28*(2), 42–49.

Archard, P. J. (2021). The psychoanalytically-informed interview in social work research. *Journal of Social Work Practice, 35*(2), 191–203.

Archard, P. J., and O'Reilly, M. (2022). Psychoanalytic therapy and narrative research interviewing: Some reflections. *Nurse Researcher, 30*(3), 28–35.

Arribas-Ayloon, M., and Walkerdine, V. (2008). Foucauldian discourse analysis. In C. Willig and W. Stainton-Rogers (Eds.), *The Sage handbook of qualitative research in psychology* (pp. 91–108). London: Sage.

Avison, D., Lau, F., Myers, M., and Nielsen, P. (1999) Action research. *Communications of the ACM, 42*(1), 94–97.

Barbour, R. (1998). Mixing qualitative methods: Quality assurance or qualitative quagmire? *Qualitative Health Research, 8*(3), 352–361.

Barker, C., and Pistrang, N. (2005). Quality criteria under methodological pluralism: Implications for conducting and evaluating research. *American Journal of Community Psychology, 35*(3/4), 201–211.

Bazeley, P. (2018). *Integrating analyses in mixed methods research*. London: Sage.

Biggerstaff, D. (2012). Qualitative research methods in psychology. In G. Rossi (Ed.), *Psychology-selected papers* (pp. 175–206). London: InTech Open Science.

Bochner, A. and Ellis, C. (2002). *Ethnographically speaking: Autoethnography, literature, and aesthetics*. Walnut Creek, CA: AltaMira Press.

Boyatzis, R. (1998). *Transforming qualitative information: Thematic analysis and code development*. London: Sage.

Braun, V., and Clarke, V. (2022). *Thematic analysis: A practical guide*. London: Sage.

Braun, V., and Clarke, V. (2019). Reflecting on reflexive thematic analysis. *Qualitative Research in Sport, Exercise and Health, 11*(4), 589–597.

Braun, V., and Clarke, V. (2006). Using thematic analysis in psychology. *Qualitative Research in Psychology, 3*, 77–101.

Brydon-Miller, M., Greenwood, D., and Maguire, P. (2003). Why action research? *Action Research*, 1(1), 9–28.

Bryman, A. (2016). *Social research methods* (5th ed.). Oxford: Oxford University Press.

Butina, M. (2015). A narrative approach to qualitative inquiry. *Clinical Laboratory Science*, 28(3), 190–196.

Burck, C. (2005). Comparing qualitative research methodologies for systemic research: The use of grounded theory, discourse analysis and narrative analysis. *Journal of Family Therapy*, 27(3), 237–262.

Caelli, K., Ray, L., and Mill, J. (2003) "Clear as mud": Toward greater clarity in generic qualitative research. *International Journal of Qualitative Methods*, 2(2), Article 1.

Cargo, M., and Mercer, S. (2008). The value and challenges of participatory research: Strengthening its practice. *Annual Review of Public Health*, 29, 325–350.

Carroll, K., and Mesman, J. (2018). Multiple researcher roles in video-reflexive ethnography. *Qualitative Health Research*, 28(7), 1145–1156.

Charmaz, K. (2006). *Constructing grounded theory: Practical guide through qualitative analysis*. London: Sage.

Charmaz, K. (2005). Grounded theory in the 21st century: Applications for advancing social justice studies. In N. Denzin and Y. Lincoln (Eds.), *The Sage handbook of qualitative research* (3rd ed., pp. 507–535). London: Sage.

Charmaz, K., and Thornberg, R. (2021). The pursuit of quality in grounded theory. *Qualitative Research in Psychology*, 18(3), 305–327.

Connelly M., and Clandinin J. (1990). Stories of experience and narrative inquiry. *Educational Researcher*, 19(5), 2–14.

Cooper, A. (2009). Hearing the grass grow: Emotional and epistemological challenges of practice-near research. *Journal of Social Work Practice*, 23, 429–442.

Cordeiro, L., and Soares, C. (2018). Action research in the healthcare field: A scoping review. *Database of Systematic Reviews & Implementation Reports*, 16(4), 1003–1047.

Cresswell, J., and Plano-Clark, V. (2011). *Designing and conducting mixed method research* (2nd ed.). Thousand Oaks, CA: Sage.

Davidsen, A. (2013). Phenomenological approaches in psychology and health sciences. *Qualitative Research in Psychology*, 10(3), 318–339.

Denzin, N. (1978). *The research act: A theoretical introduction to sociological methods* (2nd ed.). New York, NY: McGraw Hill.

Denzin, N., and Lincoln, Y. (Eds.). (2011). *The Sage handbook of qualitative research* (4th ed.). Thousand Oaks, CA: Sage.

Drew, P. (2013) Turn design. In J. Sidnell and T. Stivers (Eds.), *The handbook of conversation analysis* (pp. 131–149). Chichester, West Sussex: Blackwell Publishing.

Drew, P., and Heritage, J. (1992). Analyzing talk at work: An introduction. In P. Drew and J. Heritage (Eds.), *Talk at work: Interaction in institutional settings* (pp. 3–65). Cambridge: Cambridge University Press.

Edwards, D. (1997). *Discourse and cognition*. London: Sage.

Edwards, D., and Potter, J. (2017). Some uses of subject-side assessments. *Discourse Studies*, 19(5), 497–514.

Edwards, D., and Potter, J. (1992). *Discursive psychology*. London: Sage.

Ellingson, L. (2017). *Engaging crystallization in qualitative research: An introduction*. Thousand Oaks, CA: Sage.

Flick, U. (2017). Triangulation. In N. Denzin and Y. Lincoln (Eds.), *The Sage handbook of qualitative research* (5th ed.). London: Sage

Frosh, S. (2010). *Psychoanalysis outside the clinic: Interventions in psychosocial studies*. London: Palgrave Macmillan.

Frosh, S., and Baraitser, L. (2008). Psychoanalysis and psychosocial studies. *Psychoanalysis, Culture & Society*, 13, 346–365.

Frosh, S., and Emerson, P. (2005). Interpretation and over-interpretation: Disputing the meaning of texts. *Qualitative Research*, 5, 307–324.

Fetterman, D. (2010) *Ethnography, step-by-step* (2nd ed.). Thousand Oaks, CA: Sage.

Fetters, M., Curry, L., and Creswell, J. (2013). Achieving integration in mixed methods designs-principles and practices. *Health Services Research*, 48(6), 2134–2156.

Finlay, L. (2003). The reflexive journey: Mapping multiple routes. In L. Finlay & B. Gough (Eds.), *Reflexivity: A practical guide for researchers in health and social sciences* (pp. 3–20). Oxford: Blackwell Publishing.

Gadamer, H. (1989). *Truth and method* (2nd ed.). London: Stagbooks.

Giorgi, A., and Giorgi, B. (2003). Phenomenology. In J. Smith (Ed.), *Qualitative psychology* (pp. 25–50). London: Sage.

Glaser, B., and Strauss, A. (1967). *The discovery of grounded theory: Strategies for qualitative research*. New York, NY: Aldine.

Gray, L., Wong-Wylie, G., Rempel, G., and Cook, K. (2020). Expanding qualitative research interviewing strategies: Zoom video communications. *The Qualitative Report*, 25(5), 1292–1301.

Grbich, C. (2013). *Qualitative data analysis: An introduction* (2nd ed.). London: Sage.

Guba, E., and Lincoln, Y. (1994). Competing paradigms in qualitative research. In N. Denzin and Y. Lincoln (Eds.), *Handbook of qualitative research*. Thousand Oak, CA: Sage.

Guest, G., MacQueen, K., and Namey, E. (2012). *Applied thematic analysis*. Thousand Oaks, CA: Sage.

Haarmans, M., Nazroo, J., Kapadia, D., Maxwell, C., Osahan, S., Edant, J., Grant-Rowles, J., Motala, Z., and Rhodes, J. (2022). The practice of participatory action research: Complicity, power and prestige in dialogue with the "racialised mad". *Sociology of Health & Illness*, 44, 106–123.

Hammersley, M., and Atkinson, P. (2007). *Ethnography: Principles in practice* (3rd ed.). New York, NY: Routledge.

Heath, H., and Cowley, S. (2004). Developing a grounded theory approach: A comparison of Glaser and Strauss. *International Journal of Nursing Studies*, 41(2), 141–150.

Heikkinen, H. (2002). Whatever is narrative research? In R. Huttunen, H. Heikkinen, & L. Syrjälä (Eds.), *Narrative research: Voices from teachers and philosophers* (pp. 13–25). Jyväskylä, Finland: SoPhi.

Heritage, J. (2011). Conversation analysis: Practices and methods. In D. Silverman (Ed.), *Qualitative research* (3rd ed., pp. 208–230). London: Sage.

Hoggett, P., Beedell, P., Jimenez, L., Mayo, M., and Miller, C. (2010). Working psychosocially and dialogically in research. *Psychoanalysis, Culture & Society*, 15, 173–188.

Hollnagel, E., Wears, R., & Braithwaite, J. (2015). *Safety I to safety II: A white paper. The resilient healthcare net*. University of Southern Denmark, University of Florida, USA and Macquarie University Australia.

Hollway, W., and Jefferson, T. (2013). *Doing qualitative research differently: A psychosocial approach* (2nd ed.). London: Sage.

Holmes, J. (2013). A comparison of clinical psychoanalysis and research interviews. *Human Relations*, 66, 1183–1199.

Huang, H. (2010). What is good action research? Why this resurgent interest? *Action research*, 8(1), 93–109.

Hutchby, I., and Wooffitt, R. (2008). *Conversation analysis* (2nd ed.). Cambridge: Polity Press.

Iedema, R., and Carroll, K. (2010). Discourse research that intervenes in the quality and safety of care practices. *Discourse & Communication*, 4(1), 68–86.

Iedema, R., Carroll, K., Collier, A., Hor, S., Mesman, J., and Wyer, M. (2019). *Video reflexive ethnography in health research and healthcare improvement: theory and application*. Bocan Raton, FL: CRC Press.

Iedema, R., Forsyth, R., Georgiou, A., Braithwaite, J., and Westbrook, J. (2007). Video research in health: Visibilising the effects of computerising clinical care. *Qualitative Research Journal*, 6(2), 15–30.

Jacobs, S. (2018). A history and analysis of the evolution of action and participatory action research. *Canadian Journal of Action Research*, 19(3), 34–52.

Johnson, J., Adkins, D., and Chauvin, S. (2020). A review of the quality indicators of rigor in qualitative research. *American Journal of Pharmaceutical Education*, 84(1), 7120.

King, N. (2012). Doing template analysis. In G. Symon and C. Cassell (Eds.), *Qualitative organizational research* (pp. 426–450). London: Sage.

King, N. (2004). Using templates in the thematic analysis of text. In C. Cassell and G. Symon (Eds.), *Essential guide to qualitative methods in organisational research* (pp. 256–270). London: Sage.

Koshy, E., Koshy, V., and Waterman, H. (2010). *Action research in healthcare*. London: Sage.

Lapping, C. (2011). *Psychoanalysis in social research: Shifting theories and reframing concepts*. Abingdon, Oxfordshire: Routledge.

Lester, J.N., and O'Reilly, M. (2021). Introduction to special issue quality in qualitative approaches: Celebrating heterogeneity. *Qualitative Research in Psychology*, 18(3), 295–304.

Lester, J., and O'Reilly, M. (2019). *Applied conversation analysis: Social interaction in institutional settings*. Thousand Oaks, CA: Sage.

Lester, J., O'Reilly, M., Kiyimba, N., and Wong, J. (2018) Discursive psychology: Implications for counselling psychology. *The Counseling Psychologist*, 46(5), 576–607.

Lester, J., O'Reilly, M., and Steele, C. (2023). Promoting the value of discursive psychology for human resource development: A pedagogical guide for qualitative researchers. *Human Resource Development Review*, 22(2), 229–250.

Liegghio, M., Nelson, G., and Evans, S. (2010). Partnering with children diagnosed with mental health issues: Contributions of a sociology of childhood perspective of participatory action research. *American Journal of Psychology*, 46, 84–99.

Lingard, L., Albert, M., and Levinson, W. (2008). Grounded theory, mixed methods and action research. *British Medical Journal*, 337, 459–461.

Lopez, K., and Willis, D. (2004). Descriptive versus interpretive phenomenology: Their contributions to nursing knowledge. *Qualitative Health Research*, 14, 726–735.

Meyer, J. (2000). Using qualitative methods in health related achealth-related *British Medical Journal*, 320, 178–181.

Meyrick, J. (2006). What is good qualitative research? A first step towards a comprehensive approach to judging rigour/quality. *Journal of Health Psychology*, 11(5), 799–808.

Moccia, P. (1988). A critique of compromise: Beyond the methods debate. *Advances in Nursing Science*, 10(4), 1–9.

Moen, T. (2006). Reflections on the narrative research approach. *International Journal of Qualitative Methods*, 5(4), 56–69.

Morgan, D. (2018). *Basic and advanced focus groups*. London: Sage.

Morse, J. (2009). Mixing qualitative methods. *Qualitative Health Research*, 19(11), 1523–1524

Murray, M. (2003). Narrative psychology. In J. A. Smith (Ed.), *Qualitative psychology: A practical guide to research methods* (pp. 111–131). London: Sage.

Nair, L. (2021). From 'whodunit' to 'how': Detective stories and auditability in qualitative business ethics research. *Journal of Business Ethics*, 172, 195–209.

Neubauer, B., Witkop, C., and Varpio, L. (2019). How phenomenology can help us learn from the experiences of others. *Perspectives Medical Education*, 8, 90–97.

O'Cathain, A., and Thomas, K. (2006). Combining qualitative and quantitative methods. In C. Pope and N. Mays (Eds.), *Qualitative research in health care* (3rd ed., pp. 102–111). Oxford: BMJ Books.

O'Reilly, M., and Kiyimba, N. (2015). *Advanced qualitative research: A guide to contemporary theoretical debates*. London: Sage.

O'Reilly, M., Kiyimba, N., and Drewett, A. (2020). Mixing qualitative methods versus methodologies: A critical reflection on communication and power in inpatient care [Special Issue]. *Counselling and Psychotherapy Research, 21*, 66–76.

O'Reilly, M., & Parker, N. (2013). "Unsatisfactory saturation": A critical exploration of the notion of saturated sample sizes in qualitative research. *Qualitative Research, 13*(2), 190–197.

Patton, M. (1999). Enhancing the quality and credibility of qualitative analysis. *Health Services Research, 34*, 1189–1208.

Potter, J. (2012). Discourse analysis and disursive psychology. In H. Cooper (Ed.), *APA handbook of research methods in psychology: Quantitative, qualitative, neuropsychological, and biological* (Vol. 2, pp. 111–130). Washington, DC: American Psychological Association.

Potter, J. (1997). Discourse analysis as a way of analyzing naturally-occurring talk. In D. Silverman (Ed.), *Qualitative research: Theory, method and practice* (pp. 144–160). London: Sage.

Potter, J., and Hepburn, A. (2012). Eight challenges for interview researchers. In J. F. Gubrium and J. A. Holstein (Eds.), *Handbook of interview research* (2nd ed., pp. 555–570). London: Sage.

Potter, J., and Wetherell, M. (1987). *Discourse and social psychology*. London: Sage.

Ravitch, S., and Carl, N. (2016). *Qualitative research: Bridging the conceptual, theoretical and methodological*. London: Sage.

Reason, P., and Bradbury, H. (2001). Introduction: Inquiry and participation in search of a world worthy of human aspiration. In P. Reason and H. Bradbury (Eds.), *Handbook of action research: Participative inquiry and practice* (pp. 1–14). London: Sage.

Reiners, G. (2012). Understanding the differences between Husserl's (descriptive) and Heidegger's (interpretive) phenomenological research. *Journal of Nursing Care, 1*, 1–3.

Richards, D. A., Bazeley, P., Borglin, G., Craig, P., Emsley, R., Frost, J., Hill, J., Horwood, J., Hutchings, H. A., Jinks, C., Montgomery, A., Moore, G., Plano, Clark V. L., Tonkin-Crine, S., Wade, J., Warren, F. C., Wyke, S., Young, B., and O'Cathain, A. (2019). Integrating quantitative and qualitative data and findings when undertaking randomised controlled trials. *BMJ Open, 9*, e032081.

Richardson, L., and St Pierre, E. (2005). Writing: A method of inquiry. In N. Denzin and Y. Lincoln (Eds.), *The Sage handbook of qualitative research* (3rd ed., pp. 959–978). Thousand Oaks, CA: Sage.

Riessman, C. (2008). *Narrative methods for the human sciences*. London: Sage.

Rolfe, G. (2006) Validity, trustworthiness and rigour: Quality and the idea of qualitative research. *Methodological Issues in Nursing Research, 53*(3), 304–310.

Sacks, H. (1992). *Lectures on conversation* (Vols. I & II, G. Jefferson, Ed.). Oxford: Basil Blackwell.

Sandberg, J. (2005). How do we justify knowledge produced within interpretive approaches? *Organizational Research Methods, 8*(1), 41–68.

Sandelowski, M., and Barroso, J. (2002). Reading qualitative studies. *International Journal of Qualitative Methods, 1*(1), Art. 5.

Savin-Baden, M., & Major, C. (2013). *Qualitative research: The essential guide to theory and practice*. Abingdon: Routledge.

Shenton, A. (2004). Strategies for ensuring trustworthiness in qualitative research projects. *Education for Information, 22*(2), 63–75.

Shih, F. (1998). Triangulation in nursing research: Issues of conceptual clarity and purpose. *Journal of Advanced Nursing, 28*, 631–641.

Smith, J. A. (2004). Reflecting on the development of interpretative phenomenological analysis and its contribution to qualitative research in psychology. *Qualitative Research in Psychology, 1*, 39–54.

Smith, J. A., Flowers, P., and Larkin, M. (2009). *Interpretative phenomenological analysis: Theory, method and research*. London: Sage.

Spencer, L., Ritchie, J., Lewis, J., and Dillon, L. (2003) *Quality in qualitative evaluation: A framework for assessing research evidence*. London: Government Chief Social Researcher's Office, Prime Minister's Strategy Unit. http://www.civilservice.gov.uk/wp-content/uploads/2011/09/a_quality_framework_tcm6-38740.pdf

Staiti, A. (2012). The pedagogic impulse of Husserl's ways into transcendental phenomenology: An alternative reading of the Erste Philosophie lecture. *Graduate Faculty Philosophy Journal*, 33, 39–56.

Staller, K. (2013). Epistemological boot camp: The politics of science and what every qualitative researcher needs to know to survive in the academy. *Qualitative Social Work*, 12(4), 395–413.

Starks, H., and Trinidad, S. (2007). Choose your method: A comparison of phenomenology, discourse analysis, and grounded theory. *Qualitative Health Research*, 17(10), 1372–1380.

Stenbacka, C. (2001). Qualitative research requires quality concepts of its own. *Management Decision*, 39(7), 551–555.

Stiles, W. (1993). Quality control in qualitative research. *Clinical Psychology Review*, 13, 593–618.

Suddaby, R. (2006). What grounded theory is not. *Academy of Management Journal*, 49(4), 633–642.

Teherani, A., Martimianakis, T., Stenfors-Hayes, T., Wadhwa, A., and Varpio, L. (2015). Choosing a qualitative research approach. *Journal of Graduate Medical Education*, 7, 669–70.

Te Molder, H. (2015). Discursive psychology. In K. Tracy, C. Ilie, and T. Sandel (Eds.), *The international encyclopedia of language and social interaction* (pp. 1–11). John Wiley and Sons.

Thorne, S. (2000). Data analysis in qualitative research. *Evidence Based Nursing*, 3(3), 68–70.

Tong, A., Sainsbury, P., and Craig, J. (2007). Consolidated criteria for reporting qualitative research (COREQ): A 32-item checklist for interviews and focus groups. *International Journal for Quality in Health Care*, 19(6), 349–357.

Tracy, S. (2010). Qualitative quality: Eight "big-tent" criteria for excellent qualitative research. *Qualitative Inquiry*, 16(10), 837–851.

van Dijk, T. (1993). Principles of critical discourse analysis. *Discourse & Society*, 4(2), 249–283.

van Dijk, T. (2008) *Discourse and power*. Basingstoke, Hampshire: Palgrave.

Varpio, L., Ajjawi, R., Monrouxe, L., O'Brien, B., and Rees, C. (2017). Shedding the cobra effect: Problematising thematic emergence, triangulation, saturation, and member checking. *Medical Education*, 51(1), 40–50.

Wang, C., and Geale, S. (2015). The power of story: Narrative inquiry as a methodology in nursing research. *International Journal of Nursing Sciences*, 2(2), 195–198.

Wetherell, M. (2007). A step too far: Discursive psychology, linguistic ethnography and questions of identity. *Journal of Sociolinguistics*, 11(5), 661–681.

Wetherell, M. (2001). Debates in discourse research. In M. Wetherell, S. Taylor, and S. Yates (Eds.), *Discourse theory and practice: A reader* (pp. 380–399). London: Sage.

Willig, C. (2008). *Introducing qualitative research in psychology* (2nd ed.). Milton Keynes: Open University Press.

Wimpenny, P., and Gass, J. (2000). Interviewing in phenomenology and grounded theory: Is there a difference? *Methodological Issues in Nursing Research*, 31(6), 1485–1492.

Wooffitt, R. (2005). *Conversation analysis and discourse analysis: A comparative and critical introduction*. London: Sage.

CHAPTER 7

Working with gatekeepers, stakeholders and experts by experience

> **Learning objectives**
>
> This chapter enables the reader to:
>
> - Plan the utilisation of Public Patient Involvement and Engagement.
> - Critically assess the value of engaging stakeholders in a project.
> - Identify how to avoid tokenism when involving stakeholders.
> - Recognise the role of gatekeepers.
> - Differentiate co-design, co-production, and co-research.
> - Identify the roles of different research team members.

Introduction

The process of undertaking research in healthcare settings often necessitates the involvement of gatekeepers, stakeholders and those who utilise the services provided (patients, clients, service users). This engagement promotes the value of the research project and strengthens the applicability of the findings. When taking a more community-led approach, however, applicability will have been considered prior to the research design through those collaborative partnerships. This chapter explores the ways gatekeepers, stakeholders and those who utilise services can benefit the process of research. We also provide practical tips for working with different groups.

There are various ways in which these groups can inform and influence a research project, and this chapter examines some of these different areas. One focus is public involvement, because it is an ethical approach and considered good practice. This means that any research undertaken is not conducted to, for, or about a particular group of people, but by or with representatives of those people whom the outcomes of the research will be affected by (NHS, 2023). Typically, as is the case with research designs that prioritise Public Patient Involvement and Engagement, patients contribute their views on how the research is designed, conducted, and disseminated. This chapter also considers the role of gatekeepers in facilitating the project or bringing challenges to it. Other ways in which stakeholder involvement can matter, such as through co-design, co-production, and co-research, the role of the research team, are also discussed.

Public Patient Involvement and Engagement (PPIE)

It is now widely accepted as good practice to involve patients and the public in the design and delivery of health research (Reynolds and Beresford, 2020). Reynolds and Beresford reported that Public Patient Involvement and Engagement (PPIE) (sometimes referred to as PPI) in research reflects moral and democratic imperatives about the value and representation of the voices of those who may ultimately be affected by the research findings. To do PPIE activity well, it is necessary for researchers to ensure that the public and patients contribute either via consultation, collaboration, or leading (McMenamin, Isaksen, Manning, and Tierney, 2022). When engaging in PPIE activity, there are several key principles to consider. Liabo, Boddy, Bortoli et al. (2020) set out several of the most important, and these are summarised in Box 7.1.

Box 7.1

Principles of PPIE (Liabo et al., 2020)

The principles to remember when engaging in your PPIE activities are:

- **Inclusivity** – the involvement of a diverse group of people and promoting equality of opportunity for those people to be involved, irrespective of their social background or abilities.
- **Purposeful involvement** – clarity regarding why the public or patients are involved in the research and ensuring that this purpose is communicated to all involved.
- **Partnership** – researchers and those involved in the project having mutual respect for each other's contributions and clarity about their respective roles.
- **Transparency** – the requirement to be open and honest in communication with members of the public/patient advisers, as well as in relating information about why things are being done as they are.
- **Valuing knowledge** – valuing different kinds of knowledge by recognising that those giving advice have complementary expertise to that held by the researcher(s).
- **Support** – recognising the contributions and reimbursing them for out-of-pocket expenses.
- **Capacity building** – the co-learning that occurs between PPIE contributors and researchers.
- **Proportional involvement** – ensuring involvement is tailored to the needs of the research and any pragmatic decisions are made to balance contradictory demands.
- **Communication** – the benefits of support and the importance of the researcher being responsive and proactive by ensuring that contributors are updated on the progress

and process of a research project. The communication modality should be suitable and accessible.
- **Continuity in involvement** – the need to create opportunities for all relevant parties to be involved, whether as a patient/client, carer, public adviser, expert by experience, or other party.
- **Evaluation** – identification of good practices through communication, research, reflection, and learning.

When deciding the level and nature of your PPIE activity, consider who you will engage, what the purpose of involving specific groups or individuals will be, and the extent to which their involvement is needed. PPIE is a continuum, from simple consultation, to partnership, to full shared leadership (Ocloo and Matthews, 2016). Thus, PPIE can be considered awareness raising, informal learning, debate, sharing, or dialogue activity (Holmes, Cresswell, Williams et al., 2019). At one end of the spectrum, PPIE can be characterised by shared power and responsibility, with PPIE contributors acting as active partners involved in decision-making and shaping; at the other end, their involvement may be circumscribed to providing advice and offering views (Ocloo and Matthews, 2016).

> **Key point!**
> PPIE is often a required element of a funding application and can also be useful for identifying and addressing ethical issues within a project. PPIE needs to be meaningful, and the public contributors need to be enabled in their contributions.
> (Jackson, Pinnock, Liew et al., 2020)

When you plan and engage your PPIE group for your own research project, reflexivity is a key aspect of the process and should be a practice for the whole team. This can be operationalised through regular dialogue with the PPIE contributors and the research team, whereby all involved feel their views have been valued (Rolfe, Ramsden, Banner, and Graham, 2018). Rolfe et al. argued that this reflexivity can be promoted through ongoing dialogue and is a helpful way to address the relational dynamics that can occur between the contributors and the researchers.

As there are different reasons why you might use PPIE in your own research, we refer you to Table 7.1 where those three reasons are outlined.

PPIE will likely make a valuable contribution to the planning, design, and process of your research. Nevertheless, there are some challenges and limitations of PPIE in health research. A core issue to consider is how your PPIE might contribute to the quality and value of the project, and how it might influence the outcomes and outputs. Remember that just because you arrange some form of PPIE, this does not automatically lead to better quality or safer health care (Bergerum, Engström, Thor et al., 2020). You should be active in how you involve those contributors and carefully think about how

Table 7.1 Reasons to use PPIE in health research

Reason	Description
Normative or emancipatory	PPIE is an avenue through which patients and/or the public can exercise a right to be involved in research. On this basis, there should be effort to reduce any imbalances of power (Edelman and Barron, 2016).
Consequentialist or efficiency-orientated	This refers to the need to bring the lived experiences of patients (clients, service users) into the research plans and processes, to contribute to the efficiency and the value of the research (Greenhalgh, Hinton, Finlay et al., 2019).
Political and practical	Involving the public or patients means that research spaces can create an alliance between researchers and the contributors to facilitate accountability and transparency in the research process (Greenhalgh et al., 2019).

improvements might be made. In organising your PPIE group, think about the constitution of that group and what contributions different members might make. In the health research literature, PPIE contributors tend to be identified by a shared "role" or identity, i.e. on account of having a specific health condition or relationship, e.g. in a specific caregiving role (Bissel, Thompson, and Gibson, 2018).

> **Key point!**
>
> Be mindful that the experience of involvement in your project might be stressful or upsetting for PPIE contributors, especially if they have personal experience of the topic being studied.
>
> (Bergerum et al., 2020)

PPIE activities can be very rewarding but can also, ultimately, be challenging to manage and make progress with as well. We asked Dr Sam Little and Dr M. Farhad Peerally to reflect on their experiences of the PPIE process for their research project on gastroenterology. They outline those experiences and the lessons learnt in Box 7.2.

> **Box 7.2**
>
> **Learning about PPIE – perspective of Dr Sam Little and Dr M. Farhad Peerally**
>
> Dr Sam Little is a Clinical Research Fellow with the University of Leicester, and Dr M Farhad Peerally is an Associate Professor with the University of Leicester and Consultant Gastroenterologist in University of Leicester Hospitals Trust (UHL).
>
> The SCALE ENDO (Study of Communication and Adaptive capacity using in-situ Learning Environments based on real-life risks in ENDOscopy) project aims to explore safety issues

in gastrointestinal (GI) endoscopy. The study seeks to understand factors contributing to adverse events and how endoscopy teams adapt to maintain safety. A crucial component of this research is the involvement of patients who have undergone these procedures, helping inform and shape the study's direction by contributing their lived experiences as part of a patient advisory group.

We conducted a one-hour meeting via Microsoft Teams, bringing together three patients with experience of GI endoscopy and a charity coordinator. This session provided valuable insights into perceptions of safety, whilst also presenting certain challenges.

Patients' narratives provided rich phenomenological insights into the lived experience of endoscopic procedures, offering a nuanced understanding of safety that transcends traditional biomedical parameters. Participants emphasised aspects of procedural and psychological safety often overlooked in clinical risk assessments, underscoring the importance of a holistic approach to patient safety. The PPI meeting allowed us to explore the potential of co-producing knowledge in healthcare research, whilst also increasing our awareness of methodological and practical challenges to integrating diverse perspectives into the study design.

The virtual nature of the meeting introduced certain specific complexities. The absence of face-to-face interaction limited a thorough development of rapport and trust, crucial for eliciting candid discussions about sensitive health experiences. This digital divide risked exacerbating existing power imbalances between us as researchers and patients as participants. Time constraints also necessitated a delicate balance between allowing for the organic development of themes, whilst maintaining focus on research objectives.

Translating the patients' experiential knowledge into actionable insights for the SCALE ENDO study presented another significant challenge. This process of knowledge translation requires careful interpretation to ensure patient perspectives are meaningfully incorporated without losing their essence through over-medicalisation.

The meeting added a valuable dimension to the study, fostering professional reflection through critical insights into healthcare vulnerabilities that are often overlooked by practitioners. Despite the limitations described, the study benefits significantly from the perspectives shared by those we aim to support. To maximise the value of these insights, we have arranged further PPI meetings during the length of the study to sense-check emerging findings.

Involving experts by experience

Typically, as part of a PPIE group, you will include experts by experience to support the research. Experts by experience are individuals identified as having expert knowledge because of their lived experiences (Maguire and Britten, 2018). In the research literature and in clinical practice, you will find various terms used to refer to these individuals, including "service user", "patient", "client", or "consumer/customer". In contemporary literature, the favoured term for this group is "experts by experience", which acknowledges the epistemic value those contributors have in commenting on and helping to influence the research process as part of PPIE activity. Furthermore, the term experts by experience circumvents criticisms of the alternative term "service user", which is argued to lack an agreed definition (Beresford, 2006) and is a little vague in the context of PPIE in relation to the contribution the group make to decisions and process, as not all experts by experience are users of a service.

Although involving experts by experience is recognised as helpful for the development of all health research for PPIE, there is sometimes less clarity about *how* they can be actively and fully involved in the process (Trivedi and Wykes, 2002). Trivedi and Wykes argued that researchers need to:

- Consider the practical challenges, particularly managing the power differential between themselves as researchers and the expert by experience.
- Provide clarity about what the involvement of experts by experience will entail.
- Support experts by experience to positively influence the content of the research and identify its relevance to healthcare practice.
- Ensure there is partnership and equality in the relationship.
- Plan well and be prepared to put in the necessary effort, as the process can be challenging and time-consuming.

Advisory boards and steering groups

Alongside organising a PPIE group, you may elect to have groups with specific functions to add value to your research. That is, you might opt to have an advisory board or steering group of stakeholders to inform your decision-making. Your groups may have to be specific in their identity, such as an advisory board or steering group comprising a particular disciplinary group (e.g. oncology nurses, dentists, physiotherapists, psychiatrists) or of members with expertise in a specific topic (those with lived experience of an illness, different health professionals working in the area, carers).

The advisory board or steering group can support decision-making and steer your project by utilising their experiences, skills, and knowledge on specific topics (MIND, 2023). In bringing together this group, think about which stakeholders can provide different kinds of advice for your project, and this will diverge from the way you work with the PPIE group. Working with these advisers (or those that steer the direction of the project) can help in recognising and representing different levels of expertise (Williams, Sarre, Papoulias et al., 2020).

Depending on the project's focus, your advisory board or steering group may be made up of members of the community. These are referred to as community advisory boards, and this type of board can provide an opportunity to understand the context and community you are working with, as well as understand any risks or benefit associated with the project, which is a meaningful way to safeguard that community (Quinn, 2004). Community advisory boards serve as a source of leadership and provide structure to guide your activities in a way that reflects the best interests of the community (Newman, Andrews, Magwood et al., 2011).

The problem of tokenism

When engaging experts by experience or other PPIE contributors in your project, the involvement should be meaningful and genuine. Just because it is often a requirement in modern-day health research does not mean that it is a "box to tick". When you bring together your PPIE contributors and make use of their ideas, theories, thoughts, opinions, experiences, and perceptions, these need to be taken seriously, and opportunities for them to actively contribute need to be established. Concerns have been expressed about how the failures of research teams to actively involve PPIE contributors in the decision-making process can lead to tokenism (Morrison and Dearden, 2013). Tokenism is more likely when the competencies and abilities of contributors are underestimated, or when the methods used to engage them are superficial or condescending (Snow, Tweedie, and Pederson, 2018).

To avoid being tokenistic in your PPIE activity, think about the purpose of the group, the value of different members, and have transparency about who contributes what and when. Think about the mechanisms by which you will ensure contributors are empowered to participate and fulfil their role, bearing in mind that not all contributors will be expected to contribute equally (McLaughlin, 2009). Although individual contributions may not necessarily be equal, look for some equality of opportunity for PPIE membership. In short, a PPIE group should be of value to the research process and be constituted of members with the relevant characteristics and experiences to support the project.

Given the importance of avoiding tokenism, we encourage you to think carefully about the reasons you are engaging a PPIE group and to consider how you intend to manage this over time with your research project/area of interest. Try the reflective activity in Box 7.3 to take stock of your own PPIE plans.

Box 7.3

Reflective activity about PPIE

Consider the privilege of your position as a researcher, and the opportunity you hold to work alongside and partner with those in more marginalised communities of society to help their voices be heard through research. Perhaps a starting point for your research question might be something raised by someone who is "public or patient". Consider:

- What is the motivation driving your research? Reflect honestly on what this is about: does it stem from personal curiosity, a desire for professional advancement, empowering vulnerable people, or indeed some other reason?
- Instead of trying to "fit" your consultation partners into a predefined project by asking what their views are on an existing research question, another option is to begin by canvassing a particular group for their opinions on the kind of research that might benefit them.
- In seeking to help "liberate" or "educate" others, we sometimes misunderstand what their needs, priorities, and values are. How might you better understand what is important to your PPIE group before you do too much project planning?
- For those in a PPIE group who are invited to join a pre-existing project, how can you make provision to ensure you adjust your research plans to accommodate their suggestions?

In practice, seriously consider the process of building your PPIE group, including which experts by experience might provide a valuable critical lens on your plans as they evolve. If you have a PPIE selection process that is too rigid there is a risk that those who may gain the most from the research are excluded from decision-making (Ocloo and Matthews, 2016). Ocloo and Matthews helpfully pointed out that when research teams have a pool of PPIE membership that is overly circumscribed, there are limited opportunities to break problematic cycles of suboptimal care and services. At the same time, PPIE contributors can be difficult to recruit and reach. This relates to the question of motivation; you may need to ask yourself the hard question of whether the research is something that is interesting to you but not necessarily relevant to the PPIE population. Alternatively, perhaps the way you are going about the research process is at odds with the ways that certain cultures engage in problem-solving and knowledge generation practices. For example, there is evidence that it is less common for PPIE contributors to be recruited from minoritized backgrounds (Boote, Wong, and Booth, 2012). A potentially valuable approach could be asking members of these minority groups what it is about the *process* of integrating PPIE in research that is leading to lower levels of involvement. Hence, additional effort, time, and resources may be required to address these gaps in the field of health research.

Working with gatekeepers
As well as working with experts by experience and other PPIE contributors to support your research, it is likely that you will work with gatekeepers who facilitate your access to the participant group your research is focused on. The people who help you to access and recruit participants are known as gatekeepers and are an integral aspect of the ethicality of your research (Kay, 2019). It is therefore important that you attend to and reflect on your relationship with them as they hold some power over the success of your study.

If you start from an interest in a particular area of study or a particular health population, and then go out to find participants that relate to your research, you may find you need to convince and persuade gatekeepers of the value of your planned project. Conversely, in situations where the impetus for the direction of research inquiry has arisen from concerns grounded in practice, cooperation and collaboration with gatekeepers are more likely to be straightforward. To recruit and access the population you intend to undertake research with, there is a possibility you will need the consent, or at least the approval and support, of certain organisational representatives (gatekeepers). These representatives typically aim to act in the best interests of the population you are trying to reach and can provide useful information and advice during that process.

There are different kinds of gatekeeper, and Kay (2019) developed a stratum of potential gatekeepers. Whilst this was initially in reference to educational research, it is applicable for health research. We outline these in Table 7.2.

Gatekeepers play a crucial role in helping you to contact those who can support your project. When research involves participants who have specific vulnerabilities, for example, due to their age, their capacity to understand the research, or their health condition, gatekeepers play an especially important role. These individuals can help you to communicate with prospective participants (e.g. carers, parents of children and young people, healthcare professionals, administrative staff) and can help you ensure that mechanisms for involvement in the research are appropriate. Ultimately, the level of involvement of the gatekeeper will be influenced by their motivation and interest

Table 7.2 Strata of potential gatekeepers (Kay, 2019)

Type of gatekeeper	Description
Institutional gatekeepers	Institutional gatekeepers refer to those persons who represent organisations and support the research process. This is because seeking authorisation from an institutional gatekeeper can be an initial step in establishing the ethicality of the research in the sense that you may not be able to approach patients/clients/families without approval from the organisational representative (see also Farrimond, 2013).
Organisational gatekeepers	These gatekeepers hold a senior or authoritative role within the organisation and have a broad understanding of what it means for the organisation and individuals associated with it to be involved in research. Examples of organisational gatekeepers include a director, a headteacher, or an NHS Trust executive.
Specialist gatekeepers	These are individuals with various levels of seniority within the organisation, but who have specific responsibilities that relate to the research project (see also, Bryman, 2016). A specialist gatekeeper may have specific epistemic status or experiences that are pertinent to the research. This may be a faculty or departmental manager, consultant, or team leader.
Domain gatekeepers	These are individuals who have a leading role in the specific setting where the research will take place. These gatekeepers who can sanction the research within their domain. For example, they may be a classroom teacher or a ward manager.
Guardian gatekeepers	These are individuals who have some legal responsibility for the participants (such as parents or guardians).
Auto gatekeepers	These individuals are gatekeepers in the sense that as individual participants, they act with respect of their own participation rights and have jurisdiction over who has access to their personal lives and experiences (see also Homan, 1991).

in the project, the potential vulnerability [bear in mind this is a contested description which we discuss elsewhere in the book] of the sample group, and the sensitivity of the project. When many gatekeepers are involved, and communication and negotiations are complex, it can be more challenging, especially when seeking to engage vulnerable populations in research inquiries and when addressing sensitive topics (Kay, 2019). For instance, if participants are not able to fully consent for themselves, then others need to hold this responsibility.

An identified risk when working with gatekeepers is that they may delay or impede participant recruitment. In literature concerned with research with children and young people, it has been observed that gatekeepers have historically prevented children's voices from being heard through research, effectively silencing and excluding them without consulting them, by making decisions about their best interests in an adult-centric way (Alderson, 2004). If this is the case, gatekeepers may reduce access and delay a research project despite full institutional ethical governance being in place (McFayden and Rankin, 2016). This being so, it must also be recognised that gatekeepers have a responsibility to balance the empowerment of vulnerable participants with protection (Kay, 2019). Indeed, Kay observed that gatekeepers not only facilitate (or prevent) access, but there are also expectations that they will have a role in safeguarding.

In approaching your contact with gatekeepers, try to be reflexive and maintain professionalism as a researcher (Kay, 2019). McFayden and Rankin (2016) argued that to manage this process, there are things researchers can do to facilitate their work with gatekeepers, including:

- Engagement of the gatekeepers at an early stage of a research study and sharing decision-making to promote a positive attitude toward the research.
- Gatekeepers having clarity about the potential benefits of the research.
- Communicating clearly and transparently with a nominated point of contact on a regular basis.
- Ensuring gatekeepers have appropriate and meaningful information about the research project.
- Recognising and working to address any gatekeeper concerns about the participation of those in their care.

Alternatively, it may be that you know the gatekeepers well prior to your research starting. It may be that gatekeepers are your colleagues, manager or supervisor, or friends. In this case, it is unethical to take advantage of these existing relationships, although this insider position can provide you with knowledge of the organisation and systems, which is advantageous in approaching gatekeepers.

Engagement in research: co-design, co-production, and co-researching

In this chapter, we have shown that engaging different people at different levels and in different ways supports the trajectory and quality of your research project. Engaging experts by experience and other contributors to PPIE, constructing an advisory board or steering group and, where appropriate, working with communities are all useful when undertaking your qualitative health research project. There are different pathways you can take to involve participants with various levels of active engagement (Locock and Boaz, 2019). There are a range of allied concepts, which include:

- Co-design (see Robert, Donetto, and Williams, 2020).
- Co-production (see Smith, Williams, Bone et al., 2022).
- Co-research (see Cuevas-Parra, 2020).

Sometimes these concepts are conflated in the literature, but these different "co" terms have unique definitions (Williams, Sarre, Papoulias et al., 2020).

Co-design

When you develop a research idea, it may be with co-design in mind. Broadly, co-design denotes an approach to developing and implementing an intervention, service, or programme by meaningfully engaging and involving those for whom the intervention, service, or programme is intended to serve or help (Williams et al., 2020). It is a process of developing partnerships with users of services and other stakeholders to ensure that the intervention or programme meets the needs and preferences of those it is intended to reach (Bevan Jones, Stallard, Agha et al., 2020). A co-design approach can be beneficial as it is more likely that the service, intervention, or programme will be acceptable to the end users (Thabrew, Fleming, Hetrick, and Merry, 2018).

Co-design has become increasingly popular, especially in intervention research, as a way of developing the quality of a research project with specific regard to how user- or community-orientated it is. Co-design is not new and did not originate in health research but has been utilised by health researchers. Ideas about co-design include concerns with how it may be possible to scale the contribution of design thinking occurring within larger systems, and how it might be possible to identify appropriate roles for co-designers when addressing co-design processes and in evaluating impact to ensure the outcomes of the work (Robert et al., 2020). The idea of evidence-based co-design was originally an approach to quality improvement in healthcare but has since expanded across different clinical areas in health and research (Donetto, Tsianakas, and Robert., 2014).

> **Key point!**
>
> A co-designed piece of research harnesses the local and contextualised expertise of the "users" of the programme or service.
>
> (O'Reilly, Adams, Batchelor, and Levine, in press)

In the context of health research, increased use of co-design approaches has been aligned with an increased focus on patient-centred care (Bate and Robert, 2006). Projects incorporating co-design recognise the value of including experts by experience in the design of, or improvements to, services, programmes, and interventions. Using a co-design approach can be especially valuable in research when engaging participants from vulnerable groups, as this way of working is inherently concerned with the dynamics of power relations and actively works to transfer control to the participants (Purdy and Spears, 2020). To ensure co-design is effectively managed, Hodson et al. (2019) delineated several principles, which we have listed in Box 7.4.

> **Box 7.4**
>
> **Principles for co-design (Hodson, Dadashi, Delgado et al., 2019)**
>
> When you are developing a co-design project, it is useful to remember the following:
>
> - Engage service users who are involved in the design of the service, intervention, or programme early in the research process.
> - Planning and preparation should be prioritised before the project progresses.
> - Actively manage any perceived power differential between you and your co-designers.

- Create safe and active spaces for service users to contribute.
- Create opportunities to establish activities through which participants, service users, and experts by experience can collaborate to generate new ideas.
- You should also serve as a facilitator to develop and refine the project.
- In finalising the design, seek further collaboration with practitioners, researchers, and service users as necessary to achieve the project goals.

Evidence shows that co-design is increasingly being used for intervention development and implementation in various health-related behaviours (e.g. Champion, Gardner, McGowan et al., 2020), both inside and outside health settings. For example, co-design has become increasingly popular for use with schools to examine and explore health interventions within educational settings. Daly-Smith, Quarmby, Archbold et al. (2020) argued that the co-design approach affords a strategy and a method to work "with" schools rather than implementing interventions "on" schools. Indeed, the highly appealing premise of co-design for health researchers is that it promotes working with their participants and other stakeholders, as well as helping to manage the relationship held with them. Researchers can be flexible and work closely with the relevant individuals during the research process (Purdy and Spears, 2020).

Co-production

Another way of increasing involvement in health research is through co-production. Co-production sits on the spectrum of PPIE in health research with the aim of promoting partnerships with service users/patients/clients/experts and the public to work with researchers (Price, Clarke, Staniszewska et al., 2021). It is considered a central feature of community engagement (Tembo, Hickey, Montenegro et al., 2021). The foundation of co-production in research is to actively bring together service users/patients/clients/experts and professionals/practitioners/stakeholders to form equitable partnerships and position users of services not as marginalised individuals but rather as partners making meaningful contributions to setting the agenda, developing the research questions, and being involved in all research decisions (Williams et al., 2020). The goal of co-production is to improve services for those who use the services concerned (Tisdall, 2017).

Key point!

There is a "clear egalitarian rationale" for co-production in research, and the efforts made to be inclusive enhance research outcomes.

(Williams et al., 2020)

If research priorities are to be determined with or by the communities that research serves, and these members are to be involved throughout the whole process (Tembo et al., 2021), participants need to be considered experts and creators of knowledge, and centrally involved in decision-making (Tisdall, 2017). Equality is fundamental to co-production, as users of services, their families, practitioners, and other stakeholders are all engaged with the research (Norton, 2021). However, in promoting equality, co-production cannot function as a "one size fits all" approach, and the researcher must work to build relationships and promote engagement (Tembo et al., 2021). These relationships are not built on hierarchies but on the qualities needed for all those involved to work safely (van Leeuwen and Price, 2020). To put it another way, co-production does not refer to equality in skills or in ownership but rather to equal respect, voice, and access to shared resources (Price et al., 2021).

> **Key point!**
>
> An integral feature of co-production is the sharing of power and reduction of asymmetry between the researcher and researched.
>
> (Tembo et al., 2021)

Some scholars argue that for the health sector, co-production needs to be more highly valued so that it becomes normative and embedded in both research and care contexts (Norton, 2021; Tembo et al., 2021). To do this effectively, researchers must apply the foundational principles of a co-production approach. Slay and Stephens (2013) delineated these, and we outline them in Box 7.5.

> **Box 7.5**
> **Principles of co-production (Slay and Stephens, 2013)**
>
> There are several principles that provide the foundation of co-production:
>
> - Take an assets-based approach, in the sense that you regard participants not as passive recipients of services (and as a burden on the system), but instead as active, equal partners in the design and delivery of those services.
> - Take the opportunity to build on people's existing capabilities. In so doing, you alter the delivery model of public services away from a deficit approach towards recognition of people's capabilities by supporting them in putting their skills to use at an individual and community level.
> - Ensure there is reciprocity and mutuality. Thus, you might offer people a range of incentives to work with you by developing a reciprocal relationship with them, and with other professionals, in an ethos of mutual expectations and mutual responsibilities.
> - Develop peer support networks by engaging in networks with professionals and consider mechanisms for the transfer of knowledge.
> - Take meaningful steps to remove the distinction between researchers, professionals, and participants and reduce the possible asymmetry.
> - Facilitate rather than deliver. In other words, you take the role of a facilitator rather than being the leader of the conversation.

Co-researching

In qualitative research, participation is central, and at the most active end of the spectrum of participation is co-research (Pope, 2020). Having participants as co-researchers is a way of actively engaging and involving them in the research process. In this way, the co-researchers are "joint contributors" where their experiences and expertise are privileged as collaborators in the process of planning, data collecting, and analysis (Boylorn, 2008). By enabling participants to take on the role of researcher, an emphasis is placed on collaboration with the research team through which research outputs can be co-created to maximise their impact and inclusivity (Cumbo and Selwyn, 2022).

Involving participants as co-researchers enhances their participation and assigns those individuals a role in the research process. Ideally, co-researchers are engaged in helping identify avenues of inquiry so that a research question and aim statement can be developed collaboratively, as well as being part of the data collection process and facilitating the analysis and dissemination. Engaging participants as co-researchers is viewed as consistent with a fundamental respect for their rights and for their leadership abilities, which is particularly pertinent with certain groups, like children and young people (Dunn, 2015).

An approach involving participants as co-researchers can be highly participatory but also creates a range of practical and ethical challenges. Participants who act as co-researchers may have limited experience with research. Consequently, there may be a need for training addressing different research skills, and co-researchers can require intensive ongoing support and supervision to ensure they are comfortable with doing research and able to function in their roles. Having a team of co-researchers can thus be beneficial to ensure tasks are shared amongst a research team, as well as to enable peer support.

> **Key point!**
>
> Remember that your co-researchers may have limited research skills. To facilitate their involvement, you may need to provide some training on the practical skills of data collection and research ethics.
>
> (Van Doorn, Gielen, and Stappers, 2014)

Because co-researchers are likely to have limited, if any, research experience, designing a project together will initially mean finding a common language. As the person in the "researcher" role or with the most research training or experience, your job will be to ensure that the design of the research project fulfils all the ethical, methodological, and quality criteria necessary. Your co-researcher(s) may be more focused on the population to be studied or their hoped-for outcomes. An example of a community organisation-led research project one of the authors (Nikki) was involved in required this kind of collaboration. The co-researcher was also the gatekeeper and knew many of the would-be participants. It was necessary to be open and transparent about appropriate ways to gain informed consent for an ethical research project. At the same time, as a learning process for the researcher, it was also necessary to compromise on how much data could be collected, as the co-researchers were more aware of how many questions would be manageable for the participant group. In this case, it was agreed only three questions would be presented in an online qualitative survey.

Overlaps

We offer a short note here on how the three forms of participation discussed in this chapter (i.e. of co-design, co-production, and co-research) overlap and can be differentiated. When you engage further with the methodological literature in this area, you may find that sometimes these terms and ideas are treated as interchangeable, and in some cases they do overlap. However, as we have outlined, whilst there may be similarities and they may be based on a shared philosophical standpoint, these are different ways of engaging participants in research.

Co-design does share some similar principles to the broader concept of co-production in the sense that both stem from a desire to disrupt or subvert the traditional power relations between the researcher and the service user/patient/client (Osborne et al., 2016). Arguably though, co-design falls shorter of the more radical equalities-driven rationale of co-production (Williams et al., 2020) because co-design maintains the centrality of the researcher, who still defines the boundaries and goals of the project (O'Reilly, Adams et al., in press). O'Reilly et al. thus made a distinction between co-design and co-production in terms of the collaborative process in the development of an intervention idea with the end user, rather than the production of the research itself.

Co-research may incorporate aspects of co-design or co-production. However, the focus in co-research resides primarily with the involvement of participants as enquirers themselves, thus dismantling any rigid distinctions between researcher and researched. In the case of co-research, an emphasis is placed on co-creation in enquiry, and this should, in theory, be integrated into all aspects of a research project. In the case of co-design, co-production, and co-research in empirical research, you should carefully consider how they can be practically realised as part of a project, including reflection on barriers that may hinder or prevent this.

The research team

Unless you are undertaking a research project for the purposes of a qualification (like a PhD or master's degree), it is likely you are working as part of a research team. The collaboration of different research experts is desirable in research contexts as effective teams reach strong outcomes in ways that are less likely to be accomplished by individuals working alone (Cheruvelil, Soranno, Weathers et al., 2014). Cheruvelil et al. argued that a research team tends to be made up of people who share a commitment to the main purpose of the project, take a similar methodological approach, and are collectively accountable for the process and success of the project.

The benefits of a research team with diverse membership are the different types of expertise and experience brought to the table. Diversity includes numerous factors like gender, ethnicity, socio-economic class, and life experiences, but also in the context of research teams refers to viewpoints and skills, how people represent and solve problems, their career stage, and professional backgrounds (Hong and Page, 2004). Diversity within the research team can enhance task-related knowledge, skills, and competencies, as well as provide a basis for different perspectives and sources of information which facilitate the quality of knowledge generation (Saá-Pérez, Diaz-Diaz, Aguiar-Diaz, and Ballesteros-Rodriguez, 2015).

In leading or working with your team, or even in assembling your team initially, consider the purpose and contribution of each member. Taking a collaborative style from the outset can be helpful, as can a non-hierarchical shared leadership through engagement and commitment to the project (Bowers, Cohen, Elliot et al., 2013). This will be particularly applicable if you are working in an interdisciplinary team (as we discussed in Chapter 2). Composing an interdisciplinary team can be challenging because disciplines represent different training, knowledge bases, languages, and expertise (Curry, O'Cathain, Plano Clark et al., 2012). These are matters to consider in managing your team or working with its members and navigating any conflict that arises. It can be beneficial, therefore, to create a collaborative email exchange service for sharing thoughts and hold regular meetings via internet-mediated platforms and in person (Bowers et al., 2013). Bowers et al. argued that team meetings help foster collegiality, understanding, and trust, as well as providing a basis to discuss expectations regarding accountability and responsibility.

From our own experiences of working in research teams made up of gatekeepers/service providers, clinicians, and academics, we recognise there can be differences of opinion about many things. Instead of viewing these differences of opinion as potential problems, they can be valuable opportunities for learning and questioning some of the foundational assumptions each member of the team might hold. We provide a few examples for illustrative purposes although there are many more possible areas that may need to be navigated:

- Research team members might have different ideas about how to approach the participant group. In this scenario, conversations between team members about recruitment and consent can helpfully consider what is a clinical priority for the client/patient/service user as well as what might be in the best interests of the research agenda. As with all ethical issues in research, a balance between intrusiveness or burdening the participant must be weighed against the anticipated benefits of their involvement. In research that involves people who are also patients/clients/service users in the healthcare system, the final deciding factor in these negotiations is that care is not compromised by being involved in the research.
- Where research teams also employ meaningful collaborative partnerships with patients/clients/service users and gatekeepers, these partners may be unfamiliar with the practicalities of the research process and the pre-existing requirements for research rigour. Partners involved on the ground with running services possess valuable insight into the area of research and may be the driving force behind the research strategy. Yet, they may not understand or fully appreciate the complexities of funding applications, ethical review processes, and research protocols. Proactive and open communication, respect, and patience on all sides are essential to navigate these different expectations to ensure that your project is stronger and better for having had the difficult conversations.
- Research team members may have different views about where the findings ought to be disseminated. From a clinical perspective, reporting the findings of the research

in a practitioner journal or periodical may be deemed the best way to inform large numbers of professionals about what the outcomes were. However, these outlets may not meet the standards required by academic institutions for various research performance quality indicators, such as publishing in high-impact peer-reviewed journals. Thus, meaningful conversations between research team members, again about priorities, motivations, and access to findings, are likely to be helpful.

Author reflections and concluding remarks
From Michelle
In closing this chapter, we offer an example of our own where we have engaged children as co-researchers to co-produce an outcome with them and their teachers to promote psychosocial wellbeing and positive mental health. This research was led by Michelle, and here she describes this example to illustrate some of the practical and ethical challenges faced.

For the last few years, I have been leading a project about children's online conduct and its relationship to their mental health and well-being. This began as a project funded by the Wellcome Trust to explore young people's views on their digital media use and mental health. Using focus groups, we provided a platform for young people to voice their preferences, ideas, and opinions about digital media and mental health, also considering also the positive ways in which digital media may be harnessed for mental health promotion (see O'Reilly, Dogra, Hughes et al., 2018; O'Reilly, Levine, Donoso et al., 2023). The main outcome of that work was the development of a framework for understanding young people's moral concerns and behaviours online in relation to their mental health, a framework that we called "a digital ethics of care" (see O'Reilly, Levine, and Law, 2021). Stepping up our involvement of child experts, we believed our digital ethics of care framework could lead to a practical toolkit for schools for younger children (aged 7–11-years) but wanted that toolkit to be co-produced with children and teachers to ensure its usability. With funding from the UK Economic and Social Research Council, we therefore engaged school children as co-researchers in our project.

First, we convened a child advisory board as part of our PPIE activity to ensure our ideas and plans were sound, that our ethical information was accessible and appropriate, and that the questions we were asking had relevance to the age group. This child advisory board offered us lots of useful advice, and we followed their guidance in the project. It was agreed that if these young children were going to interview each other as part of the data collection for the project, they needed some training to develop their interview skills. Thus, the school's deputy head teacher and a research team member who was an educationalist co-designed a lesson plan for the teachers to use in class to train the children in research and interviewing.

The co-research approach worked very well. The research associate facilitated the interviews online via Microsoft Teams (due to severe acute respiratory syndrome coronavirus 2 [SARS-CoV-2] COVID-19 related social distancing restrictions at the time). A teaching assistant was present in the room for safeguarding, and the pairs of children (n = 18) interviewed each other with some guidance. They rose to the challenge and asked some great questions, showing active listening skills and allowing each other space to answer the questions (see O'Reilly, Adams et al., in press). Part of the interviewing process was to discuss ways in which teachers could teach digital citizenship,

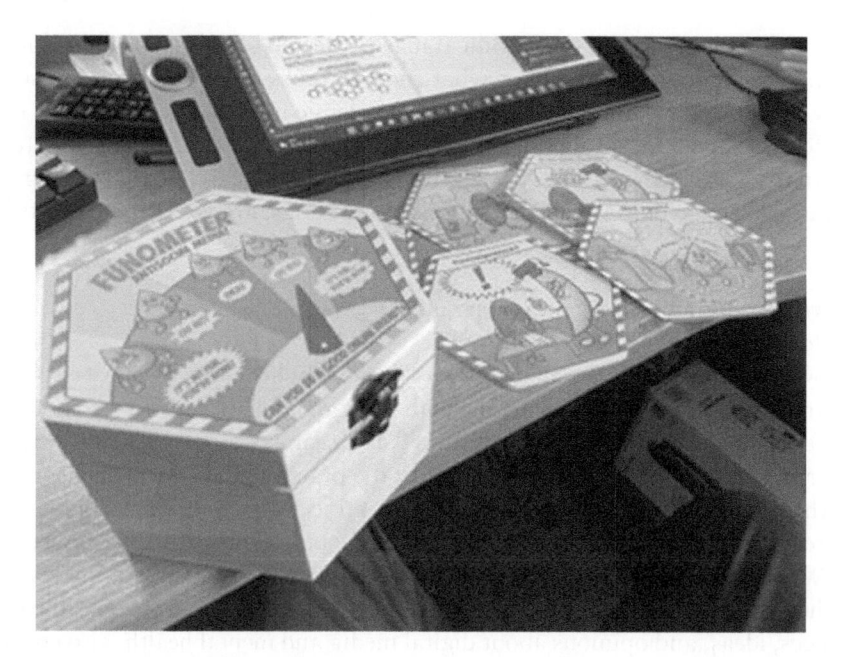

Figure 7.1 Digital ethics of care game

including by storyboarding ideas for a game to promote moral thinking online. The children had some creative, innovative, and interesting stories and were able to convey their own experiences to their peer interviewers.

The research team collated all their ideas and passed these to a professional artist to create the final game. Through collaboration with our child advisory board and teachers, the game pieces were finessed and finalised (see Figure 7.1). To complete the game output, we collaborated with teachers to co-produce the lesson plans needed to enable other teachers to implement the dialogical activity in class as part of teaching digital citizenship. Thus, teachers, child co-researchers, and the child advisory board, with the research team and the artist, created a storyboard game that can now be used by schools (see O'Reilly, Levine, Batchelor, and Adams., in press, for an overview of the project and details of the analysis and game).

References

Alderson, P. (2004). Ethics. In S. Fraser, V. Lewis, S. Ding, M. Kellett, and C. Robinson (Eds.), *Doing research with children and young people*. London: Sage.

Bate, P. and Robert, G. (2006). Experience-based design: From redesigning the system around the patient to co-designing services with the patient, *Quality & Safety in Health Care, 15*(5) 307–310.

Beresford, P. (2006). A service-user perspective on evidence. In M. Slade and S. Priebe (Eds.), *Choosing methods in mental health research: Mental health research from theory to practice* (pp. 223–230). Hove: Routledge.

Bergerum, C., Engström, A., Thor, J., and Wolmesjö, M. (2020). Patient involvement in quality improvement – a "tug or war" or a dialogue in a learning process to improve healthcare? *BMC Health Services Research, 20*, 1115.

Bevan Jones, R., Stallard, P., Agha, S., Rice, S., Werner-Seidler, A., Stasiak, K., Kahn, J., Simpson, S., Alvarez-Jimenez, M., Rice, F., Evans, R., and Merry, S. (2020). Practitioner review: Co-design of digital mental health technologies with children and young people. *The Journal of Child Psychology & Psychiatry, 61*(8), 928–940.

Bissel, P., Thompson, J., and Gibson, B. (2018). Exploring difference or just watching the experts at work? Interrogating Patient and Public Involvement (PPI) in a cancer research setting using the work of Jurgen Habermas. *Sociology, 52*(6), 1200–1216.

Boote, J., Wong, R., and Booth, A. (2012). Talking the talk or walking the walk? A bibliometric review of the literature on public involvement in health research published between 1995 and 2009. *Health Expectations, 18,* 44–57.

Bowers, B., Cohen, L., Elliot, A., Grabowski, D., Fishman, N., Sharkey, S., Zimmerman, S., Horn, S., and Kemper, P. (2013). Creating and supporting a mixed methods health services research team. *Health Services Research, 48*(6), 2157–2180.

Boylorn, R. (2008). Participants as co-researchers. In L. Given (Ed.), *The Sage encyclopedia of qualitative research methods* (pp. 600–601). Thousand Oaks, CA: Sage.

Bryman, A. (2016). *Social research methods* (5th ed.). Oxford: Oxford University Press.

Champion, K., Gardner, L., McGowan, C., Chapman, C., Thornton, L., Parmenter, B., and Newton, N. C. (2020). A web-based intervention to prevent multiple chronic disease risk factors among adolescents: Co-design and user testing of the Health4Life school-based program. *JMIR Formative Research, 4*(7), e19485.

Cheruvelil, K., Soranno, P., Weathers, K., Hanson, P., Goring, S., Filstrup, C., and Read, E. (2014). Creating and maintaining high-performing collaborative research teams: The importance of diversity and interpersonal skills. *Frontiers in Ecology & the Environment, 12*(1), 31–38.

Cuevas-Parra, P. (2020). Co-researching with children in the time of COVID-19: Shifting the narrative on methodologies to generate knowledge. *International Journal of Qualitative Methods, 19,* 1–12.

Cumbo, B., and Selwyn, N. (2022). Using participatory design approaches in educational research. *International Journal of Research & Method in Education, 45*(1), 60–72.

Curry, L., O'Cathain, A., Plano Clark, V., Aroni, R., Fetters, M., and Berg, D. (2012). The role of group dynamics in mixed methods health sciences research teams. *Journal of Mixed Methods Research, 6*(1), 5–20.

Daly-Smith, A., Quarmby, T., Archbold, V., Corrigan, N., Wilson, D., Resaland, G., Bartholomew, J., Singh, A., Tjomsland, H., Sherar, L., Chalkley, A., Routen, A., Shcikle, D., Bingham, D., Barber, S., van Sluijs, E., Fairclough, S., and McKenna, J. (2020). Using a multi-stakeholder experience-based design process to co-develop the creating active schools framework. *International Journal of Behavioral Nutrition & Physical Activity, 17*(13), Article 13.

Donetto, S., Tsianakas, V., and Robert, G. (2014). *Using experience-based co-design (EBCD) to improve the quality of healthcare: Mapping where we are now and establishing future directions.* London: Kings College.

Dunn, J. (2015). Insiders' perspectives: A children's rights approach to involving children in advising on adult-initiated research. *International Journal of Social Research Methodology, 18*(1), 91–104.

Edelman, N., and Barron, D. (2016). Evaluation of public involvement in research: Rime for a major re-think? *Journal of Health Services Research & Policy, 21,* 209–211.

Farrimond, H. (2013). *Doing ethical research.* Basingstoke, Hampshire: Palgrave Macmillan.

Greenhalgh, T., Hinton, L., Finlay, T., Macfarlane, A. Fahy, N., Clyde, B., and Chant, A. (2019). Frameworks for supporting patient and public involvement in research: Systematic review and co-design pilot. *Health Expectations, 22,* 785–801.

Hodson, E., Dadashi, N., Delgado, R., Chrisholm, C., Sgrignoli, R., and Swaine, R. (2019). Co-design in mental health: Mellow: A self-help holistic crisis planning mobile application by youth for youth. *The Design Journal, 22,* 1529–1542.

Holmes, L., Cresswell, K., Williams, S., Parsons, S., Keane, A., Wilson, C., Islam, S., Joseph, O., Miah, J., Robinson, E., and Starling, B. (2019). Innovating public engagement and patient involvement through strategic collaboration and practice. *Research Involvement & Engagement*, 21(5), 30.

Homan, R. (1991). *The ethics of social research*. London: Longman.

Hong, L., and Page, S. (2004). Groups of diverse problem solvers can outperform groups of high-ability problem solvers. *Proceedings of the National Academy of Sciences of the United States of America*, 101, 16385–16389.

Jackson, T., Pinnock, H., Liew, S., Horne, E., Ehrlich, E., Fulton, O., Worth, A., Sheikh, A., and De Simoni, A. (2020). Patient and public involvement in research: From tokenistic box ticking to valued team members. *BMC Medicine*, 18, 79.

Kay, L. (2019). Guardians of research: Negotiating the strata of gatekeepers in research with vulnerable participants. *Practice*, 1(1), 37–52.

Liabo, K., Boddy, K., Bortoli, S., Irvine, J., Boult, H., Fredlund, M. Joseph, N., Bjornstad, G., and Morris, C. (2020). Public involvement in health research: What does 'good' look like in practice? *Research Involvement & Engagement*, 6, 11.

Locock, L., and Boaz, A. (2019). Drawing straight lines along blurred boundaries: Qualitative research, patient and public involvement in medical research, co-production and co-design. *Evidence & Policy*, 15, 409–421.

Maguire, K., and Britten, N. (2018). 'You're there because you are unprofessional': Patient and public involvement as liminal knowledge spaces. *Sociology of Health & Illness*, 40(3), 463–477.

McFayden, J., and Rankin, J. (2016). The role of gatekeepers in research: Learning from reflexivity and reflection. *GSTF Journal of Nursing & Healthcare*, 4(1).

McLaughlin, H. (2009). Keeping service user involvement in research honest. *British Journal of Social Work*, 40(5), 1591–1608

McMenamin, J., Manning, M., and Tierney, E. (2022). Distinctions and blurred boundaries between qualitative approaches and public and patient involvement (PPI) in research. *International Journal of Speech-Language Pathology*, 24(5), 515–526.

MIND. (2023). Working and steering groups – deciding together. https://www.mind.org.uk/workplace/influence-and-participation-toolkit/how/methods/working-and-steering-groups/

Morrison, C., and Dearden, A. (2013). Beyond tokenistic participation: Using representational artefacts to enable meaningful public participation in health service design. *Health Policy*, 112(3), 179–186.

National Health Service (NHS). (2023). What is public involvement in research? https://www.hra.nhs.uk/planning-and-improving-research/best-practice/public-involvement/NHSUK.

Newman, S., Andrews, J., Magwood, G., Jenkins, C., Cox, M., and Williamson, D. (2011). Community advisory boards in community-based participatory research: A synthesis of best processes. *Preventing Chronic Disease*, 8(3), A70.

Norton, M. (2021). Co-production within child and adolescent mental health: A systematic review. *International Journal of Environmental Research & Public Health*, 18, 11897.

Ocloo, J., and Matthews, R. (2016). From tokenism to empowerment: Progressing patient and public involvement in healthcare improvement. *BMJ Quality & Safety*, 25, 626–632.

O'Reilly, M., Adams, S., Batchelor, R., and Levine, D. (in press). Exploring the practice of 10-11-year-olds as co-researchers: Using a hybrid approach in educational research to promote children as interviewers. *International Journal of Social Research Methodology*.

O'Reilly, M., Levine, D., Batchelor, R., and Adams, S. (in press). Digital ethics of care and digital citizenship in UK primary schools: Children as interviewers. *Journal of Children & Media*.

O'Reilly, M., and Parker, N. (2014). *Doing mental health research with children and adolescents: A guide to qualitative methods*. London: Sage.

Osborne, S., Radnor, Z., and Strokosch, K. (2016). Co-production and the co-creation of value in public services: A suitable case for treatment? *Public Management Review*, 18, 639–653.

Pope, E. (2020). From participants to co-researchers: Methodological alterations to a qualitative case study. *The Qualitative Report*, 25(10), 3749–3761.

Price, A., Clarke, M., Staniszewska, S., Chu, L., Tembo, D., Kirkpatrick, M., and Nelken, Y. (2021). Patient and public involvement in research: A journey to co-production. *Patient Education & Counseling*, 105(4), 1041–1047.

Purdy, N., and Spears, B. (2020). Co-participatory approaches to research with children and young people. *Pastoral Care in Education*, 38(3), 187–190.

Quinn, S. (2004). Ethics in public health research. *American Journal of Public Health*, 94(6), 918–922.

Reynolds, J., and Beresford, R. (2020). 'An active, productive life': Narratives of, and through, participation in public and patient involvement in health research. *Qualitative Health Research*, 30(14), 2265–2277.

Robert, G., Donetto, S., and Williams, O. (2020). Co-designing healthcare services with patients. In E. Loeffler and T. Bovaird (Eds.), *The Palgrave handbook of co-production of public services and outcomes*. Cham, Switzerland: Palgrave Macmillan.

Rolfe, D., Ramsden, V., Banner, D., and Graham, I. (2018). Using qualitative health research methods to improve patient and public involvement and engagement in research. *Research Involvement & Engagement*, 4, 49.

Saá-Pérez, P., Diaz-Diaz, N., Aguiar-Diaz, I., and Ballesteros-Rodriguez, J. (2015). How diversity contributes to academic teams performance. *R&D Management*, 47(2), 165–179.

Slay, J., and Stephens, L. (2013). *Co-production in mental health: A literature review*. London: New Economics Foundation – with MIND.

Smith, B., Williams, O., Bone, L., and the Moving Social Work Collective. (2022). Co-production: A resource to guide co-producing research in the sport, exercise, and health sciences. *Qualitative Research in Sport, Exercise & Health*, 15(2), 159–187.

Snow, M., Tweedie, K., and Pederson, A. (2018). Heard and valued: the development of a model to meaningfully engage marginalized populations in health services planning. *BMC Health Services Research*, 18(1), 181.

Tembo, D., Hickey, G., Montenegro, C., Chandler, D., Nelson, E., Porter, K., Dikomitis, L., Chambers, M., Chimbari, M., Mumba, N., Beresford, P., Ekiikina, P., Musesengwa, R., Staniszewska, S., Coldham, T., and Rennard, U. (2021). Effective engagement and involvement with community stakeholders in the co-production of global health research. *British Medical Journal*, 372, n178.

Thabrew, H., Fleming, T., Hetrick, S., and Merry, S. (2018). Co-design of eHealth interventions with children and young people. *Frontiers in Psychiatry*, 9(481).

Tisdall, K. (2017). Conceptualising children and young people's participation: Examining vulnerability, social accountability and co-production. *The International Journal of Human Rights*, 21(1), 59–75.

Trivedi, P., and Wykes, T. (2002). From passive subjects to equal partners: Qualitative review of user involvement in research. *British Journal of Psychiatry*, 181, 468–472.

Van Doorn, F., Gielen, M., and Stappers, P. (2014). *Children as co-researchers: More than just a role-play*. Proceedings of the conference on Interaction design and children, pp. 237–240.

van Leeuwen, D., and Price, A. (2020). Everyone-included research podcast and blog. https://www.health-hats.com/everyone-included-research.

Williams, O., Sarre, S., Papoulias, S., Knowles, S., Robert, G., Beresford, P., Rose, D., Carr, S., Kaur, M., and Palmer, V. (2020). Lost in the shadows: Reflections on the dark side of co-production. *Health Research Policy & Systems*, 18, 43–53.

CHAPTER 8

Ethics and integrity

Learning objectives
This chapter enables the reader to:

- Identify ethical parameters relating to qualitative health research.
- Critically assess how qualitative research can approach ethical principles in specific ways.
- Recognise how different ethical theoretical frameworks influence thinking in health research.
- Identify how to implement different principles in research practice.
- Evaluate the meanings of ethical principles in relation to sensitive topics and populations who may need greater levels of protection.
- Translate and extrapolate ethical thinking in relation to different kinds of project.
- Appreciate the role of ethical governance in research.

Introduction
As a healthcare practitioner you will likely be familiar with the importance of practising in a way that is ethical, respectful of those you seek to help, and which upholds the integrity of your profession. Your clinical work will also likely be underpinned by specific standards of ethical conduct, through alignment with a professional body that oversees these. Qualitative health research is also regulated, with a wide set of ethical principles in place to guide researchers. In ensuring that research is conducted ethically, three fundamental issues are considered important:

1. Whether the potential benefits of undertaking the research are meaningful, useful, and well-articulated.
2. How well risks are ameliorated, mitigated and/or managed.
3. The extent to which any potential benefits justify any residual risks.

In simple terms, ethical parameters guide a research study to promote benefits and minimise harm to the participants and researchers (we discuss researcher safety in detail in Chapter 12). We also acknowledge that the act of asking anyone to participate in research, and the time commitment thereof, can be considered a "harm" – as it is an imposition on and variation from daily life. In healthcare settings where clinical coercion can be a factor, such a commitment of time may be considered more burdensome. In this chapter we provide practical guidance to help you develop your own thinking about research ethics, the implementation of core principles for your research project, and thoughts on ways in which you can produce a high-quality application for institutional ethical review where this governance is necessary.

Ethics in qualitative research

When undertaking research most codes of conduct follow an approach grounded in certain ethical principles; that is, a set of basic rules that require translation and implementation to the specifics of the work. Such an approach is founded in ethical philosophy and reflects one of three major debates in relation to this, which we outline in Table 8.1.

Deontology is the most common approach to research ethics. This is not to discount the importance of the values of the researcher nor the importance of consequences, but in developing codes of conduct for researchers to follow they are founded on rules to guide practice. The deontological approach to ethics promotes four main principles for you to follow, which we detail in Table 8.2 (based on an outline provided by Beauchamp and Childress, 2019).

Although the deontological principles of ethics are useful, you need to be mindful of how they are implemented. Ethical codes of conduct in health services and universities have frequently been founded on these four principles. Yet, there remain tensions in the ways these are specifically applied to promote ethical research. Reflections on the deontological principles and the pragmatics of application are different for qualitative

Table 8.1 Three philosophies of ethics

Philosophy	*Description*
Consequentialism	This derives from utilitarianism in the sense that it emphasises the potential and actual consequences of one's actions. It is founded on the premise that the "rightness" or "wrongness" of actions is determined by their consequences (Driver, 2011).
Virtue ethics	This derives from Aristotle's philosophical ideas, emphasising the moral character of individuals, the moral aspects of actions, and the moral basis of communities. In research, the area of importance is the moral character of the researcher and assumes we acquire virtue through practice (see Athanassoulis, 2013).
Deontology	This derives from Kant's philosophy and is based on the idea of principles guiding morality. This philosophy proposes that actions can be determined as good or bad according to a predetermined set of rules. Deontology is a theory that guides and assesses choices of what ought to be done (that is, deontic theory) (Alexander and Moore, 2020).

Table 8.2 Deontological principles (Beauchamp and Childress, 2019)

Principle	Description
Respect autonomy	This refers to the researcher accounting for a research participant's capacity to make decisions for themselves and act in ways that safeguard their own best interests.
Advocate justice	This refers to the researcher's obligation to treat research participants equitably and fairly. It relates to considerations to avoid bias when sampling and not exposing participants to procedures or experiences that may disadvantage them in some way.
Promote beneficence	This refers to engaging rules or performing actions that seek to benefit others and relates to the need for researchers to consider the welfare of all individuals involved in a research study.
Assure non-maleficence	This refers to the researcher's obligation not to inflict harm on participants or others involved in the research (or minimise the level of harm incurred).

research projects because qualitative methods raise ethical concerns in slightly different ways than other forms of research.

Ethical principles in detail

Qualitative health research typically has a goal of benefiting certain population groups or society more generally, and in achieving that goal, researchers need to manage any risks that arise. When participating in your research, participants are putting their trust in you to involve them in a manner that protects their best interests and safeguards them from harm. Your conduct will also reflect on the institution you represent and the public image of "research" and "science". There are, therefore, a range of practices through which deontological principles are realised in research. Whilst there are many nuances in the implementation of ethical principles, we offer here an overview of these principles to help you to map your project and consider how you will manage the ethical complexities involved.

> **Key point!**
>
> In considering the implementation of deontological principles through ethical practices, think of the specific issues attendant to your own project and to have a clear plan of action for how you will attend to these in your research.

Informed consent and the right to withdraw

Informed consent is one of the fundamental ways in which respect for autonomy is secured in research. Indeed, the recognition that participants possess free will to make decisions for themselves has become a cornerstone of ethical guidelines and regulations across the globe (Beach and Arrazola, 2019). This is founded on a respect for dignity and the person's right to self-determination, with an aim to ensure participants can decide whether to participate or not (Miller and Boulton, 2007). There are, however, caveats. Specifically,

- The individual must be able to give their consent voluntarily, free from coercion.
- All risks and benefits must be clear for the participants to make their decision.
- Informed consent is a process and is more than a written signature on a form. It is, in fact, a lot more than that and is an ongoing process. Even more care should be taken where individuals may lack capacity.
- The nature of the research relationship must be reflected upon to ensure participants do not misunderstand or are led to the wrong assumptions about the research or researcher.

When designing methods for implementing a process around informed consent, be mindful of your role, status, and title and how these might influence your participants. In the next chapter we discuss the challenges of occupying dual or multiple roles, and this is especially important when you seek informed consent from your participants. Power is not inherent in people or fixed, but rather an aspect of the process and social interactions you have with your participants (Christensen, 2004). It may not be possible for you to fully achieve a balance in the power relations (Aluwihare-Samaranayake, 2012), at the same time, you can take steps to recognise your influence and prevent risks that you may unduly coerce your participants to consent. Given your role as a healthcare practitioner, this is especially important when taking consent for your own research project, and we encourage you to think through the reflective activity in Box 8.1.

Box 8.1
Reflective activity on taking informed consent

When seeking participants' consent to involvement in a qualitative health research project, clarity in information is key. A matter that participants need to be clear about is the difference between your role as their healthcare provider (if you hold that role) and your role as researcher. Often clients/patients/service users can find it confusing to keep track of the different professionals involved in their care and may not be sure about which things they are required to do and which things are optional. It is your responsibility to clarify these differences with your would-be participant to ensure they have all the information they need to freely decide whether they want to be involved in the research project or not. The following questions are provided to help you think through a few of the ways that you can make sure you are clear in your communication.

- In what role do your research participants currently know you? (Have they met you before, do they know you in your clinician role, or some other role?)
- Are they clear that being involved in the research is not required of them as part of their treatment/support/service?

- Are they clear that they can say no to the research project and still receive the same clinical treatment/support/service?
- Is there any other potential confusion they may experience in relation to what the research is for? (Some individuals might, for instance, think that the research is a way to access benefits or services).

In research, you need to recognise that requesting consent from participants is not a singular isolated event but a process (Barnett, 2007). Qualitative research does not always unfold in ways that were anticipated (Flewitt, 2005), and thus consent should be treated as iterative and revisited frequently at various junctures (O'Reilly, Parker, and Hutchby, 2011). Furthermore, informed consent is best thought of as a relationally constituted process and is not static (Klykken, 2022). Klykken noted that the formalised approach to informed consent is usually described as giving information to and obtaining consent from participants, suggesting that understanding is accomplished because of this transference of information. Yet, knowledge is developed throughout the research by a social collective and is thus a joint process activity. As such, the increasingly standardised ways of "performing" research ethics do not straightforwardly align with the complex nature of qualitative research. Approaching consent as socially constructed, changing, and multi-layered is more appropriate (Miller and Boulton, 2007).

When managing the process of informed consent in your research, do not view this as a one-off event but reflexively revisit the process throughout. In practice, this means checking at several points (for example, before collecting data, after collecting data, and offering another date before research findings are amalgamated for them to contact you if they change their mind). In designing your consent procedures, you will need to account for the specific parameters of your own project. For example, your consent procedures will need to accommodate all the individuals you plan to include, who may be from different social, educational, and cultural backgrounds or have certain vulnerabilities (Field and Behrman, 2004; Moriña, 2021). You will also need to attend to the capacity of your participants to provide informed consent. This is to say the participants must be able to understand and process the information you provide them with about your project. This may involve more than one occasion of checking with the participant to ensure they know what is expected, perhaps in both verbal and written forms. Some population groups may not have full capacity to do this. For example, children do not have the legal capacity to consent for themselves and may rely on a parent to act in their best interests, or an older adult with dementia or an adult with intellectual disabilities may struggle to fully understand the information provided to them and rely on a carer. In these types of situation, consent is taken from a representative, and assent from the individual.

In Box 8.2, we outline things for you to think about when planning your consent process.

Box 8.2
Informed consent processes

There are several steps to take when planning and obtaining consent from participants:

- It is essential that you have a detailed information leaflet about the project. This leaflet should include what is expected of participants and the time commitment anticipated of them. It should contain contact details so participants can ask questions about the project and participation in advance. The leaflet should outline the possible benefits and risks so an informed decision can be made. Any safeguarding steps should be clear, and sources of support (should they be needed) outlined.
- A consent form that is accessible should be available for participants to sign. This refers to the information leaflet and contains a series of statements pertinent to the boundaries of the research study and participation.
- Information should be accessible, clear, and age appropriate. Any disabilities, capacity issues, or health conditions that may impair understanding should be accounted for in the way the information is presented and related (e.g. visual format, larger font, and audio versions).
- Information is made available to participants in advance of taking signed consent to allow sufficient time to make an informed decision. One way to do this is to email or post the information ahead of the data collection session, and then remind the participant again when you meet to confirm they received, read, and understood the information before they sign.
- For participants with limited literacy, reading the information about the study to them and ensuring they have understood the information you have relayed (perhaps by checking and asking questions) may be an alternative or addition to the written information sheet.
- For some participants, it may be appropriate for them to have a family member with them when you explain consent to them, so that the participant is additionally protected.

In relation to consent, participants can withdraw their consent to participate at any point before engaging, during the data collection, or for a specified time after data collection. Any limits of withdrawal need to be outlined to participants, so they are properly aware that they can only fully withdraw up to the point of formalisation (provide a date on the information sheet). This means that once you have published your first report, conference presentation, or academic article, you cannot withdraw published quotations as these are already (albeit anonymously) in the public domain. Participants can withdraw from any further involvement, however, if they choose to. Indeed, some participants may opt to withdraw whilst a project is ongoing (for example, with multiple interviews or diary entries completed) and consent for you to keep the material or data you have collected up until that point for your research. Alternatively, participants may request that a certain portion of what they have shared is removed from the research project. This can be achieved either by allowing the participant to review a transcript of their oral contribution, or they can request verbally or in writing to exclude the portion of data covering a particular topic (such as an extract that includes information about a third party, or part of their data they later consider too personal or that it might make them potentially identifiable because of its specificity).

Confidentiality and anonymity

Vital in relation to protecting participants from possible harm is to maintain a level of privacy regarding what they reveal. This means affording participants a level of confidentiality and ensuring any quotation of them in dissemination is anonymous. As described by Tilley and Woodthorpe (2011):

- **Confidentiality** – refers to managing the personal and private information of the individuals involved in your research.
- **Anonymity** – refers to the removal and alteration of any identifying information about the participants to protect their identities in any documents, reports, or other outputs from the research.

Anonymity thus is one form of confidentiality as it conceals the identity of the participants, but confidentiality also means that what is revealed by participants is kept private and careful decisions about what from the data are shared (Saunders et al., 2015).

It may not be possible to fully anonymise qualitative research data as to manage the data corpus may require the research team or other partners to have information about the participants. In qualitative research complete anonymity is rarely possible as some people will be privileged to know who the participants are (Scott, 2005), and time and cost of digitally removing identities from the original recordings may be too difficult (albeit possible with the right resources). Thus, the limits of both anonymity and confidentiality should be explained to participants (Saunders, Kitzinger, and Kitzinger, 2015). Article 4 of the General Data Protection Regulation (GDPR) [associated with Europe] (2018) offered this:

- **Pseudo-anonymity** – refers to the processing of data in a way that personal data cannot be attributed to a person without using additional information, with that additional information being stored separately with organisational measures to ensure these are not identifiable outside of the research team.

Notably, then, a transcript can be made anonymous and quotations in dissemination can have all identifying details removed, but you and your team will likely have access to the original recordings and any collected personal data from the participants. Whilst the transcripts are possible to anonymise, the level of detail in them means there is a risk of deductive disclosure (Tilley and Woodthorpe, 2011).

> **Key point!**
>
> Deductive disclosure refers to the possibility of others identifying the participant, particularly by those who know the participant well and recognise unique characteristics or features in the data. That is, someone known to the participant can deduce who they are based on the details in the transcript.
>
> (Sieber, 1992)

The possibilities of deductive disclosure that may occur in your research should be considered, alongside the steps you can take to mitigate against it occurring. The quotes from participants that you cite may contain clues about the identity of the participant, and the more detail provided, the more likely this is (Sieber, 1992). It can be a challenge to consider how identifiable a participant may be from what you are revealing about them. Indeed, it has been suggested that qualitative researchers tend to underestimate the extent to which known persons from the same community or organisation may be able to work out who participants are (Stein, 2010). Further, if a participant's identity is revealed, this might result in sanctions, stigma, prejudice, or reprisals (Kylma et al., 1999). A balance therefore needs to be achieved to maintain the rich and detailed accounts (Kaiser, 2009) and not blunt the power of the story or the incisiveness of the analysis (Stein, 2010), but also sufficiently disguising and anonymising the data so that deductive disclosure is unlikely (Richards and Schwartz, 2002).

In addition to this, when reflecting on your plan to anonymise the transcripts and other aspects of the data, you can consider that whilst this tends to be the default position in ethics, it may not be the one your participants prefer. Some discussion amongst qualitative researchers has critically questioned whether anonymity and confidentiality are always needed. For example, evidence suggests some participants do want to be empowered to reveal (and "own") their identity in print (Bass and Davies, 2002; O'Reilly, Karim, Taylor, and Dogra, 2012). Given that qualitative health researchers frequently seek to use their positions of privilege as a platform for the voices of their participants, there is an argument that participants should be afforded the opportunity to waive the ethic of anonymity, and, by the same token, that it is problematic if researchers impose anonymity upon them (Kelly, 2009), even preferable to support participants to make decisions on these particular ethical matters (Giordano, O'Reilly, Taylor, and Dogra, 2007). This being so, there are arguments that promote anonymity as the default position, and any alternative framing needs a clear rationale and safe way to waive it (Kelly, 2009). Furthermore, the ethic of confidentiality also has limits. It is the case that absolute confidentiality cannot be guaranteed (Taquette and Borges da Matta Souza, 2022). Limits mostly relate to safeguarding and protection from wider harms.

Safeguarding

Defined broadly, safeguarding participants in research means protecting them from potential harms by taking appropriate measures to ensure their safety. This means that there may be limits to the ethic of confidentiality where participants may reveal information that alerts the researcher to possible risks of harm in their lives. Thus, there is likely to be a duty of care on the researcher to take formal steps to safeguard the participants if they reveal:

- **Risk of harm to self** – which may include self-harm, suicidal ideation, or risk-taking behaviours.
- **Risk of harm to others** – which may be a revelation of the disclosure of actual or intended aggressive behaviour, weapons use, or researching violent acts online.
- **Risk of harm from others** – which may include disclosure of adverse childhood experiences, trolling, grooming, or intimate partner violence.

When evaluating these risks and the need to take steps, you should consider the nature and type of harms that may need to be included. Livingstone (2013) discerned different harms along three dimensions:

1. **Type** – which includes physical, psychological, and social harms.
2. **Severity** – this relates to the impact on the individual and/or others.
3. **Longevity** – refers to how long the impact influences the person.

In the case of safeguarding when undertaking your research, it may be possible that you have to breach a participant's confidentiality. If you have founded concerns, then you may need to report those risks to an authority that can take action to protect persons from harm. For example, the General Medical Council (UK) (GMC, 2017), reports that there is a basis for breaching confidentiality where protecting the individual or public interest supersedes the rights of privacy for the person.

> **Key point!**
>
> The limits to confidentiality should be discussed with participants as part of the consent process and should be outlined in the participant information leaflet. It should be the case that the information leaflet indicates who will be informed should the need arise and the process that would be followed.

There are two populations who may need closer consideration in relation to the risk of harms, which are children and young people and vulnerable adults. For children, this is because of child protection obligations, and for vulnerable adults because their vulnerability may mean they are at greater risk in relation to safeguarding. Hence, the likelihood of a confidentiality breach is arguably higher in these two groups.

Child protection – the welfare and protection of children is well-founded in most countries, and there is typically legislation that sets out the interests of children to be protected from harm and neglect. In England and Wales, the Children Act (1989, 2004) provides a legislative framework that offers statutory guidance for child protection (NSPCC, 2021) and in New Zealand similarly, the Children's Act (2014) describes legal parameters for safeguarding children from harm. This legislation provides a structured approach to aid collaborative working between agencies to promote the welfare of children and to support children who are at risk from harm (NSPCC, 2021). Whilst it is contentious to assume children are inherently vulnerable, and we discuss this tension of vulnerability elsewhere in the book, it is possible that "red flags" about possible safeguarding issues may arise during data collection. If you have serious concerns about the welfare of one of your child participants, you can disclose your concerns to a designated safeguarding person in your organisation or to social services. As a healthcare practitioner, you are likely to also be governed by the safeguarding policies of your organisation and relevant safeguarding policy, practice guidance, and legislation relating to this.

Vulnerable adults – some populations are conceptualised as vulnerable by virtue of specific characteristics. Ordinarily competent adults are deemed to be able to safeguard their own interests satisfactorily, and those who are unable to do this fully need to have their interests safeguarded by others (Nickel, 2006). Adults with vulnerabilities (e.g., older adults with medical conditions like dementia, adults with intellectual disabilities) can be at increased risk of harm, and it may be the case that a researcher may become privy to information that reveals or suggests this. In such cases, it may be necessary to breach confidentiality to ensure they receive support. Recognise that going into the research project the adult you are working with may not be obviously vulnerable, and this may become more apparent as you progress through the data collection process. Working with trusted individuals connected to a vulnerable adult during the process of them taking part in research can help to mitigate some of the risks around this and ensure that appropriate support is in place should any disclosures of concern be made. With this type of scenario, having a protocol in place and being transparent with the participant about what you may need to share with others due to concerns that arise is vital.

Safeguarding any of your participants, regardless of whether they are vulnerable or not, is important. It needs to be clear to the participants the circumstances under which you may need to breach confidentiality. Notably, the need to breach confidentiality may occur within any form of project, and often unexpectedly – it is how this is done, and how the individual may be informed or affected that needs to be carefully considered before you start collecting data. NHS England (2014) offered some procedural principles to support practitioners in safeguarding, which are also relevant to research activity, and we outline these in Table 8.3.

The NHS principles were conceived with clinical practice in mind rather than research, and although translatable and useful, context is relevant. In your clinical practice, your professional responsibility for safeguarding will be clear from your organisational and professional codes of conduct and safeguarding policies (Williamson, Goodenough, Kent, and Ashcroft, 2005; O'Reilly and Kiyimba, in press). However, as we have previously argued, as a clinician researcher, your obligations will be less clear and the boundaries between confidentiality and safeguarding less transparent (O'Reilly and Parker, 2014).

Table 8.3 Safeguarding principles (NHS England, 2014)

Principle	Description
Empowerment	Supporting the person in their decision-making and ensuring sufficient information for informed consent.
Prevention	Trying to act prior to the occurrence of any harm, or any further harm.
Proportionality	Managing any risk in the least intrusive way possible.
Protection	Advocating and representing those who are vulnerable in society.
Partnership	Working collaboratively with professional services and community agencies in the prevention, detection, and reporting of any abuse or neglect.
Accountability	Having transparent and accountable practices in terms of safeguarding procedures.

Data protection and privacy statements

There are legal frameworks in many countries that guide the use of data collection and storage, so familiarise yourself with these to understand the context of research. It is likely that your organisation will have a code of conduct or guidance about data collection and data storage, which will probably have specific guidance on data gathered for research purposes. When undertaking a research project, you will need to familiarise yourself with the guidance provided by the organisation and you will need to comply with any legal obligations in your country. Data management is necessary, and this relates to protecting your participants from any harms that may result from their data being compromised. Thus, in practical terms, these relate to confidentiality (as discussed earlier), data storage, record keeping, data ownership, and data sharing (Li-Chen, 2009).

Prior to data collection, participants should be provided with information about how you intend to gather and make use of their data. It is helpful if you provide your participants with a privacy statement, showing:

- Why the data are needed and the purpose.
- How the data will be collected.
- Where those data will be stored.
- How long data will be stored for.
- When data will be deleted or destroyed.
- Who will have access to that data and with whom will the data will be shared. For example, in the UK, the Data Protection Act 2018 incorporates General Data Protection Regulation (GDPR). According to this, there needs to be a named data controller and data processor.

In addressing these questions, you will need to be clear about which data you are referring to. Remember, you may have visual or audio recordings. You are likely to have a document containing names, email addresses, telephone numbers, and other demographic details. You might have photographs or artwork, diary entries, or similar data, and you will probably have an anonymous transcript representing the data (and potentially an identifiable version too). Anonymised transcripts, though less sensitive than the recordings and personal details, would still benefit from being password-protected because of the risk of deductive disclosure we outlined earlier.

If there are multiple members of your research team from different locations and representing different organisations, then the participants need to be made aware of that also. Furthermore, if you involve professionals from other organisations in the dissemination process later, you need to ensure that this is contained in the privacy document and/or information sheet. It may be the case that a written data-sharing agreement is instituted between the different organisations so all members are aware of their responsibilities, and it can be helpful to draft a data management plan so all parties are clear about issues related to data from the early stages of a research project.

Thinking ethically about qualitative research

Anecdotally, qualitative research is sometimes represented as less ethically risky than quantitative research, for example, in the sense that qualitative researchers do not undertake invasive physical procedures with participants, such as taking blood tests or dealing with medications. However, this does not mean that there are no serious risks of harm imposed by using qualitative methods, and it is a misconception that qualitative work is less risky, meaning researchers may overlook or underestimate possible harms (Hedgecoe, 2008). We have therefore argued that there are various ethical domains that present in slightly different ways in qualitative research, which are crucial to consider if your topic is sensitive and/or your population is vulnerable (see Chapter 11) (O'Reilly and Kiyimba, 2015). These domains are depth, researcher involvement, iterative process, visibility, and data management.

Depth: Qualitative research, especially in relation to health, requires the researcher to probe deeper into people's lives to capture information about their opinions, experiences, values, ideas, beliefs, and so forth. In analysing these elements of a participant's life, it is possible, if not probable, that the researcher will be privileged to hear some sensitive and personal things, hearing narratives that can be emotional or difficult for those participants to express (O'Reilly and Kiyimba, 2015). In some ways, then, qualitative research can be experienced as intrusive by the participant as the researcher delves deeper into their experiences, and this means that the application of ethical principles needs greater thought and attention (Hewitt, 2007). This needs special consideration if the participants are also within a vulnerable group because of the greater risk of additional stigmatisation, misrepresentation, and/or the invitation of voyeurism (Malacrida, 2007). There is indeed a history of unethical research on marginalised communities, and therefore qualitative researchers need to be mindful of the complexities of implementing research among those communities already subject to stigma so as not to reinforce or reify such views (Gabbidon and Chenneville, 2021). Certain populations may also be at risk of being "over researched", as many different research teams take an interest in the same relatively small sample of participants.

Researcher involvement: As we acknowledged earlier, the researcher is an integral part of the work. Because of this, the researcher will have an impact on the process, which can raise ethical concerns, such as power, risks of coercion, and positionality (issues we return to in more detail in Chapter 9). Inherent in the qualitative research relationship is the challenge of the power held by the researcher, which may connect to status, gender, race, or age. To achieve depth in data collection, the researcher needs to build a level of rapport with the participants where they can actively and gently encourage the participants to reveal a high level of detail. However, through this rapport and encouragement, it is possible that the participants reveal more than they feel comfortable with, and the researcher may create an environment where a participant finds it difficult to withdraw (Dahal, 2024; Duncan, Drew, Hodgson, and Sawyer, 2009). In health research, especially where the researcher is a known clinician to the participants, this can be especially challenging, and so careful reflection is essential, and keeping the participant's best interests in mind always will serve as a valuable guiding principle.

Iterative process: Qualitative research is iterative, evolving over time, and the research can have an impact on participants in ways that are difficult to predict. By its very nature, there is not a simple linear process of doing a qualitative project as research questions are refined and modified, and the practices of understanding the issues at stake are attended to. This means that researchers must be responsive to changes in the research environment, participants, and processes. In other words, ethical implementation of research also must be iterative, and researchers constantly need to renegotiate this aspect of the project. Information provided to participants, the consent processes, confidentiality practices, and the nature of questions asked may need to be modified to suit the specific participant or the group, and researchers need to translate and alter the ways in which they work to suit the situation. This iterative process can be challenging as possible changes to questions or subtleties in the consent processes may increase risks to the participants (Hadjistavropoulos and Smythe, 2001), and any risk assessment conducted will therefore need to be reflexive and iterative too (Morse et al., 2008).

Visibility: There are risks in qualitative research that participants may be identified from the sound of their voice (in audio), their image (in photo or video), or from phrases they use, roles they occupy, or other unique features. Because of the in-depth nature of data collection and the nature of the tools used to collect information, participants are identifiable from the raw data. In quantitative research, for example, using surveys, participants can fill in the forms anonymously, and even in more substantial forms of data collection such as in RCTs, the data is often separated from the person's identity using a number instead. In qualitative research, the data collection process is typically personal in terms of the audio-visual materials used and the use of rich narratives in publications in the form of direct quotations. Care and attention therefore need to be dedicated to the process of data protection, data storage, and data representation in dissemination.

Data management: In qualitative research, the researcher will be processing and disseminating large amounts of data, and data management is crucial. This is a particularly salient issue in relation to the way in which those data are collected, in that it is not ethical to gather more data than necessary, and the way in which those data are disseminated to sufficiently protect the identities of participants.

These five broad domains of ethical interest for the qualitative researcher can be connected to implementing the four deontological principles in research practice (set out above). We therefore invite you to extrapolate these broad and general messages we have conveyed to your own specific research project by considering the reflective activity on the matter in Box 8.3.

Box 8.3

Reflective activity on the domains of ethical interest

Based on the five domains of ethical concern qualitative researchers need to be mindful of, we invite you to think about how these might be relevant in your research. In your research diary, we encourage you to answer the following questions:

1. How deeply will you need to probe participants' experiences and perspectives to be able to adequately address your research question?
2. To what extent is your research sensitive or your population vulnerable, and how might this intersect with the depth of the investigation?
3. In what ways might your role or other aspects of your identity influence the data collection process?

4. What are the risks of power and coercion that may operate in your project?
5. How will you manage the iterative process of your research?
6. What are the risks related to the visibility of your participants and how might this relate to the nature of your data collection methods?
7. How will you go about creating a data management plan to assure the ethicality of your data management process?

Ethical governance and applying for institutional ethical review approval
There is usually a formal process associated with research ethics where researchers illustrate how they will attend to the principles in the specific context of their own research project. The ethical governance process will vary across countries, but most researchers will require a formal structure to their ethical proposals. The necessity for an ethical authority over ethical principles and practices is founded in wider global events in history.

Broad debates and practices in ethics in health research are largely attributed to the Nuremberg trials (Ashcroft, 2003). The research scandals associated with Nazi experiments during World War II led to the development of three major documents, which were the Belmont Report, the Declaration of Helsinki, and the Nuremberg Code, creating expectations for medical researchers to conform to in terms of the application of ethical principles (Hunter, 2008). During the 1960s, medical research came under the spotlight and in many countries, such as the UK and US, ethics committees were set up as a requirement for research funding (Hedgecoe, 2008). Consequently, in the history of health research, ethics committees are a quite recent development, and these are formed to assess the potential benefits against any plausible harms (Shaw and Barrett, 2006).

Ethics committees (sometimes referred to as Institutional Review Boards) play an important role in assessing ethicality and work in partnership with researchers to support research quality. Whilst largely appreciated by researchers, tensions sometimes occur between researchers and ethics committees who decline approval for some research projects. The reason put forward by some researchers is that ethics committees, during the decision-making processes, are often largely risk-averse (McGuinness, 2008) and that they can be overly paternalistic (Smith, 2008). It has also been posited as problematic for qualitative research, as some ethics committees may not have sufficient methodological expertise (Morse, 2003) nor do they necessarily fully appreciate the iterative, cyclical, or inductive nature of the approach (Morse, Niehaus, Varnhagen et al., 2008). Although some researchers are critical of the practices of ethics committees, it is arguable that some oversight is necessary and that committees offer useful insights and support to research teams. The value, or not, of ethics committees seems to link to the quality of the communication between them and the team, the systems around the committee, and the research culture of the organisation to promote mutual learning (Brown, Spiro, and Quinton, 2020).

When developing, reviewing, and revising an ethics application, both the researcher and the committee have responsibilities for ethical research. Researchers need to ensure that they show an awareness of the practical and philosophical issues in relation to implementing any ethical guidelines, and committees need to support the needs of those research teams (Brown et al., 2020). A challenge for qualitative researchers is that the decisions and processes tend to evolve throughout the duration of the project, and it is difficult to anticipate the specifics (O'Reilly and Kiyimba, 2015). Researchers do hold accountability for their practices, and they are arguably not best placed to judge the ethicality of their own proposed ideas (Hedgecoe, 2008). Thus, in terms of researchers playing a central role in illustrating and specifying to the ethics committee that their research project is ethically viable and showing that their practices are informed by broader principles, there are several key issues to consider in the application, and we outline these in Box 8.4.

Box 8.4

Developing an ethics application

There are several steps to take in developing your application:

- Make sure you read through the application form questions a couple of times to ensure you are clear on what is expected.
- Do some reading of the research ethics literature to help you understand the common ethical issues in relation to your topic, research population, and broader deontological principles.
- Seek support from more experienced researchers, especially those who have conducted research on similar topics or with similar populations.
- Your organisation may have an ethics officer or a similar role dedicated to helping researchers with their ethics applications that you can call upon.
- Alternatively, you may have an allocated supervisor who can help you navigate this process efficiently.
- Take the time to address each question properly and with the relevant detail that is needed. It is better to ensure to complete the form fully for your first submission, to avoid time-consuming resubmissions.
- Use evidence where appropriate to support your answer to the question. Referencing a few key articles may be appropriate.
- Take note of how many words are required in each section, and do not exceed the word limits; remain succinct.
- Be consistent across your application and be careful not to contradict previous answers. Consistency is one of the biggest reasons for ethics applications to require re-submission. Remember, if you change something in one place – change it everywhere, including your participant information sheet.
- Ensure that you proofread all your answers to avoid spelling errors and typos.
- Where you have identified potential risks to participants or researchers, be clear about exactly what you will do to ameliorate or mitigate those risks.
- Account for any vulnerabilities in your research population.
- Show how you will manage any sensitivity in your topic.
- Check that you have the researcher contact details on your documents and that these are correct and consistent.

One of us (Michelle) takes on several roles relating to ethics. She sits in a deputy chairing capacity on her university-level ethics committee, dealing with the ethical governance structures and escalated applications. Additionally, she supports clinical practitioners in constructing their ethics applications in the context of UK health research governance. From these experiences, she has found there are several common errors or problems seen in applications. Based on this experience, there are various things we would recommend you remember in drafting your application, which we outline in Box 8.5.

> **Box 8.5**
> **Important things to remember in ethics applications**
>
> There are several common problems seen with applications, and the most pertinent are listed here:
>
> - A common error seen in many ethics applications is that researchers will say clearly what they intend to do (e.g. take informed consent, safeguard participants from harm, and so on) but frequently fail to illustrate the step-by-step process of *how* they will do those things in practice in the context of the recruitment and the setting.
> - Researchers report that their decisions are underpinned by a code of conduct (like the British Psychological Society's or the General Medical Council's code of ethics), and yet simply saying this or illustrating an awareness does not provide the committee with evidence of which aspects of the code are relevant or why those are relevant.
> - When outlining the inclusion and exclusion criteria, researchers may not be clear enough in explaining the differences.
> - It is sometimes the case that researchers will say that the research is valuable and has the potential to be beneficial. However, these vague sweeping statements are not especially meaningful if there is no detail as to how they will be valuable, the types of benefits that may be realised, and the mechanisms that will be needed to ensure there is benefit.
> - Some applications received do not fully account for the risks that may be incurred through the project. Whilst it is not necessarily possible to account for every eventuality, many risks are visible and obvious based on the topic, the vulnerabilities of the population, the methods to be used, the context of recruitment, and so on. Try to be transparent about the possible and probable risks, and to show how these will be managed practically.
> - Some applications have clear inconsistencies across documents, for instance, saying one thing in an information sheet and something different in an application.
> - Some applications are light on details, making it difficult for the committee to make a judgement.

In the field of health there are many professionals who support and promote ethical research practices. In our own health service work context (Michelle [and formerly Philip]), we have a helpful Research and Development department with an excellent Head of Research Operations (Dr Dave Clarke) in an NHS Trust who provides support for clinicians submitting ethics applications and ensuring the application is relevant to the local environment of the research. In the box below, Dr Dave Clarke discusses his years of experience promoting the ethicality of research in the local organisation, in Box 8.6.

Box 8.6

Practitioner perspective – Dr Dave Clarke

Dr Dave Clarke is the Head of Research Operations in Leicestershire Partnership NHS Trust, supporting the Research and Development Department in its daily tasks. Here, Dave talks about the importance of ethics in qualitative health research and his history of working in this field.

When I joined the NHS in the mid-1990s it was quite a culture shock! The power dynamics of NHS professional hierarchies were far worse than anything I had previously encountered. To be honest, I found some researchers in the system at the time were more inclined to do research on or to people, rather than with them, with some having a spectacularly cavalier attitude towards ethical principles, informed consent, or any form of oversight. Their funding sources and indemnity were equally opaque. It felt a little bit like a wild west frontier town at times!

Against considerable resistance I created internal systems from scratch to find out first what was going on, and second to ensure that it was being done *ethically*. This also started to get a grip on when income was received, how it was managed, and where it went. Many of these system principles were later adopted into the UK Research Governance Framework in 1997.

In the years since I have guided many individuals, teams, and leading academics through the changing regulatory landscape. The fundamental ethical principles remain consistent throughout, but the greatest challenge is getting applicants to think ethically. The development of NRES (National Research Ethics Service) eliminated many "rogue" ethical committees (they were closed as non-compliant), also introduced the first bureaucracy reduction systems, and developed a small number of specialist committees, to whom particular sorts of studies would be sent. NRES proceeded to quality-assure ethics committees, introduce robust governance, and consistency management.

In line with the "busting bureaucracy" agenda, the idea was to make the UK a great place to do research by identifying issues at an early stage, becoming part of a supportive regulatory system designed to *support* good, ethical research, to modify and improve where necessary, and to reduce rogue activity.

Author reflections and concluding remarks
From Nikki

In my experience as Chair of an Ethics Committee that reviewed student and staff research projects, I noted that sometimes both students and supervisors can find the ethics process daunting. Perhaps, because there are often time limits on the whole research process, "getting through ethics" can be viewed as a difficult process fraught with "red tape" and frustrating hold-ups. I agree that sometimes it can feel a bit overwhelming when initially faced with an ethics application form. From a certain perspective, it can also feel like ethics committees are a barrier to getting on with the research itself – an obstacle to overcome so that you can get the "green light" to get started with data collection. However, what I have learnt over my time as a researcher, supervisor, and ethics committee Chair, is that engaging well with the ethics process can be a real gift and a blessing in the research process if approached with the right attitude. No one wants to spend months or years on a research project, only to find that the results are not really viewed as valuable in the rest of the research community because of design flaws or ethical questions. What we would all love is for our research to be respected by our peers, and valuable for the population that the research has represented. To achieve this, allowing our peers, our supervisors, and those on the ethics committee who review the research proposal to comment on and help us refine the research project at an early stage is invaluable. If we can rectify any problems at this early stage, then our research will be more respected and useful in the end. The idea of having "critical friends" review our ideas may be one that we find a bit irritating at first, but if we can manage to put aside our impatience and self-doubt, and embrace the feedback of others, we will no doubt be pleased that we listened to their wisdom further down the line.

References

Alexander, L., and Moore, M. (2020). Deontological ethics, revised. In E. Zalta (Ed.), *Stanford encyclopedia of philosophy*. https://plato.stanford.edu/entries/ethics-deontological/

Aluwihare-Samaranayake, D. (2012). Ethics in qualitative research: A view of the participants' and researchers' world from a critical standpoint. *International Journal of Qualitative Methods*, 11(2), 64–81.

Ashcroft, R. (2003). The ethics and governance of medical research: What does regulation have to do with morality? *New Review of Bioethics*, 1(1), 41–58.

Athanassoulis, N. (2013). *Virtue ethics*. London: Bloomsbury.

Barnett, J. (2007). Seeking an understanding of informed consent. *Professional Psychology: Research & Practice*, 38(2), 179–182.

Bass, E., and Davis, L. (2002). *The courage to heal: A guide for women survivors of child sexual abuse*. London: Vermilion.

Beach, D., and Arrazola, B. (2019). Ethical review boards. Constitutions, functions, tensions and blind spots. In H. Busher and A. Fox (Eds.), *Implementing ethics in educational ethnography: Regulation and practice* (pp. 32–47). New York, NY: Routledge,

Beauchamp, T., and Childress, J. (2019). *Principles of bioethics* (8th ed.). New York, NY: Oxford University Press.

Brown, C., Spiro, J., and Quinton, S. (2020). The role of research ethics committees: Friend or foe in educational research? An exploratory study. *British Educational Research Journal*, 46(4), 747–769.

Children Act. (1989). https://www.legislation.gov.uk/ukpga/1989/41/contents.

Children Act. (2004). https://www.legislation.gov.uk/ukpga/2004/31/contents.

Christensen, C. (2004). Children's participation in ethnographic research: issues of power and representation. *Children & Society*, 18(2), 165–176.

Dahal, B. (2024). Participants' right to withdraw from research: Researchers' lived experiences on ethics of withdrawal. *Journal of Academic Ethics*, 22(1), 191–209.

Driver, J. (2011). *Consequentialism*. London: Routledge.

Duncan, R., Drew, S., Hodgson, J., and Sawyer, S. (2009). Is my mum going to hear this? Methodological and ethical challenges in qualitative health research with young people. *Social Science & Medicine*, 69, 1691–1699.

Field, M. and Behrman, R. (2004) (Eds). *Ethical conduct of clinical research involving children.* Washington: Institute of Medicine.

Flewitt, R. (2005). Conducting research with young children: Some ethical considerations. *Early Child Development & Care*, 175(6), 553–565.

Gabbidon, K., and Chenneville, T. (2021). Strategies to minimize further stigmatization of communities experiencing stigma: A guide for qualitative researchers. *Stigma & Health*, 6(1), 32–42.

General Data Protection Regulation (GDPR) (2018). Article 4: Definitions. https://www.privacy-regulation.eu/en/article-4-definitions-GDPR.htm

General Medical Council (GMC). (2017). *Confidentiality: Good practice in handling patient information.* London: GMC.

Giordano, J., O'Reilly, M., Taylor, H., and Dogra, N. (2007). Confidentiality and autonomy: The challenge(s) of offering research participants a choice of disclosing their identity. *Qualitative Health Research*, 17(2), 264–275.

Hadjistavropoulos, T., and Smythe, W. (2001). Elements of risk in qualitative research. *Ethics & Behaviour*, 1(2), 163–174.

Hedgecoe, A. (2008). Research ethics review and the sociological research relationship. *Sociology*, 42(5), 873–886.

Hewitt, J. (2007). Ethical components of researcher-researched relationships in qualitative interviewing. *Qualitative Health Research*, 17(8), 1149–1159.

Hunter, D. (2008). The ESRC research ethics framework and research ethics review at UK universities: Rebuilding the tower of Babel REC by REC. *Journal of Medical Ethics*, 34(11), 815–820.

Kaiser, K. (2009). Protecting respondent confidentiality in qualitative research. *Qualitative Health Research*, 19(11), 1632–1641.

Kelly, A. (2009). In defence of anonymity: Rejoining the criticism. *British Educational Research Journal*, 35(3), 431–445.

Klykken, F. (2022). Implementing continuous consent in qualitative research. *Qualitative Research*, 22(5), 795–810.

Kylma, J., Vehvillainen-Julkunen, K., and Lahdevirta, J. (1999). Ethical considerations in a grounded theory study on the dynamics of hope in HIV-positive adults and their significant others. *Nursing Ethics*, 6(3), 224–239.

Li-Chen, L. (2009). Data management and security in qualitative research. *Dimensions of Critical Care Nursing*, 28(3), 132–137.

Livingstone, S. (2013). Online risk, harm and vulnerability: Reflections on the evidence based for child internet safety policy. *Journal of Communication Studies*, 18(35), 13–28.

Malacrida, C. (2007). Reflexive journaling on emotional research topics: Ethical issues for team researchers. *Qualitative Health Research*, 17(10), 1329–1339.

McGuinness, S. (2008). Research ethics committees: The role of ethics in a regulatory authority. *Journal of Medical Ethics*, 34(9), 695–700.

Miller, T., and Boulton, M. (2007). Changing constructions of informed consent: qualitative research and complex social worlds. *Social Science & Medicine*, 65, 2199–2211.

Moriña, A. (2021). When people matter: The ethics of qualitative research in the health and social sciences. *Health & Social Care in the Community*, 29(5), 1559–1565.

Morse, J. (2003). A review committee's guide for evaluating qualitative proposals. *Qualitative Health Research*, 13(6), 833–851.

Morse, J., Niehaus, L., Varnhagen, S., Austin, W., and McIntosh, M. (2008). Qualitative researchers' conceptualizations of the risks inherent in qualitative interviews. In N. Denzin and M. Giardina (Eds.), *Qualitative inquiry and the politics of evidence.* Walnut Creek, CA: Left Coast Press.

National Society for the Prevention of Cruelty to Children (NSPCC) (2021). Child protection system in England. https://learning.nspcc.org.uk/child-protection-system/england

NHS England. (2014). Safeguarding adults. https://www.england.nhs.uk/wp-content/uploads/2017/02/adult-pocket-guide.pdf

Nickel, P. (2006). Vulnerable populations in research: The case of the seriously ill. *Theoretical Medicine & Bioethics*, 27, 245–264.

O'Reilly, M., and Kiyimba, N. (2015). *Advanced qualitative research: A guide to contemporary theoretical debates*. London: Sage.

O'Reilly, M., Karim, K., Taylor, H., and Dogra, N. (2012). Parent and child views on anonymity: 'I've got nothing to hide'. *International Journal of Social Research Methodology*, 15(3), 211–224.

O'Reilly, M., and Parker, N. (2014). *Doing mental health research with children and adolescents: A guide to qualitative methods*. London: Sage.

O'Reilly, M., Parker, N., and Hutchby, I. (2011). Ongoing processes of managing consent: The empirical ethics of using video-recording in clinical practice and research. *Clinical Ethics*, 6(4), 179–185.

Richards, H., and Schwartz, L. (2002). Ethics of qualitative research: Are there special issues for health services research? *Family Practice*, 19(2), 135–139.

Saunders, B., Kitzinger, J., and Kitzinger, C. (2015). Anonymising interview data: Challenges and compromise in practice. *Qualitative Research*, 15(5), 616–632.

Scott, C. (2005). Anonymity in applied communication research: Tensions between IRBs, researchers, and human subjects. *Journal of Applied Communication Research*, 33(3), 242–225.

Shaw, S., and Barrett, G. (2006). Research governance: Regulating risk and reducing harm? *Journal of the Royal Society of Medicine*, 99, 14–19.

Sieber, J. (1992). *Planning ethically responsible research: A guide for students and internal review boards*. Newbury Park, CA: Sage.

Smith, L. (2008). How ethical is ethical research? Recruiting marginalised, vulnerable groups into health services research. *Journal of Advanced Nursing*, 62(2), 248–257.

Stein, A. (2010). Sex, truths, and audiotape: Anonymity and the ethics of pulbic exposure in ethnography. *Journal of Contemporary Ethnography*, 39(5), 554–568.

Taquette, S. R., and Borges da Matta Souza, L. M. (2022). Ethical dilemmas in qualitative research: A critical literature review. *International Journal of Qualitative Methods*, 21.

The Royal New Zealand College of General Practitioners. (2014). The *Children's Act*. Te Whare Tohu Rata o Aotearoa. https://www.rnzcgp.org.nz/running-a-practice/the-foundation-standard/whare-haumanu-the-practice/151-childrens-act-2014/#:~:text=Children's%20Act%202014-,The%20Children's%20Act%202014%20strengthens%20the%20safety%20of%20children%20in,may%20be%20vulnerable%20to%20abuse

Tilley, L., and Woodthorpe, K. (2011). Is it the end for anonymity as we know it? A critical examination of the ethical principle of anonymity in the context of 21st century demands on the qualitative researcher. *Qualitative Research*, 11(2), 197–212.

Williamson, E., Goodenough, T., Kent, J., and Ashcroft, R. (2005). Conducting research with children: The limits of confidentiality and child protection protocols. *Children & Society*, 19, 397–409.

CHAPTER 9

Dual roles – the clinician and researcher roles

> **Learning objectives**
>
> This chapter enables the reader to:
>
> - Identify different roles occupied in research.
> - Recognise how researcher positionality impacts research.
> - Critically assess how occupying dual or multiple roles can be advantageous and/or disadvantageous to a research project.
> - Consider the importance of reflexivity in qualitative research.
> - Critically assess the role of power and the risks of coercion in research projects.

Introduction

For the clinician-researcher, there are many critical questions about the interaction between clinical and research roles, particularly with respect to insider and outsider status. Questions arise such as whether they recruit their own clients/patients, i.e., people who use their services, and how challenges of managing asymmetry might be addressed. As a practitioner involved in qualitative health research there are salient areas of consideration to think about doing research, in relation to the roles you occupy and the type of person you are. These issues intersect and cannot be separated from each other in the way the structure of this chapter would indicate. In introducing one aspect, it necessarily relates to others, albeit for clarity we treat them separately.

In this chapter we introduce you to applicable concepts such as positionality, reflexivity, insider–outsider positions, dual roles, and how they connect to research considerations of power and asymmetry, the challenge of coercion, and how your endeavours as a researcher might shape your clinical practice. As a clinician-researcher, you should consider these concepts because your research is likely to be intrinsically linked to your motivations and experiences (Schostak and Schostak, 2013) and it is necessary to understand how such concepts shape the process of research, as in qualitative inquiry, the researcher is the research instrument (Geddis-Regan, Exley, and Taylor, 2021).

Because this chapter relates so closely to issues of subjectivity, personal and professional motivation, professional roles, and reflexivity, we begin our discussion by encouraging you to reflect on some hypothetical examples. The idea is to give you some stimulus material to help you identify some of the reasons why this discussion is important to your understanding of research. We encourage you to work through the reflective activities in Boxes 9.1, 9.2, and 9.3 before you engage with the content of the chapter.

Box 9.1
Reflective activity on the oncologist as researcher

Imagine a scenario where a consultant oncologist has been leading a mixed-methods research project about cancer care and medical treatments. The qualitative aspect of this project is focused on the personal experience of undergoing chemotherapy. The oncologist has opted to recruit her own patients and their family members to understand their perspectives in depth and is directly involved in the recruitment of her patients to the interview phase of the study. However, she has employed a qualitative interviewer to conduct the interviews.

- What do you think the main issues are in the consultant recruiting her own patients to the study?
- What other challenges can you imagine with this study?
- What do you see as the main ethical considerations with this kind of research? Refer to the previous chapter on ethics to help your thinking.

Box 9.2
Reflective activity on the psychiatrist as researcher

Imagine a scenario where a trainee psychiatrist is undertaking a PhD project. As part of this doctoral study, he is going to recruit patients from the mental health hospital he practices in. The patients are all adult service users, but some of them do not currently have the mental capacity to make informed decisions. He wants to do individual interviews with them to ascertain their views on their treatment programme and hospital care more generally.

- How might his role as a trainee psychiatrist influence the recruitment of participants?
- How might having a role as a student researcher be important in this project?
- Why might the issue of patient capacity be relevant in terms of researcher power?

> **Box 9.3**
>
> **Reflective activity on the dentist as researcher**
>
> Imagine a scenario where a dentist is completing a master's degree programme which includes a research dissertation. The dentist is interested in child patients and the levels of anxiety regarding visits to dental practices. She wants to facilitate focus groups to gain ideas from children on how dental practices can help manage their anxieties about appointments more effectively. She plans to run the focus groups herself as there are limited resources, and she is conducting the project for an educational qualification.
>
> - How is her role as a dentist important for the recruitment of children to the study?
> - What challenges might be raised by having participants in the study under the age of 18 years?
> - What steps can she take to reduce the risk of coercion?

It is not our intention here to provide you with example answers to the questions we have posed in these reflective activities. Rather, as you read through this chapter, we encourage you to develop original answers in your diary, add new salient information, and revisit any initial ideas you may have had as you go along.

Researcher positionality

Positionality is all about you, and acknowledgement of this is necessary in qualitative research. Positionality refers to your worldview, that is, the position you take in relation to your research task (Savin-Baden and Major, 2013) and the extent to which you are a member of the group you are researching. Thus, your positionality will be shaped by many different personal characteristics, like your gender, sexuality, political affiliation, ethnicity, culture, age, social class, and so forth. To put it a different way, your worldview reflects your ontological assumptions (your beliefs about the nature of social reality), your epistemological assumptions (your beliefs about the nature of knowledge and how new knowledge is generated), and your assumptions about human nature and agency (that is, the way persons interact with the surrounding social environment) (Grix, 2019).

> **Key point!**
>
> You might find it useful to revisit Chapter 3 where we first introduced you to some of these concepts related to theory and qualitative research.

Qualitative research examines participants' lives as embedded, complex, and socially meaningful (Reich, 2021). Qualitative research does not sit simply in contrast to quantitative research but involves concepts (theory), data, and evidence through an iterative process where understanding is deepened or enriched by getting closer to the phenomenon being studied (Aspers and Corte, 2019). At the same time, it is also not simply getting close to the phenomenon that makes qualitative research qualitative, but the issue that research is anchored by a "methodological obligation" on researchers to critically reflect on how and why the closeness is important (Reich, 2021). Reich argued that qualitative research is qualitative because of the explicit ways researchers consider their positionality and the position of the participants as part of its inquiry. This means researchers must make sense of their roles and the boundaries of the researcher–participant relationship (Fenge et al., 2019). Fenge et al. observed that being mindful of one's positionality means that the researcher actively negotiates the insider–outsider perspectives within that relationship and considers how they locate themselves within that continuum and how much of their position they share with the participants.

Actively "doing" positionality
Positionality is a matter to attend to on an ongoing basis as you work through the process of your project. There is some overlap with reflexivity, and researchers sometimes get the two concepts confused. Reflexivity is a tool for researchers to use to explore the impact of their positionality on the research process and to examine any subconscious motivations or beliefs (Finlay, 2002). For positionality, then, you need to acknowledge your own views, values, and beliefs through self-reflection and identify and critique your position (Manohar, Liamputtong, Bhole, and Arora, 2017). By way of this reflection, you can critically question how knowledge and experience are situated, co-constructed, and historically and socially located (Reich, 2021). You can also recognise your own subjective experiences of the phenomenon, which can help you think through power relations and your position in relation to others and consider the extent to which you have similarities or differences from your research participants across relevant domains (Mohler and Rudman, 2022).

Acknowledging your positionality also means that people reading your research can draw their own conclusions about how your position may have had an influence on the way the data were gathered, analysed, and interpreted. There are three ways in which you can accomplish positionality (as identified by Savin-Baden and Major, 2013):

1. You can locate yourself in relation to the subject – that is, it is helpful to acknowledge how your personal position can influence your interest in the research topic.

Example
If you have personal experience of the topic area you are doing a qualitative health research project on, in addition to your clinical role and your researcher role, it is helpful to be transparent about the insider position you share with your participants, that is, about both having experienced the same life experience.

2. You can situate yourself in relation to your participants – think about how you view yourself and how your participants view you.

Example
Consider if you are a clinician and researcher involved in work representing a particular group in the country where you practice. Consider any differences in your position

within your worldview compared to your participants' position, and how they might experience the way that you engage in research, how you interpret what they say, and what you do with the findings of the work.

3. You can locate yourself in relation to the broader research context and process – that is, you need to think about how your work is influenced by the wider social context.

Example
As a feminist clinician-researcher, it would be helpful to make it clear that you are approaching your research from that perspective. You may contextualise your research within a body of feminist literature on a similar topic.

Holmes (2020) added a fourth way, that is, thinking about time in the sense that acknowledging and clarifying your positionality will take time.

> **Key point!**
>
> In mapping your positionality, you need to think about your identity and recognise that you will have many different identities that overlap.

Your positionality is intrinsically connected to your identity as a clinician, as a researcher, and through other relevant attributes (e.g. gender, in an age group, and so on). Establishing your positionality in research is complex because of the fluidity of changing social identities, their abstract nature, their temporality, and how they impact the research process (Jacobson and Mustafa, 2019). Jacobson and Mustafa have, however, provided a practical method to help you map your positionality for the project via a "social identity map", which is a visual representation serving as a starting point. We outline the practical steps of creating this map in Box 9.4.

> **Box 9.4**
>
> **Practical steps for creating a social identity map (Jacobson and Mustafa, 2019)**
>
> This map is created through three tiers:
>
> 1. Identifying broader facets of social identity, like socio-economic status, age, race, gender, sexual orientation, and so forth.
> 2. Questioning how this impacts our lives, and reflecting on how social identities might broadly, specifically, or socially impact research.
> 3. Reflecting on these elements of positionality and identifying emotions that you feel might be tied to your social identity.

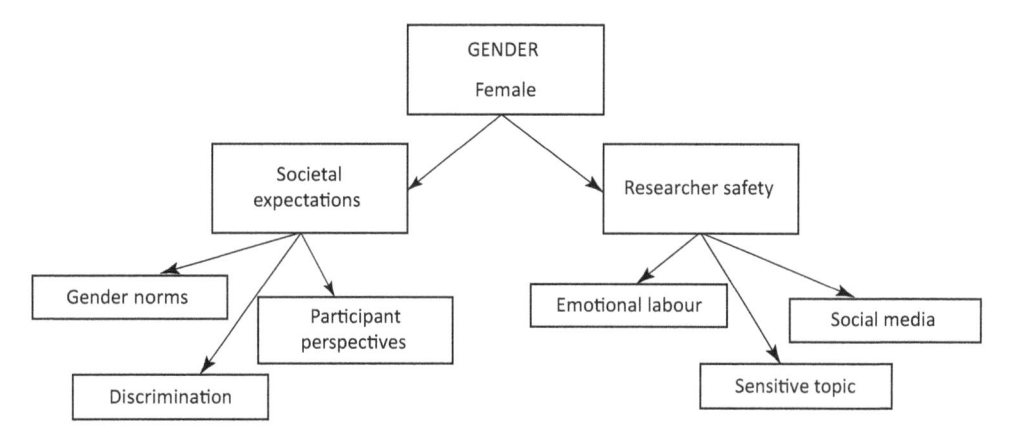

```
                    GENDER
                    Female
         ↙                      ↘
    Societal                  Researcher safety
  expectations
   ↙    ↓                      ↙    ↓      ↘
Gender  Participant       Emotional  Sensitive  Social
norms   perspectives       labour     topic     media
  ↓
Discrimination
```

Figure 9.1 Social identity map

We present a visual example of one aspect of this in Figure 9.1. This figure represents a hypothetical example and is intended only as an illustration.

Mapping positionality in this way can start to unearth or create additional branches of influence on the research process that mean something to the worldview, personal experiences, and individual characteristics of the researcher. By representing these visually, you can iteratively change the boxes as you reflect on the aspects of your research, your participants, society, methods, and who you are as a person, which influences and shape the way in which you are working.

We encourage you to critically reflect on this approach to positionality and consider the extent to which the three tiers might represent a reductionist style of thinking about your position in the research. Furthermore, there is a risk in developing a map whereby assumptions about identity categories may be made, especially when working in a team. For example, you may not want to accept presuppositions that you belong to a particular category and that within that category there are other presuppositions about what people belonging to that category feel or think. Engaging in reflection about what you consider to be your own positionality is important, and a framework like this can be helpful to some extent, or you may choose to take a different approach. If you want to start thinking about your own positionality and how it relates to your research, have a go at attempting the reflective activity in Box 9.5.

Box 9.5

Your positionality

Think about your own positionality and start to create your own social identity map. In our example, we used the three tiers recommended. However, you may choose to do your social identity map in a different way. The point of this exercise is to encourage you to reflect on your position, as this will impact the way in which you do your research and interpret your findings.

Dual roles – insider–outsider positions

Closely related to positionality is the issue of insider or outsider status. In a basic sense, insider research is when the researcher is working with populations where they are also a member of that group; that is, they share a language, identity, or experiential base (Dwyer and Buckle, 2009). Outsider research involves the researcher working with a population with whom they are unfamiliar and with whom they do not share characteristics or experience of the phenomenon (Gair, 2012). Whilst insider–outsider research exists on a continuum, the greater the level of insider status, the greater the level of shared experience and knowledge. Thus, insider positionality is often considered a privilege, as in-group membership can provide a foundation for trust and acceptance with the group or community being researched (Dwyer and Buckle, 2009).

> **Key point!**
>
> Whilst positionality is often considered in relation to insider–outsider positions, this dichotomy is thought to be too simplistic when identity categories are fluid and flexible, and thus positionality is intersectional.
>
> (Tinker and Armstrong, 2008)

Insider and outsider positions have sometimes been constituted in paradigmatic framings described in relation to emic and etic accounts (see Chapter 3 for details). The insider position has been viewed as an *emic* account, whilst the outsider position as *etic*. The emic description is an insider's view of reality (Fetterman, 2008) and is situated within a relativist framing that recognises behaviour and actions as relative to the individuals' culture (Holmes, 2020). The etic account is situated within a realist perspective and thus attempts to discern differences across cultures and assumes a predefined reality in terms of the researcher–participant relationship (Nagar and Geiger, 2007). Thus, this account seeks to be culturally neutral and written using terminology appropriate to externally imposed "scientific" standards rather than those within the culture (Holmes, 2020). Arguably however, in seeking to be "culturally neutral", this is, in its own right, a form of cultural imposition that may be alien to the cultural group that is the interest of the research project.

Put simply, then, emic and etic refer to the ontological positions of insider and outsider researchers, respectively, referring to whether that person is an insider or outsider to the culture they are investigating. However, it does not necessarily mean they are operating from an etic or emic position (Holmes, 2020). Insider researchers are those that are already members of a specific group with specified social status, and outsiders are non-members (Merton, 1972). In other words, insiders can potentially better understand the experiences of those inside the culture due to similar biographical experiences, shared gender, race, or sexual orientation, and this provides a lived familiarity with the group being researched (Holmes, 2020). An example is the methodology of Kaupapa Māori research (Cram and Adcock, 2022). Emerging from a critical response to dominant culture, largely Western researchers *doing research on* the indigenous peoples of Aotearoa New Zealand, the Kaupapa Māori research framework was developed to resist this imposition of a culturally incongruent "etic" or outsider logic. The premise was to treat participants with respect and engage in research that was meaningful to participants rather than researchers. By allowing participants control over interpretation and dissemination of findings, any research involving Māori participants should be conducted "by Māori for Māori". The argument was that only emic, insider research would be an appropriate way to understand Māori worldview and experiences, especially in qualitative health research.

Many researchers in health are practising in a clinical speciality and are therefore considered to be insider researchers. This is because they possess insider insight and access to certain settings or populations as they are part of the participants' cultures and have a physical and psychological proximity to them. Other researchers may be considered outsider researchers when they work for an outside organisation and do not have that practice-based knowledge in the field.

There are many advantages and disadvantages of an insider position, and some of the main ones are listed in Table 9.1. Please note, however, that although we have presented the two positions as dichotomous, there are arguments that the insider versus outsider position is on a continuum (Mercer, 2007). Thus, distinguishing between insider status and outsider status can involve blurred distinctions, and consequently it can be preferable instead to define the position of the researcher in terms of physical and psychological distance from the research phenomenon and not in relation to paradigmatic position (Holmes, 2020).

Table 9.1 Advantages and disadvantages of insider positions

Advantages	*Disadvantages*
Easier access to the culture being studied and alignment with the population (Sanghera and Thapar-Bjokert, 2008).	The researcher may be unknowingly biased or identify with participants and their experience to the extent they struggle to adopt a more independent position in the research (Holmes, 2020).
The researcher can ask more insightful questions due to a priori knowledge (Holmes, 2020).	The researcher might be too familiar with the culture, which inhibits their ability to raise questions that are provocative or probing (Holmes, 2020).
There is potentially an established trust between the researcher and participant leading to more candid responses as they can build rapport (Hayfield and Huxley, 2015).	Participants may assume that the researcher has more knowledge than they do (Holmes, 2020).
It is possible to produce more truthful or authentic understandings of the culture (Geertz, 1973).	The researcher is unlikely to bring an external perspective to the process (Holmes, 2020).
The likelihood of disorientation due to "culture shock" is reduced (Holmes, 2020).	Participants might be inhibited by the knowledge status of the researcher and feel they cannot ask questions (Naaek et al., 2010).
The researcher can better understand the language, including both colloquial language and professional terminology used by participants (Holmes, 2020).	There is a risk that participants are less willing to reveal sensitive information to an insider than to an outsider (Holmes, 2020).

Holding more than one role

> The dual role is not seen as intrinsically unethical, but as a phenomenon – like other conflicts of interest – that should be carefully managed.
>
> *(Bell, 2019, p. 11)*

Linked to the concepts of insider or outsider positions is the nature of the roles occupied. As a clinical practitioner undertaking a qualitative health research project, you have at least two roles: that of clinician and that of researcher. This means that there are at least four areas of possible concern that you need to reflect on and consider in how you recruit participants to your research project, as we previously identified (O'Reilly and Parker, 2014):

1. You may choose to undertake research with your own clients or patients (service users).
2. You may choose to undertake research with clients or patients who are using the services to which you are affiliated.
3. You may choose to undertake research with clients or patients from another service or organisation and may or may not reveal your clinical status to them.
4. You may choose to undertake research with your own colleagues within your organisation or those from another setting.

Each of these domains prompts different considerations, depending on whether you are recruiting your own patients/clients or not, researching within your organisation or not, revealing your clinical identity or not, or doing work involving other practitioners known to you or not. If you do decide to reveal your clinical identity to your participants, you may do that with an open declaration at the outset on all associated paperwork, you may do this at the point of data collection (rather than recruitment), or you may only disclose if you are directly asked about it (Geddis-Regan et al., 2021). Geddis-Regan et al. noted that declaring your clinical role promotes transparency, but the researcher role needs to be clarified, including informing the participant about the limits of the clinical role in the research. They also recognised that leaving this information to the point of data collection might be problematic as it may negatively impact that process as participants may hold unrealistic expectations about possible help or support.

We encourage you to reflect on how you are going to do your project and who you are recruiting by engaging with the activity detailed in Box 9.6. We will be returning to the issue of recruitment and sampling more specifically later in the book, so in this chapter we are simply inviting you to think about how your clinical role might be influential in this process.

Box 9.6

Reflective activity on your dual role

As we have reminded you throughout this book, you need to be reflective as a researcher, and we encourage you here to start asking yourself some questions about recruitment in terms of your roles. Think about the benefits or possible challenges that this may cause.

- Who are you recruiting to your study, and how is your role an influence on decision-making around who this is?
- What are the benefits of your roles in the recruitment process?
- What challenges and/or ethical complexities might your clinical identity raise in the recruitment process, and how can you mitigate them?

When considering how your role might be important if you are recruiting your own patients or colleagues, or even how it might be influential if you are working with patients/clients from another service or region, you will hopefully have thought about some of the challenges. This may include things like:

- **Boundary drift** – when the clinician-researcher and their participants find it difficult to maintain the boundaries of the activity as research without the researcher slipping into engaging in clinical practice (e.g. providing therapy or giving medical advice) (Dickson-Swift, James, Kippen, and Liamputtong, 2006).
- **Incompatibility of expectations** – if the participants are aware of your clinical expertise, they may have unrealistic expectations about what they can expect in the research setting. For example, they may believe that you can offer some form of diagnosis, medication, or a clinical opinion.
- **Excessive or inappropriate disclosure** – clinicians are trained in communication skills and are used to speaking with patients/clients where highly sensitive and personal information is disclosed. In mental health, for example, practitioners are experienced in discussing sensitive topics, and the skills professionals develop in this area can be advantageous in qualitative research practice (Lakeman, McAndrew, MacGabhann et al., 2013). However, in research, stronger boundaries about the degree of emotional depth sought are needed, as researchers are not seeking to help participants work through trauma or difficulty, and their involvement in research tends to be a one-off event in many cases or at least short-term (Long and Eagle, 2009).
- **Coercion** – whilst we will be detailing this challenge further shortly in the chapter, it is a consideration for you when you recruit people known to you and the power your role identity may convey. A clinical title can lead to a greater level of trust and may unduly influence your participants to agree to participate.

There are things you can do to manage some of these challenges, and we provide you with some practical steps to take in Box 9.7.

Box 9.7
Practical steps to mitigate the challenges of dual role

There are some steps you can take to manage the challenges associated with your clinical role and identity:

- You should be clear about the boundaries of the research relationship and clarify from the initial communication with potential participants what your research role is and what you can and cannot do for them. Be clear that you will not be giving clinical advice.
- For some participant groups who do not know you, it may be possible to identify yourself in your other role (e.g. PhD student, academic researcher, etc.). You need a clear rationale for how you identify yourself and what the implications are for that in your project.
- Ensure that you provide information in simple and accessible ways.
- Try to give your participants some control over the research process and reduce power differentials wherever possible, ensuring that they are aware of their rights.
- Be mindful when communicating with participants and when collecting data from them to ensure that they remain cognisant to only revealing stories they are comfortable sharing. Revisit consent afterward and remind participants of their rights to withdraw all or some of their data.
- Be reflective during the process of data gathering and continually ask yourself questions about how you are interacting with your participants. Check that you are staying in the role of researcher and are aware of any pressures acting on you to be pulled out of this role.
- Reflect on how your background, training, and skills may be influencing the relationships that develop with participants.
- Check that there is nothing about how you have presented your role as a clinician-researcher that might mislead them into thinking that their participation in the research will have a bearing on their clinical treatment.
- Check that your participants are freely volunteering and do not feel obliged to take part because of your position. Make sure they know what the research is for and how it will be used.

To help you consolidate your thinking about your own roles and how they overlap and impact your own research project, we offer the experienced voice of Dr Samuel Tromans. In Box 9.8, Dr Tromans talks about how his role as a Consultant Psychiatrist and Researcher influenced and shaped his own research on autism.

Box 9.8

The views of Dr Samuel Tromans on holding a dual role

Dr Samuel Tromans is a Consultant Psychiatrist working for Leicestershire Partnership NHS Trust and an Associate Professor working for the University of Leicester, UK. He specialises in neurodevelopmental conditions.

I am a white British male who is an academic psychiatrist, working in both university and healthcare trust settings. I grew up in a working-class family where my father was an environmental health officer and my mother a housewife supporting me and my two brothers. I attended state primary and secondary schools. I had a longstanding interest in human behaviour, particularly enjoying psychology at college, and applied to medical school with the intention of becoming a psychiatrist. At medical school and as a junior doctor, I also had enjoyable training experiences in other specialities, including infectious disease and nephrology, leading to being briefly uncertain about which type of medical training to undertake as a postgraduate doctor. I ultimately chose psychiatry and soon realised I had made absolutely the right decision for me, based on my strong interest and skillset.

I was fortunate enough to be funded by my healthcare trust to undertake a PhD towards the end of my psychiatry training. My project involved interviewing adult patients who had been admitted to acute mental health wards. The nature of this project caused me to reflect on my dual role as a clinical academic, recognising that it was necessary to be sensitive to the position of power that psychiatrists hold. For example, patient participants may feel more inclined to consent to take part in a study if asked to take part by a psychiatrist, making it is particularly important to emphasise the voluntary nature of research. Over recent years, I have thought more about how I view myself. As a medical student and junior doctor, I considered myself a bit of an underdog, having come through the state school system and having no doctors in my family. Whereas now I recognise that whilst this self-conceptualisation is not entirely inaccurate, many of my peers and patients have faced significant adversities and forms of discrimination that I have never experienced, and I think I have a more balanced perspective of myself. Additionally, at medical school and as a doctor, I have had the opportunity to meet friends, colleagues, and patients from a much wider range of cultures than in my earlier life, and I feel this has significantly influenced both my modern-day professional practice as well as my personality more generally.

Reflexivity and (self-)reflection

Up until this point in the chapter we have introduced you to the concept of positionality and discussed the influence of your clinical identity and how that interacts with your researcher role. Aligned with this is reflexivity, which we referred to earlier. Reflexivity informs your positionality as it requires an explicit and conscious self-assessment by you as the researcher about how your views or positions may directly or indirectly influence the design, execution, and interpretation of the research (May and Perry, 2017). As such, ideas regarding reflexivity informing positionality stand in opposition to the idea that research is separate from a wider sociocultural context or the researcher's biography. This means that being reflexive is not about not trying to eliminate the effect of the researcher's position, but rather researchers seeking to be transparent in their work to understand and (to differing degrees) apprehend their influence on and in the research process (Holmes, 2020).

When we introduced you to reflexivity, we did so alongside the concept of reflection, a skill you are likely familiar with from your clinical training. Sometimes, reflexivity is confused with reflection, but they are different skills on a continuum (Finlay, 2002). Reflexivity has similarities with Schön's (1983) idea of "reflection-in-action" (see Chapter 1), that is, where the thinking is immediate, in situ, continuous, and dynamic self-awareness (Finlay, 2002).

> **Key point!**
> Reflexivity refers to the process of exploring how you are impacting and transforming the process of the research.
>
> (Finlay, 2002)

Inevitably you will be influencing the idea formation, planning, collection of the data, selection and recruitment of participants, analysis, and interpretation of the data (Finlay, 2002). There are different kinds of reflexive practice, and we outline two of the main types as outlined by Willig (2008) in Table 9.2.

We encourage you to use your research diary to help you with the reflexive process, as this provides a mechanism for you to keep track of your thoughts, feelings, decisions, and so forth.

The importance of reflexivity

In qualitative health research conducted by clinician-researchers, reflexivity is useful as the challenges presented by the dual role are openly recognised and discussed (Geddis-Regan et al., 2021). However, doing reflexivity in practice does require a level of sensitivity to your cultural, social, and political context (Bryman, 2016) and illustrates how your personal integrity and social values, as well as your clinical competencies, may influence the way you conduct your project (Bourke, 2014). There are, therefore, many reasons why being reflexive is part of qualitative research, and we previously identified some of the most salient (O'Reilly and Parker, 2014):

1. Being reflexive embraces and acknowledges the influence that you have over your research project.
2. Being reflexive helps render transparent your theoretical and epistemological positions.
3. Being reflexive serves to promote quality in your qualitative project.

Table 9.2 Two main types of reflexivity

Personal reflexivity	*Epistemological reflexivity*
This requires you to reflect on your attitudes, political alliance, values, beliefs, experiences, and social identities. Here, you reflect on the ways that these have impacted your research and shaped the process (from initial ideas and question identification through to data gathering, analysis, and dissemination).	This requires an engagement from you with your research question and thinking about how your worldview is influencing the study design and how the research question is designed. This kind of reflexive practice requires you to reflect on the theoretical assumptions you bring to the inquiry and how they shape the analysis and findings.

Reflexivity is fundamental to your positionality, to critical insights into the impact of your dual role as clinician and researcher, and to the quality of your project. We therefore note the important things you need to remember about reflexivity in Box 9.9 to help you summarise this aspect of the work.

Box 9.9

Important things to remember about reflexivity

We list here some important things to remember about reflexivity, but also invite you to add to this list from any additional reading you do:

- Reflexivity and reflection are similar and related but different.
- Your reflexivity should start from the beginning when you first conceive your research idea, with you considering the genesis of the idea for the research and how involved your participant group was in shaping your research focus.
- Reflexivity remains essential throughout the process, from the design, data collection, and interpretation through to dissemination, impact, and the sustainability of your work.
- Reflexivity is an iterative process that makes you visible in your research. You will need to take a critical perspective on yourself, your role, and your work (Finlay, 2002).
- A way to facilitate your reflexive practice is to keep your research diary up to date and write your thoughts, feelings, beliefs, practices, ideas, and so forth down as you experience them.
- Often, it is challenging to reflect on our own assumptions because we take for granted our own cultural lens. It can be helpful, therefore, to talk to others in your research or clinical team, to ask them to help you see any "blind spots".

You need to be continuously reflexive as you do your research, particularly as you interact with your participants at various points in the project, noting the effect you appear to have on them and how they respond to you, and how this shapes the insights obtained through the research (Finlay, 2002). This kind of critical reflexive engagement is necessary as without this there is a risk of iatrogenic difficulties where there might be unintended harmful impact because of unfounded claims of neutrality or objectivity, with reflexivity being both an issue of quality and ethics (O'Reilly and Parker, 2014). In relation to ethics, then, your reflexive practice provides insights into the power you hold within the research process (Reich, 2021).

Asymmetric relations and power

Part of your reflexivity will be to iteratively and critically question how your role might hold influence or be perceived as powerful by research participants. Understanding your position in comparison with the social position of your participant is necessary to help you identify the power relations that can operate within your research project and affords you space to be reflexive about what you can do to address them (Day, 2012). Your status as a clinician and as a researcher will lead to various perceptions on the part of your participants about how they see you and how they respond to you and any requests you make of them.

Power dynamics

There are many different possible power dynamics that operate whilst you are undertaking research. In the following pairings, we propose that as a clinician-researcher, you may hold different positions of privilege in comparison to participants. These are a few types of relational dynamics to consider, and we deal with each in turn.

- **Researcher versus participant**

The most obvious power dynamic operating is the roles occupied in the research. It is well-established that researchers typically hold power as they usually direct the research, set the agenda, ask the questions, design the project, convey the information, undertake analysis, and control dissemination pathways. Whilst participants can decline participation, they may find it difficult. A way to manage this is to consider engaging in research that has relevance to your participant group and allows them to have a lot of input into the design of the research focus, questions, and methodology. Participants who have more influence over this stage will potentially gain more "power" than the researcher, who could legitimately occupy a role of serving the participants and helping them to generate knowledge about issues important to them. Similarly, where participants have more control over how the findings are analysed, interpreted, and disseminated, the balance of power is shifted.

- **Clinician versus patient/client/service user**

Whilst you are undertaking a research project, you also occupy a clinical role, and it is this dual role status that has been the subject of this chapter. We have already discussed how revealing a clinical identity might sway patients or clients to agree to participate or prompt them to take to greater risks in participating as they misunderstand the possible benefits to them. Clinical practitioners hold a lot of power in the field of health, and whilst levels of seniority can be influential, the clinical expertise and position you hold are likely to influence participation decisions and engagement. To manage this, ensure your participants are clear about what they are consenting to, and how the information will be used. Specifically, they need to understand that the research is not connected to their clinical treatment or care, and involvement in the research will not mean that they receive a better or worse clinical service. Also, they need to understand that the questions asked are not for the purpose of clinical assessment, and that the research interview is not a clinical interview. Managing participant expectations and answering their questions is essential.

- **Resilient versus vulnerable**

Given that you are researching an area of health, it is possible that the participants have a vulnerability by virtue of their health condition, experiences, or certain characteristics.

For example, they may have a physical condition, a mental health condition, or a disability. The characteristics of these conditions may make them vulnerable in various ways, or their dependency on care may leave them feeling it is difficult to decline the opportunity to participate. An advantage of being a clinician as well as a researcher is that you are likely able to assess their suitability to be involved in research as participants. You may have "insider" knowledge about their level of vulnerability or their ability to understand what is being asked of them. This is where both clinical and research ethics come into effect. It is an ethical obligation as a researcher to ensure your participants have understood what they are consenting to and have the requisite capacity to do so.

- Having capacity versus impaired capacity

The nature of your research and the characteristics of your participants may lead to some questions about the capacity of your participants to consent. For example, some conditions impair an individual's ability to act in their own best interests (e.g. older adults with dementia), and for some their cognitive development may influence their understanding (e.g. young children). If you are doing your research with populations that may not be able to fully make decisions that safeguard their own interests, then the power relationship will be especially important to manage. As mentioned in the previous section, one advantage of holding the dual role of clinician and researcher is that you have the potential to be aware of matters of capacity and impairment, so you may be able to utilise that skill to make ethical decisions about the involvement of certain individuals or populations in the research process.

- Privileged versus under-privileged

There are certain social groups that hold a greater level of power in society. Whilst the ways in which these groups are conceptualised may be contested, the demographics of the researcher and those of the participants might intersect in ways that mean one is perceived as more powerful. Gender is an example of this, as men are often positioned as more powerful than women, and when combined with hierarchical organisational positions this can be strengthened. For example, consider an experienced senior male consultant dermatologist who has a leadership role in an organisation and has worked there for ten years asking a female receptionist who has been with the organisation for three weeks to be a participant in his project. Another example may be the difference in privilege between a middle-aged white male Consultant Psychiatrist asking a South Asian, disabled, female adolescent with an eating disorder to participate in a focus group for his research. These are strong hypothetical examples for the purposes of illustrating the point, but nonetheless, we encourage you to consider your own work context for further examples and to critically question the notion of vulnerability as we have encouraged you to do at various points in the book.

Power and the ethics of care
An important step in managing the power you hold in the research relationship with your participants is to be continuously reflexive and actively navigate ways to achieve balance, or even tip it in favour of participants. In qualitative research, there is a

methodological obligation to embrace an ethics of care (Reich, 2021). Simply stated, an ethics of care is the human capacity to care for others, to be kind, respectful, empathic, and responsible. The ethics of care philosophy centralises attentiveness to need and responsibility to respond to need (Tronto, 1994). The ethics of care emphasises empathy and moral reasoning, as well as the obligation toward the alleviation of suffering of others (Slote, 2007), which also translates to a digital ethics of care in online interactions (O'Reilly, Levine, and Law, 2021).

So, in the context of qualitative research, the ethics of care is foundational so that researchers are aware of the potential to cause harm to individuals and communities, as well as to the researcher (Hanson and Richards, 2017). By reflexively operating within a framework of an ethics of care, you can critically explore how inequalities of power between you and your participants are managed and consider how to protect participants from harm (Reich, 2021), even if the harm is unintended. The concept of iatrogenesis designates the potential to cause harm unintentionally in the process of trying to do good. If we apply this principle of iatrogenesis to the research context, it is possible to cause unintended harm to participants and the populations they represent, by simply being insufficiently attentive and insufficiently reflexive about the kinds of power dynamics that we have raised here.

The risk of coercion

We introduced you to the idea of coercion in the previous chapter on ethics. It is especially important in relation to role and power. Power is not inherent within people, nor is it fixed or absolute; rather, it resides within the research process, the interactions you have with your participants, and others involved (Christensen, 2004). Thus, the power operating within your research is relational. It takes form in how you interact with others, the types of information you reveal to them, the strategies you use to illustrate what is expected of everyone in the process, and how you work with the data once collected.

Intrinsically related to the challenge of managing your potentially privileged position as a clinician-researcher is the risk that you may inadvertently (hopefully not deliberately) coerce your participants into agreeing to participate. Your access to participants with the right characteristics for your study, your familiarity with patient care pathways, direct clinical contacts, and networks with possible other gatekeepers can be advantageous, but also risk coercion (Hiller and Vears, 2016). As we noted earlier, the closeness you may have to your patients/clients, or the epistemic status you hold as a clinician, likely means that potential participants may have expectations that decisions and requests you make are in their best interests.

It is, of course, difficult, if not impossible, to completely separate your clinical role from your researcher one, but maintaining reflexivity, taking a critically inquisitive position on all decisions, and actively taking steps to redress the power differential are aligned with research integrity. Moreover, whilst it is necessary to consider how some patients/clients may feel disempowered to refuse participation, one needs to be mindful not to make too many assumptions that they necessarily feel undue pressure or obligation (Wilson, Draper, and Ives, 2008). These are assumptions you need to pursue and check out, providing your participants with sufficient time to think things through, have clear information about the balance of benefits and risks of taking part, and being reminded that they are permitted to decline without this affecting your relationship with them.

Practitioner profile

Something we have not said anything about in this chapter is how the activity of engaging in qualitative health research can shape one's practice as a healthcare professional. There are some aspects that are general. For example, research experience can be helpful for the application of research evidence to practice, particularly for thinking more critically about this evidence and how it can be utilised in different areas of care delivery in one's organisation or team. There are also other ways in which doing research can shape one's practice. Having the experience of listening and thinking in-depth about what research participants say during interviews can hone one's listening skills as a practitioner. It can help one to listen to different levels of communication, for example, to be more inclined to consider what is not being said (or seems as though it cannot be said) as well as what is manifest in dialogue. Equally, a clinician-researcher may become more keenly aware of how particular social discourses are invested in by professionals and users of services they work with and the structuring effect that these wider discourses can have on the things they say.

Practitioners who undertake research may also refine their understanding of issues of consent and nonmaleficence in the delivery of care, having had to consider them closely when undertaking research. Their awareness of different organisational processes and dynamics of interprofessional relationships develops, having had to consider these as part of empirical inquiry or having been led to reflect on how they have impacted their research.

In these different respects, (clinician-)researcher reflexivity is part and parcel of a research project, i.e. in its design, the gathering and analysis of data, and writing up. However, it also extends beyond this and relates to the ways one thinks about and approaches one's clinical practice.

Author reflections and concluding remarks

In the interest of transparency and in the spirit of being reflective and reflexive authors, we bring this chapter to a close by talking about our own positionality in research. As clinicians and academics writing this chapter, we have undertaken a great deal of qualitative health research, sometimes with populations we have worked with, sometimes with those of our colleagues, and sometimes with those unknown to us. We have also engaged in research that involved clinical practitioners as participants, some who were colleagues and some with whom we were not acquainted. We grappled with the power dynamics, the ethical parameters, the intention of beneficence and empowerment, and with promoting high-quality research that can be applied and make a difference. We navigated partnerships, networks, and challenged how our identities were influential in undertaking those projects. To draw this chapter to a close, each of the three authors provides a brief insight into who we are, the positions we take in doing qualitative research, and a reflection on how that is helpful to reveal to you how our positionality may have shaped our work.

From Michelle

I identify as a white British female, with some Irish heritage, who is an academic researcher working in a university undertaking the traditional academic roles of teaching and research, and working in an NHS Trust as a supervisor, mentor, and research adviser. I grew up in a working-class environment with a mother who stayed at home looking after her children and a father working in a blue-collar role. This changed in my early childhood following my father's stroke, when my mother then went to university and trained to be an educator. This shift in my family dynamic helped me to develop a different way of thinking about women in the workplace as I strove to develop a career pathway for myself. From a young age, I had an interest in psychology, mental health, and children's lives, inevitably shaped by the challenges of having an autistic brother who struggled to fit in and displayed externalising behaviours in his special needs school. These childhood and adolescent experiences shaped my early views of mental health as well as of healthcare and educational practitioners. Whilst these views have shifted and evolved as I have become more educated, more experienced, and more knowledgeable, they nonetheless still influence the way in which I conduct health research, identify with participants, and my ambitions to showcase their narratives and voices to promote change. I also feel that these experiences, alongside my training, help me to connect with my participants and get close to their lives.

From Philip

As a practitioner-researcher or clinical academic, I have held various roles since finishing my professional training and PhD – for example, a practice-based role in a child and adolescent mental health service in one NHS Trust, a role lecturing and supervising health and social care professionals engaged in research in another, and an additional leadership role with a national organisation of health and care research.

I am white, male, English, and middle class in terms of my social identity. My parents have, respectively, middle- and working-class backgrounds. I attended state primary and secondary schools and, after school, drifted into employment in different helping roles in youth and play work and learning support. Whilst undertaking my first full-time job (as a youth advocate), I was advised to train as a social worker, which I did. Through exposure to research and then relationships I was fortunate to develop during a practice placement as part of this training, I applied for a studentship to complete a master's in research methods and a PhD. I commenced this shortly after qualifying, completing it on a part-time basis so as to care for my young son, who was born just before I finished my social work degree. I would say that this experience, of becoming a father and parenting whilst studying, has had perhaps the most far-reaching influence on my work as a qualitative researcher, particularly in relation to my preoccupation (in terms of the topics I've studied) with the use of psychoanalytic ideas for understanding how parents experience being parents.

From Nikki

In Aotearoa New Zealand, where I am now a permanent resident, the importance of connection and understanding who someone is and where they are from is essential to the Māori worldview. In practice, although I have lived most of my life in the UK in accordance with quite Western ways of relating, I now attend far more thoughtfully to this aspect of professional life. Whakawhanaungatanga is the process of connecting, relating, and learning about one another. As part of that process, each person shares their whakapapa, or heritage. In tracing mine, I have discovered that I am of Roma

Gypsy descent. So, my lineage is Roma, my family or whānau background is working-class white British, and my current turangawaewae, or place that I now call home, is the North Island of Aotearoa New Zealand. As a researcher, I have always felt most comfortable taking a social constructionist position that allows me to value several different perspectives as equally "true" and to see that reality is not a fixed, pre-determined entity but something we co-create.

References
Aspers, P., and Corte, U. (2019). What is qualitative in qualitative research. *Qualitative Sociology, 42*, 139–160.
Bell, K. (2019). The "problem" of undesigned relationality: Ethnographic fieldwork, dual roles and research ethics. *Ethnography, 20*(1), 8–26.
Bourke, B. (2014). Positionality: Reflecting on the research process. *The Qualitative Report, 19*(33), 1–9.
Bryman, A. (2016). *Social research methods* (5th ed.). Oxford: Oxford University Press.
Christensen, C. (2004). Children's participation in ethnographic research: Issues of power and representation. *Children & Society, 18*(2), 165–176.
Cram, F., and Adcock, A. (2022). Kaupapa Māori research. In P. Liamputtong (Ed.), *Handbook of qualitative cross-cultural research methods* (pp. 56–84). Cheltenham, Gloucestershire: Edward Elgar Publishing.
Day, S. (2012). A reflexive lens: Exploring dilemmas of qualitative methodology through the concept of reflexivity. *Qualitative Sociology Review, 8*, 60–85.
Dickson-Swift, V., James, E., Kippen, S., and Liamputtong, P. (2006). Blurring boundaries in qualitative health research on sensitive topics. *Qualitative Health Research, 16*(6), 853–871.
Dwyer, S., and Buckle, J. (2009). The space between: On being an insider-outsider in qualitative research. *International Journal of Qualitative Methods, 8*(1), 54–63.
Fenge, L., Oakley, L., Taylor, B., and Beer, S. (2019). The impact of sensitive research on the researcher: Preparedness and positionality. *International Journal of Qualitative Methods, 18*, 1–18.
Fetterman, D. (2008). Emic/Etic distinction. In L. Given (Ed.), *The Sage encyclopedia of qualitative research methods*. London: Sage.
Finlay, L. (2002). "Outing" the researcher: The provenance, process, and practice of reflexivity. *Qualitative Health Research, 12*(4), 531–545.
Gair, S. (2012). Feeling their stories: Contemplating empathy, insider/outsider positionings, and enriching qualitative research. *Qualitative Health Research, 22*(1), 134–143.
Geddis-Regan, A., Exley, C., and Taylor, G. (2021). Navigating the dual role of clinician-researcher in qualitative dental research. *JDR Clinical & Translational Research, 7*(2), 215–217.
Geertz, C. (1973). *The interpretation of cultures*. New York, NY: Basic Books.
Grix, J. (2019). *The foundations of research*. London: Macmillan International.
Hanson, R., and Richards, P. (2017). Sexual harassment and the construction of ethnographic knowledge. *Sociological Forum, 32*(3), 587–609.
Hayfield, N., and Huxley, C. (2015). Insider and outsider perspectives: Reflections on researcher identities in researcher with lesbian and bisexual women. *Qualitative Research in Psychology, 12*(2), 91–106.
Hiller, A., and Vears, D. (2016). Reflexivity and the clinician-researcher: Managing participant misconceptions. *Qualitative Research Journal, 16*(1), 13–25.
Holmes, A. (2020). Researcher positionality – a consideration of its influence and place in qualitative research: A new researcher guide. *International Journal of Education, 8*(4), 1–10.

Jacobson, D., and Mustafa, N. (2019). Social identity map: A reflexivity tool for practicing explicit positionality in critical qualitative research. *International Journal of Qualitative Methods, 18*, 1–12.

Lakeman, R., McAndrew, S., MacGabhann, L. et al. (2013). "That was helpful… no one has talked to me about that before": Research participation as a therapeutic activity. *International Journal of Mental Health Nursing, 22*(1), 76–84.

Long, C., and Eagle, G. (2009). Ethics in tension: Dilemmas for clinicians conducting sensitive research. *Psycho-Analytic Psychotherapy in South Africa, 17*(2), 27–52.

Manohar, N., Liamputtong, P., Bhole, S., and Arora, A. (2017). Researcher positionality in cross-cultural and sensitive research. In P. Liamputtong (Ed.), *Handbook of research methods in health social sciences*. Singapore: Springer.

May, T., and Perry, B. (2017). *Reflexivity: The essential guide*. London: Sage.

Mercer, J. (2007). The challenges of insider research in educational institutions: Wielding a double-edged sword and resolving delicate dilemmas. *Oxford Review of Education, 33*(1), 1–17.

Merton, R. (1972). Insiders and outsiders: A chapter in the sociology of knowledge. *American Journal of Sociology, 78*(1), 9–47.

Mohler, E., and Rudman, D. (2022). Negotiating the insider/outsider researcher position within qualitative disability studies research. *The Qualitative Report, 27*(6), 1511–1521.

Naaeke, A., Kurylo, A., Grabowski, M., Linton, D., and Radford, M. (2010). Insider and outsider perspective in ethnographic research. *Proceedings of the 68th New York State Communication Association*. https://docs.rwu.edu/cgi/viewcontent.cgi?article=1017&context=nyscaproceedings

Nagar, R., and Geiger, S. (2007). Reflexivity and positionality in feminist fieldwork revisited. In A. Tickell, E. Sheppard, J. Peck, and T. Barnes (Ed.), *Policy and practice in economic geography* (pp. 267–278). London: Sage.

O'Reilly, M., Levine, D., and Law, E. (2021). Digital ethics of care philosophy to understand adolescents' sense of responsibility on social media. *Pastoral Care in Education, 39*(2), 91–107.

O'Reilly, M., and Parker, N. (2014). *Doing mental health research with children and adolescents: A guide to qualitative methods*. London: Sage.

Reich, J. (2021). Power, positionality, and the ethic of care in qualitative research. *Qualitative Sociology, 44*, 575–581.

Sanghera, G., and Thapar-Bjorkert, S. (2008). Methodological dilemmas: Gatekeepers and positionality in Bradford. *Ethnic & Racial Studies, 31*(3), 543–562.

Savin-Baden, M., and Major, C. (2013). *Qualitative research: The essential guide to theory and practice*. Abingdon: Routledge.

Schön, D. (1983). *The reflective practitioner*. New York, NY: Basic Books.

Schostak, J., and Schostak, J. (2013). *Writing research critically: Developing the power to make a difference*. London: Routledge.

Slote, M. (2007). *Ethics of care and empathy*. London: Routledge.

Tinker, C., and Armstrong, N. (2008). From the outside looking in: How an awareness of difference can benefit the qualitative research process. *The Qualitative Report, 13*(1), 53–60.

Tronto, J. (1994). *Moral boundaries: A political argument for an ethic of care*. New York, NY: Routledge.

Willig, C. (2008). *Introducing qualitative research in psychology* (2nd ed.). Milton Keynes: Open University Press.

Wilson, S., Draper, H., and Ives, J. (2008). Ethical issues regarding recruitment to research studies within the primary care consultation. *Family Practice, 25*(6), 456–461.

CHAPTER 10

Sampling and recruitment

> **Learning objectives**
>
> This chapter enables the reader to:
>
> - Identify different sampling approaches in qualitative research.
> - Recognise some of the challenges of determining sample size.
> - Critically assess the quality indicator – sampling adequacy.
> - Identify the benefits and challenges related to participant recruitment.

Introduction

For your qualitative health research to be successful, you are likely reliant on collecting data from human participants. These participants will be central to informing you about their perceptions, experiences, thoughts, views, opinions, and life events – the analysis of which will provide the empirical insights of your study. Typically, those accounts from a "sample", that is, a small group that represents the whole population of people who fall within the category of your research, are collected and analysed. To do this, you will need to think carefully about your sampling approach, your sample size, the adequacy of that sample size, and the methods of recruitment for your study. In this chapter, we address these decisions and consider some of the benefits and challenges of different methods. We conclude the chapter by reflecting on the issue of participation in research, which has received considerable attention in the research literature, and consider how this connects to certain kinds of proposed vulnerabilities associated with specific populations who may be involved in your project.

Approaches to sampling

On first impressions, sampling in qualitative research can appear complex because of the various ways in which it can be accomplished. Sampling strategy and sample size are typically decisions that funders, ethics committees, journals, and academics often expect to know about in advance of participant recruitment. However, these decisions are complicated as they are often decided over time during the completion of a research project. Problematically, some advice about sampling and sample sizes is derived from standards relating to quantitative research that are not directly applicable to qualitative research which has different criteria as it is not numerical in nature (Nakkeeran, 2016). Whilst sampling is often something that is figured out during a project, it is nonetheless a focal part of the project that requires dedicated consideration.

> **Key point!**
> Sampling has been defined as a process of selecting persons to participate in a research investigation by considering the information they might provide relating to the research problem.
>
> (Oppong, 2013, p. 203)

The sampling approach adopted for a research study needs to be suitable for the research question. This is because, in qualitative research, participants are often sampled deliberately, and additional questions may be generated throughout the process, meaning that sampling approaches may be modified or changed (Moser and Korstjens, 2018). There are many different approaches to sampling available, with a seminal contribution on the subject proposing at least 24 approaches, classified as random/probabilistic or non-random/non-probabilistic schemes (Onwuegbuzie and Leech, 2007).

Onwuegbuzie and Leech argued that the selection of participants for a qualitative study is tied to the goals of qualitative research of gaining insights into phenomena, events, or experiences and usually not to generalise from the findings. In this way, in qualitative research, the sampling approach is determined by conceptual requirements more so than the representativeness of the population (Moser and Korstjens, 2018) and is broadly categorised as either purposeful, convenience, or theoretical sampling (Oppong, 2013).

Purposeful sampling

> **Key point!**
> Purposeful sampling is sometimes referred to as purposive sampling or judgement sampling, and there are different purposeful sampling approaches.

Purposeful sampling is perhaps the most common sampling approach in qualitative research. This type of sampling is especially helpful for the identification and selection of information-rich cases as it allows researchers to identify individuals or groups who have knowledge or experience of the phenomena being explored (Cresswell and Plano-Clark, 2011). The researcher therefore categorises participants in terms of them fulfilling criteria relevant to the goals of the project and the topic explored (Mack, Woodsong, Macqueen et al., 2005). There are different ways in which purposeful sampling can be undertaken, as detailed by Palinkas et al. (2015):

- **Typical case sampling** – when the researcher selects participants to highlight what is average or typical.
- **Homogeneous sampling** – when the researcher selects a sample to represent a subgroup of a population in depth, to simplify analysis or reduce variation (commonly used in focus group research).
- **Snowball sampling** – when a researcher identifies individuals who are known to them or other participants and have similar characteristics or knowledge of the topic or area of investigation.
- **Extreme or deviant cases sampling** – when the researcher selects individuals who can illuminate the atypical as well as the typical.
- **Stratified purposeful sampling** – when a researcher wants to capture variations as opposed to the common characteristics, as each stratum constitutes a homogenous sample (to some extent).
- **Purposeful random sampling** – when a researcher designs a sampling strategy as a means of ensuring the credibility of results by selecting participants from a random sample.
- **Opportunistic sampling** – when the researcher takes advantage of opportunities to collect data from participants who are available and willing.

Convenience sampling

Convenience sampling is also a common approach to sampling in qualitative research projects. This kind of sampling approach is used where researchers recruit individuals who are easily accessible to the researcher but in a way that is neither strategic nor purposeful in the way other sampling approaches are (like opportunistic sampling) (Palinkas et al., 2015). Another way of representing this is that convenience sampling is a non-probabilistic form of sampling whereby participants are conveniently situated to take part in a research study and are willing to support the researcher in their endeavour.

> **Key point!**
>
> Convenience sampling is generally viewed as the least demanding or difficult of the sampling approaches, as participants are available and less is required by the researcher or team in terms of cost, time, or effort to recruit them.
>
> (Oppong, 2013)

Convenience sampling can be advantageous in qualitative research as the goal is, typically, not generalisability. This sampling strategy is generally cost-effective and provides a simple mechanism for recruiting participants (Jager, Putnick, and Bornstein, 2017). Jager et al. further suggested that where the convenience sample has some homogeneity, there are greater benefits to this kind of approach than when the population is more diverse. As they noted, homogeneous convenience samples are those that are intentionally recruited because of specific sociodemographic characteristics, and thus are homogeneous on one or more of those sociodemographic factors. The challenge for convenience sampling is that because of the low demand and the low effort required to reach participants and recruit them to a study, there is a greater risk of poorer quality data, which has implications for the quality of the analysis and findings (Oppong, 2013).

Theoretical sampling
Theoretical sampling is the third category of sampling approach in qualitative research commonly deployed by researchers. Its use follows the researcher formulating a tentative explanatory theory that is tied to the information obtained through the data, and a new sample is selected and recruited to test this configured theory (Oppong, 2013). As such, when using theoretical sampling, researchers select participants based on the potential of their accounts, or observations of them, and use these accounts/observations to contribute to developing and refining theoretical concepts. Theoretical sampling is often associated with grounded theory methodology (we discuss this approach later in the book), where sampling is viewed as more than simply data generation and the sampling approach is used to contextualise data to build concepts and theory (Conlon, Timonen, Elliott-O'Dare et al., 2020). In relation to grounded theory, theoretical sampling allows data collection for the purpose of generating theory, whereby the researcher can collect, code, and analyse data to refine theory as it emerges through the process (Glaser and Strauss, 1967).

Now that you have a better understanding of the three main categories of approaches to sampling in qualitative research, we encourage you to reflect on these and consider which might be most appropriate or practically possible for your own research (using the reflective activity in Box 10.1).

Box 10.1

Reflecting on sampling approaches

In this activity you will need to reflect on the notes you have already made in your research diary about the specific area/s of interest for your research project and the research questions that you have been formulating. The questions for you to consider in deciding which sampling approach to take have been offered to you in four categories:

- From a pragmatic point of view, consider your financial resources as well as your time frame. This may influence which of these three sampling strategies you choose. For example, do you have the resources to travel to different locations to collect data if your

sample participants are geographically spread out? Also consider what avenues you have to recruit potential participants; for example, where will you advertise, and how will you identify and contact gatekeepers?
- From an idealistic point of view, consider what your aspirations are for your research. Are you starting from a position of "unmotivated looking" without a particular idea of what you intend to find, or do you already have an idea or theory that you would like to test out?
- From the point of view of generating evidence, you may want to consider what knowledge has already been generated in your field of interest. Consider what approach may be most effective to gather data that will add a unique contribution to what is already known.
- From an ethical point of view, consider which sampling strategy offers the most appropriate balance between inconveniencing your participants and providing useful data that will extend the knowledge base on the topic of your enquiry.

Recruiting participants

Sampling relies heavily on your recruitment process, and this can be challenging for health research. Recruitment can be difficult to plan in detail as this is dependent on others who support the process and is, to some degree, unpredictable; therefore, you will need to put in the effort to recruit (Kristensen and Ravn, 2015). Furthermore, recruitment can be especially challenging if your population is considered vulnerable and/or your topic is sensitive (Gibson, 2022) (see Chapter 11). When approaching participants, you need to think about the issues of dual role (see Chapter 9), ethics and the issues of power and coercion (see Chapter 8), how many participants are required (as noted above in this chapter), and whether you need the support of gatekeepers (see Chapter 7), as well as what might be motivating your participants, your inclusion and exclusion criteria.

In the process of recruitment, you need to identify, approach, and motivate people to participate, and you will also need to think about the medium through which you will reach those people (Kristensen and Ravn, 2015). Whilst the internet or advertisements in public spaces like cafes or universities may be helpful in terms of ensuring visibility, a more direct approach in person can also work. McCormick, Crawford, Anderson et al. (1999) described four phases involved in the process of recruitment:

1. **Locating your sample** – you will likely have specific needs in terms of recruitment and the sites you may recruit through, such as hospitals, hospices, schools, mental health outpatient and primary care services, and dental practices.
2. **Screening** – you will have specific interests and goals for your research, so you need to define who is relevant for your sample and screen the larger population for those who meet your needs.
3. **Consent** – there is an ethical dimension to recruitment, and you will need the consent of gatekeepers, participants, and possibly others.
4. **Incentives** – you need to decide whether you are going to incentivise to promote increased recruitment, for example by using gift vouchers or monetary payment.

Recruitment can seem challenging, especially if you are working within tight time constraints and need to complete your project by a specific date.

Reasons why people participate in research

There are different reasons why people agree to participate in health research. There is some evidence that suggests that there are two central ones, which are those that are self-rewarding (like financial reward, experimental treatment that may be beneficial, curiosity, and a sense of self-satisfaction) and those that are altruistic and for the benefit of society (the benefit of future others, help for groups or certain populations, and the advancement of knowledge) (DuBois, 2008). This remains the case with sensitive topics, where participants can report that taking part led to self-understanding and they wanted others to benefit from their experiences (Littlewood, Harris, Gooding et al., 2019). Whilst participants mostly reported participation as a positive experience stemming primarily from a sense of altruism, for some topics of research, there could also be reported dips in mood following participation (Gibson, Boden, Benson, and Brand, 2014).

Incentives are also used in research projects sometimes as a way of compensating participants for the burden of participation. This can also be a motivating factor for some participants as they are directly rewarded in monetary value or entered in a prize draw (Monshat, Vella-Brodrick, Burns, and Herrman., 2011) or in the form of a charity donation. Incentives are necessary to consider as participants sacrifice their time to take part in research. Although the prospect of a voucher to spend at a particular shopping outlet or online may seem attractive, researchers need to consider how much this will sway a decision to participate. However, providing a reward recognises the input from participants and shows an appreciation of their time. In a similar way to considerations in clinical ethics, care must be taken to consider what an appropriate token or incentive would be so that it does not unduly influence prospective participants to take part, for example to overlook any potential risks in taking part in a study. The incentive must be consistent with the commitment expected of the participant to ensure it does not function as a form of soft coercion to take part. Considering the experiences and needs of the population with whom you are undertaking research is vital (see, for example, Afkinich and Blachman-Demner, 2020), as is consistency with international, national, and institutional ethical standards in determining the nature and value of an incentive or payment for taking part (see, for example, Polacsek, Boardman, and McCann, 2017). It also essential to accept that the participant has the right to refuse this if they wish to.

Where the initiative for the research starts

Thinking about recruitment and initiatives is based on the premise that the research project or agenda originated with the research team, and that secondary to that is the process of recruiting suitable participants to fulfil that agenda. Another way of thinking about the research process, and one which has field integrity, is that the impetus or initiation of the project begins with the would-be participants. In other words, a particular group or organisation approaches a potential research team with an idea for a research topic or question that they have already formulated, and requests support in achieving some desired outcomes. This participant-led approach negates the potentially challenging arena of recruitment and incentives because the motivation for the project exists intrinsically in the participant group without any need for extrinsic motivators, and some PPIE activity can help understand this (see Chapter 7).

Inclusion and exclusion criteria

In the recruitment process, you will need to clarify who should be included and excluded from your research project, specifically regarding your inclusion and exclusion criteria. Clarifying these criteria will help you narrow down who you need to approach and where you might recruit those people from. Simply stated, inclusion criteria are those characteristics and conditions that the participants must meet to be able to participate in your project. Your exclusion criteria are those criteria that disqualify certain people from participating in your research. We provide an example below.

Example: The research topic is to explore the levels of satisfaction with their insurance provider among people who have made physical injury claims in the past 12 months.

When thinking about *inclusion* criteria, we want to specify the factors or conditions a person must fulfil to be eligible to be a participant. In this case, these might be:

- Has a health care insurance plan.
- Has made a claim in the past 12 months.
- Is over 18 years old.
- Has had a physical injury.

Now that we have a potential pool of people who could be participants on the basis that they respond "yes" to each of the above questions, we need to think about what additional factors might *exclude* them from being suitable participants. These factors will vary considerably depending on your research context, but the following suggestions are aimed at giving you an idea of some of those exclusion criteria.

- Has also made a mental injury claim in the past 12 months.
- Has a current legal case against their insurance company.
- The injury occurred in another country.
- Does not have any medical evidence related to the injury.

If the pool of potential participants who said "yes" to the inclusion criteria also say "yes" to any of the exclusion criteria, then they will be excluded from the research study.

Sampling adequacy and sample size

Sample size and the markers for sampling adequacy can be somewhat controversial in qualitative research. As you begin to engage with the literature in this area, you will see that there are various kinds of guidance for researchers in terms of deciding how many people would be appropriate or adequate to recruit to a project (see, for example, Dodd and Epstein, 2012, pp. 114–130). Part of the problem is that it is generally accepted that qualitative research requires "small" or "modest" sample sizes without much determination of what constitutes "small", and in terms of assessing sampling adequacy, there are different criteria, and the methodological approach and design are also relevant (Lester and O'Reilly, 2021). There are, however, reasons for keeping a sample size relatively small, and these were outlined by Ritchie, Lewis, McNaughton Nicholls, and Ormston (2014) as being:

- The in-depth nature of the analysis of data means that at some point, little new evidence will be obtained from each additional participant or group.
- It is not the goal of qualitative research to report incidence or prevalence, and so the sample does not need to be used to determine statistically significant discriminatory variables.
- The purpose of qualitative research is to collect data that is rich in detail, and each unit of data will be comprised of interesting information. Thus, the sample size needs to be reasonably small so the researcher can make "good" or full use of the data.
- Qualitative research can be intensive and requires sufficient resources. It would be unmanageable to recruit large numbers of participants for data collection because of time and cost.

A fundamental challenge of sampling is that sample sizes are difficult to determine in advance of a study because qualitative approaches are interpretative, and yet, funders, ethics committees, and educational requirements often expect a clear indication of anticipated sample size from the outset (Sim, Saunders, Waterfield, and Kingstone, 2018). There are, however, some useful things to remember when thinking about your sample size, as suggested by Ritchie et al. (2014), which we outline in Box 10.2.

Box 10.2

Important things to remember about sample sizes (Ritchie et al., 2014)

According to Ritchie et al. (2014), there are several things you can do to help you reflect on the number of participants you need to recruit for your project:

- The heterogeneity of your population will be applicable in your planning. The more diverse the sample, the greater likelihood that you will need to increase your sample size. If the population that you are recruiting is reasonably homogeneous, then a smaller sample will be more acceptable in terms of sampling adequacy.
- The selection criteria will be influential in your decision-making. The relevant criteria need to be considered, as the more criteria you are adhering to, the more participants you are likely to need.
- You will need to consider which nesting of criteria is needed. In other words, when criteria need to be nested, that is, controlling the representation of one criterion within another, the reasons for interdependency between characteristics or need for diversity will necessarily increase your sample size.

- Some groups of special interest will require more intensive study, and to ensure some level of representation and diversity, a larger sample will be needed.
- Some projects require multiple samples, for comparison or to represent different stakeholders to address the question, and a sufficient number of participants from each population is needed.
- The data collection method you are using will influence the sample size needed.
- Pragmatically, the budget and resources available to you will influence how many participants you can afford to recruit.

Data saturation, thematic saturation, and theoretical saturation
Probably the most commonly deployed marker of sampling adequacy in academic research circles is that of saturation. There has been growing acceptance that the adequacy of a qualitative sample is when "saturation" has been reached, which means that both depth as well as breadth of information have been achieved (Bowen, 2008). Problematically, however, the development of the concept of saturation, and the way it is understood and implemented are varied, and we have raised the issue that the value of this as a marker in qualitative research is disputed in the qualitative community regarding its usefulness and appropriateness as a marker (O'Reilly and Parker, 2013). In its simplest conception, saturation is defined as the continuation of data collection from new participants until nothing new is generated (Green and Thorogood, 2009), or until the point where there are no new patterns yielded from the data (Gaskell, 2000). Some researchers have argued that it is not the data that reach a point of saturation; rather, it is the themes and codes that are important; it is these that become saturated as different participants will always use different words (Morse, 2015).

However, these somewhat simplistic views of saturation and the critiques of its usability as a quality indicator have been discussed by researchers in recent years. There are now different types of saturation with different meanings to guide researchers in their thinking. These are generally conceptualised in the following ways (see Favourate, 2020; Saunders et al., 2018):

- **Theoretical saturation** – the generation of conceptual or theoretical categories, typically associated with grounded theory, refers to the point at which the concepts are fully reflected in the data.
- **Thematic or code saturation** – inductive thematic saturation refers to the point where no new codes or themes are identifiable from the data. *A priori* thematic saturation refers to the extent to which the determined codes or themes represent the data.
- **Code saturation** – refers to the point in data collection where no new codes are identifiable.
- **Data saturation** – is the level at which new data simply repeats codes and themes already generated by the analyst.
- **Meaning saturation** – relates to the quality of the data in terms of depth and richness; meaning saturation is the point where no additional information comes from the data, and the researcher can conclude that detailed data have been gathered and meaning has been adequately generated in the analysis.

As different forms of saturation have been discussed in the literature, new ideas about the value of saturation as a marker for sampling adequacy have been appraised. Note that the original meaning of saturation resides with theoretical saturation and was associated with grounded theory. Within this methodological approach, the value of theoretical saturation has retained its central importance where it does not refer to the point at which no new ideas emerge, but illustrates a point at which categories are fully accounted for, the variability between them is explained, and the relationships between them are valid so that a theory can emerge (Glaser and Strauss, 1967; Green and Thorogood, 2009). Although theoretical saturation is tied to grounded theory methodology and in turn a specific meaning and purpose linked to the approach, other conceptualisations of saturation are not intrinsically connected with a specific methodology and have therefore been subject to debate.

In qualitative research more broadly, it has been recognised the term saturation captures "no new information being generated", and this is often considered the gold standard to assure sampling adequacy (Guest, Bunce, and Johnson, 2006). In this qualitative literature, saturation tends to be considered in relation to determining sample size (Guest, Namey, and McKenna, 2017) and research quality (Hancock Amankwaa, Revell, and Mueller, 2016). In determining the point of saturation, according to Guest (2015), there are five factors that influence it being realised:

1. The degree of instrument structure.
2. Sample homogeneity or heterogeneity.
3. Complexity of the study topic.
4. The purpose of the study.
5. Analyst categorisation style.

Additionally, it has been argued that it is necessary to differentiate between coding saturation and meaning saturation, as this relates to the depth of the analysis (Hennink, Kaiser, and Weber, 2017). Hennink et al. argued that code saturation is the point where no new information is identified, and the coding framework is stabilised. They delineated four kinds of codes:

1. **Inductive codes** – those which are content-driven and raised by participants.
2. **Deductive codes** – those that are researcher-driven and developed from the interview guide and literature.
3. **Concrete codes** – those codes referencing explicit and definitive issues.
4. **Conceptual codes** – those that capture the abstract constructs.

(Note that we cover much more about coding later in the book when we come to the matter of data analysis.)

Hennink et al. contended that meaning saturation is different. They defined this as the point at which the issues are fully understood and where there are no additional dimensions, insights, or nuances about those issues to be made. Code saturation is typically achieved much sooner than meaning saturation. Reaching a saturation point and following a strategy to do so has not been fully explored in the literature, one of the more recent procedural approaches was developed by Guest, Namey and Chen (2020) and we outline the steps involved in Box 10.3.

> **Box 10.3**
> **A practical approach to reaching saturation (Guest et al., 2020)**
>
> Guest et al. (2020) have outlined some practical steps for determining the saturation point in research. This is founded on the definition of saturation being when the data produce little or no new useful information in relation to the objectives of the study and are connected to:
>
> - **The base size** – for base size saturation to be assessed, the incoming information must be weighed against the information gathered. Thus, base size is the minimum number of data collection events needed to calculate the information already yielded.
> - **The run length** – refers to the set of consecutive events or data collection points (e.g. number of interviews).
> - **The new information threshold** – this is in terms of what level of information is indicative of saturation.
>
> These steps involved are as follows:
>
> 1. You need to find the theme number for the base size – this requires looking at the first four interviews and identifying the number of unique themes in each interview and then adding them together.
> 2. You then find the number of themes for the first run, using a run length of two, so you include the data for your next two interviews (that is, 5 and 6), and identify how many new themes are evident in each of those.
> 3. At this point, you can calculate your saturation ratio by dividing the new themes in the run length by the number of unique themes in the base set and ascertain if it meets the saturation point that you set.
> 4. If at this point, it does not meet that threshold, then add a further run of two more interviews, 7 and 8, and repeat.
> 5. Now you can update your saturation ratio by taking the number of themes in the new run and dividing it by the number of themes in your base set.
> 6. Repeat steps four and five until you reach your threshold. You can then identify your actual saturation point.

It is necessary to recognise that there are different ideas about the meaning of codes and themes, which are often associated with the different kinds of thematic analysis (we return to this later in the book in Chapter 18). Consequently, saturation tends to rely on an understanding of codes and themes as fixed entities pre-existing the analysis and residing in the data to be found, which is arguably inappropriate, especially for certain methodologies (Braun and Clarke, 2019). Saturation and the point at which it might be reached have been subject to critique, which is especially pertinent for some methodological approaches. It has long been argued that the idea of saturation is not congruent with all methodologies in qualitative research (O'Reilly and Parker, 2013), with some arguments that the very notion of "no new information" is a logical fallacy as there are always possible novel insights to be accomplished from new participants (Low, 2019).

For some methodological approaches, like some forms of discourse analysis, conversation analysis, and reflexive thematic analysis (discussed later in the book, in Chapters 18 and 19), the coding and analytic process does not reach a fixed endpoint. Instead, in approaches like reflexive thematic analysis, the researcher engages in an interpretive and situated judgement about when to conclude sampling, when to stop coding, and when the themes in the data are exhaustive so they can map the thematic relationship and write up the findings of the project (Braun and Clarke, 2019). Furthermore, in terms of sampling adequacy, saturation as a marker is typically discussed in relation to orthodox data collection methods, such as interviews and focus groups, and is arguably less appropriate for other forms of data, for example, naturally occurring data, observation, text, and so forth (see Chapter 13 for a full discussion).

Now that you have had an opportunity to think about when and how saturation may or may not be a useful marker for sampling adequacy, we encourage you to align this learning with your own project and answer the questions in Box 10.4.

Box 10.4

Reflective activity on sampling adequacy

There are critiques of saturation as a marker for sampling adequacy. However, there are circumstances wherein it can be a useful way of determining appropriate sample sizes, especially for interviews or focus groups with relatively homogeneous samples and using certain analytic approaches. We now encourage you to think about the following questions in relation to your learning and your own project.

- What do you see as the benefits of using saturation as a marker for sampling adequacy?
- What do you see as the main criticisms of using saturation as a marker for sampling adequacy?
- How appropriate (or not) is saturation as a marker for sampling adequacy in your own project?

Information power

While saturation may be considered a gold standard for sampling adequacy, we have shown that this is arguably a less appropriate marker for studies not using interviews or focus groups as data collection methods, and for specific methodologies whereby theory and epistemology are contrary to the principles of saturation. For methodologies and data collection methods that do not neatly align with saturation, an alternative way of thinking about sampling adequacy is that of analytical sufficiency. This involves a greater focus on the rigour of the analytic process and the richness of the data (LaDonna, Artino, and Balmer, 2021). LaDonna et al. argued that, unlike saturation which is premised on the idea of an objective saturation point, the notion of sufficiency acknowledges the uniqueness of human experience and the socially constructed nature of qualitative data, as well as the iterative development of using interview questions and sampling new participants with multiple, overlapping stages of analysis.

> **Key point!**
>
> Research studies cannot go on indefinitely with recruitment and sampling having to stop at some point. The notion of analytical sufficiency helps consider parameters in relation to this process focussing on analytic rigour and the richness of data.
>
> (LaDonna et al., 2021)

Because of the iterative nature of qualitative research, the importance of depth rather than breadth, and the relevance of epistemologies that challenge or reject the idea of an objective reality or neutral perspective, information power can provide a more meaningful way of deciding on sample sizes and recruitment. Information power refers to the idea that the more relevant information that a sample of people may hold, the fewer participants are necessary (Malterud, Siersma, and Guassora, 2016). In this respect, the notion directly challenges the idea that larger samples equate to better data, as this is not the case given that in qualitative research, it is the quality that is more meaningful than the quantity (LaDonna et al., 2021). As Malterud et al. (2016) reported, in determining information power, there are five dimensions to account for:

1. **The aims of the research** – narrower aims require fewer participants. Studies with broad aims will need a larger sample size, so researchers can make their aims more focused and precise to ensure sufficient information power with smaller samples.
2. **Specificity of the sample** – studies involving unique types of participants warrant smaller sample sizes. Where participants have characteristics specific to the aim of the study, a smaller sample is beneficial.
3. **Established theory** – studies that are theoretically informed require fewer participants. Therefore, the level of theoretical background is relevant as where there is a limited theoretical perspective, a larger sample is necessary to provide sufficient information power as theory serves to "synthesise existing knowledge" and expand the source of knowledge beyond empirical data.
4. **Quality of dialogue** – research involving high-quality dialogue needs fewer participants. This relates to communication between the researcher and the participant as data are co-constructed.
5. **Analytic strategy** – research projects that require greater depth necessitate fewer participants.

Additionally, the length and depth of the interview or focus group (or nature of other kinds of data) will have an impact on information power, as studies involving shorter interviews will need more participants than when longer, in-depth interviews are used (LaDonna et al., 2021).

Determining sample size

Using saturation or information power in qualitative projects can, to some extent, help you determine how many participants you need for your research. When we talk about sample size in this section, we are referring mostly to the number of participants you recruit for your project, which aligns well with interviews and focus groups, and to some extent, case studies and observations, but less well with other methods of data collection (see Chapter 14 for further discussion).

> **Key point!**
>
> The method of data collection should be considered in relation to sample size, as some methods rely more on the volume of data (number of minutes, number of events recorded, etc.) than they do the number of people recruited.

Arguably, estimating in advance the number of people required for a study can be advantageous, as this reduces the likelihood of wasted funds, additional burdens on the study population, and wasted data left unanalysed. It ensures the sample is sufficient to capture the phenomenon investigated (Hennink et al., 2017). It is, however, challenging to think about how many people you need to recruit in advance, and an interesting series of articles was presented by Baker and Edwards (2012) where various propositions are made by different authors, and recognition that the number is dependent on the scope of the study, the nature of the research question, and the epistemological framework. We argue also that the method and its style, as well as the methodology, are essential to consider. We invite you to contemplate the hypothetical scenarios in Box 10.5 and think about how these might influence the sample size needed for those projects.

> **Box 10.5**
>
> **Reflective activity on sample size**
>
> In each example below, think about how sample size and sample homogeneity/heterogeneity might affect choices about sample size. Consider these hypothetical propositions:
>
> - An interviewer recruits ten 11-year-old-girls from one school and interviews each of them for 20 minutes individually about their physical activity levels. The participants are all the same age and gender, and all from the same geographic area, and so there is some homogeneity in the sample, and the interviews are relatively short.
> - Interviews are conducted with adults aged between 18 and 85, male and female, from different ethnic backgrounds from five different countries, and each interview lasts about one hour. Here you have heterogeneity in the sample and longer interviews.
> - University students from one university participate in an interview where all participants are asked the same ten questions about the impact of academic pressure on their well-being. Interviews last approximately 30 minutes each, and all the participants are male. Again, there is relative homogeneity in the sample, and the interviews are quite short with the same questions asked of all participants.

While it is difficult to anticipate in advance how many people you will need to recruit for your study, the guidance in this chapter so far should give you some impression. There is also research that has provided general markers for thinking about how you might provide this information for your funder, educational institution, and/or ethics committee (see, for example, Mason, 2010). Clarke and Braun (2019) found that the number of participants recruited for qualitative interview-based studies tended to be between 21 and 25. In terms of saturation of a single population sample (e.g. female children, patients with epilepsy, older adults with Parkinson's disease), proposals have been put forward for determining the number at which saturation is likely to be reached, thus predicting the sample size.

One example that is widely cited was that offered by Francis, Johnston, Robertson, et al. (2010) who considered sampling for interview studies. They argued that researchers can have an *a priori* impression of the sample size in interview-based research where the sample is relatively homogeneous and, from their work, suggested the saturation point is approximately ten people, but that up to three more interviews should be conducted to check that no new ideas or material are evident. They referred to this point as the "stopping criterion" (Francis et al., 2010). If new ideas are then identifiable in the data, then a further three are required, and the researcher keeps adding three as appropriate. Arguably, this is needed for each population included. So, for example, if you are recruiting young people with learning disabilities and their carers, you essentially have two populations and need to ensure saturation for both. Heterogeneity is heavily influential on the choice of sample size. Research has shown, for example, that for cross-cultural research, saturation can be achieved at 16 interviews, but this is not sufficient to identify the meta-themes that are pertinent across sites, where 20–40 interviews were warranted (Hagaman and Wutich, 2017).

> **Key point!**
>
> It can still be challenging for researchers to know when to stop recruiting additional participants despite guidance in the literature.
>
> (Constantinou, Georgiou, and Perdikogianni, 2017)

As mentioned above, much of the literature around saturation and information power refers to interviews and focus groups, but notably, the discussions around focus groups (and indeed other data collection methods) are more limited, and it can be challenging to determine how many focus groups to conduct and how many participants to include in each (see Chapter 14 for this discussion). In terms of saturation, discussions have focused on an adequate number of focus groups conducted. For example, in a review, Guest et al. (2017) found that many textbooks did not provide guidance for focus groups, and those that did tended to use saturation as the marker. There are fewer papers that discuss the saturation point of focus groups, but those that have considered this for sampling adequacy recommended approximately five (Coenen et al., 2012) to eight focus groups suffice (Kirchberger et al., 2009). Yet, more recent work has suggested that 2–3 focus groups are likely to capture at least 80% of the themes if the sample is reasonably homogeneous (Guest et al., 2017).

As we have discussed in this chapter, there are multiple factors to bear in mind when making decisions about sampling strategy and sampling adequacy. This is illustrated by Linda Homan, who describes her experience of recruiting participants for health research in Box 10.6.

> **Box 10.6**
>
> **Linda Homan's experience of making sampling decisions in health research**
>
> > Linda Homan is a qualified social worker and has worked in adult and child protection, and Mental Health Act Assessments as part of an Emergency Duty Team. She has also worked as a Senior Practitioner in a CAMHS Home Treatment team. Linda is currently a lecturer in social work.
>
> Sampling in qualitative research can be a dynamic tension between the availability of participants, opportunities for participant involvement, sign-up, and location of the sample as the practical aspects; and getting enough participants to achieve "saturation" in terms of when enough data collected, and what constitutes the right data. To illustrate this, I draw on examples from a study I am planning and a previous study I undertook across a wide geographical area, which used both individual interviews and focus groups.
>
> You need a rationale for decisions made in sampling choices. For a county-wide project exploring youth smoking uptake, the sample had to be multi-site and purposive. This was to ensure that the geographical areas were represented in the study, and that the young people chosen had actually experienced smoking or had definite views on smoking. I also narrowed this to a specific limit (13–17-year-olds). My lower age limit was set at 13 upwards in the smoking study because it allowed them to reflect on smoking at an earlier age and allowed for the possibility of those taking up smoking later on also having opportunities to contribute. Using mixed methods, quantitative data which went out to a wider youth population, alongside the qualitative narratives, provided key insights into the prevalence of smoking, key reasons for smoking uptake or refusal, and socioeconomic impact.
>
> In the study I am planning, I have identified two groups who meet separately on a single site. These two groups represent a group of young people who are at risk of not being engaged within the community, and a group that is involved in community projects. Using contrasting groups can provide limitations and benefits. Being aware of stigmatisation, oversimplification, and selection bias, the benefits of these contrasting groups' insights could yield rich insights into any key similarities or differences related to engagement and disengagement. To ensure a better understanding in this process, key socioeconomic and contextual factors will also be examined. I think the researcher has to immerse themself in the scenarios and use a "sociological imagination" to think through sampling and how the best quality data can be reached. A desire to explore and some awareness of the lived experiences of the population to be studied are also important when planning the sample.

Author reflections and concluding remarks

From Philip

Working on this chapter with my co-authors, I am struck by just how much researchers (have to) account for in developing a sampling and recruitment strategy – and am reminded of the common questions novice clinician-researchers can ask, of "How many participants is enough?" and "How much material do I need?" Of course, the short answer to these questions, which one can discern from this chapter, is that it depends… and it depends on lots of different things.

Inevitably, when seeking to undertake research, alongside other commitments and constraints on one's time as a practising professional, pragmatism can be important. Moreover, there are issues that arise during research that are unanticipated. In my own doctoral research, an interview-based study with child welfare professionals, I had an unfortunate experience (or fortunate – depending on how one looks at it). I believed I had access to interview professionals within one local authority team, in the form of an initial agreement from a senior manager, only to be told some months later that it would not be possible to facilitate access due to other demands on practitioners' time. The same manager then informed me, some months later again, that they could facilitate the research, and this was after I had secured access to professionals from another local authority and completed interviews there. In all, I ended up doing about ten more interviews than I had initially planned to. Whilst this was beneficial for the research, there was a lot of data to work with, and I spent about two months just transcribing the interviews.

For me, this experience reinforces how sampling strategies and issues of recruitment and data saturation are essential to consider from the very outset of a project, that is, in developing a proposal and protocol for a study. Whilst challenges with recruitment are difficult to predict, planning well affords an opportunity to reduce the material costs and time expended in undertaking research; this process of reflection, which can seem quite abstract, serves to ensure one is more efficient as a researcher. It also supports ethical practice as it reduces the potential burden on prospective participants and services involved in the research.

References

Afkinich, J., and Blachman-Demner, D. (2020). Providing incentives to youth participants in research: A literature review. *Journal of Empirical Research on Human Research Ethics*, 15(3), 202–215.

Baker, S., and Edwards, R. (Eds.). (2012). *How many qualitative interviews is enough? Expert voices and early career reflections on sampling and cases in qualitative research*. Working paper. National Centre for Research Methods: ESRC.

Bowen, G. (2008). Naturalistic inquiry and the saturation concept: A research note. *Qualitative Research*, 8(1), 137–142.

Braun, V., and Clarke, V. (2019). To saturate or not to saturate? Questioning data saturation as a useful concept for thematic analysis and sample-size rationales. *Qualitative Research in Sport, Exercise & Health*, 13, 201–216.

Clarke, V., and Braun, V. (2019). Feminist qualitative methods and methodologies in psychology: A review and reflection. *Psychology of Women & Equalities Review*, 2(1), 13–28.

Coenen, M., Coenen, T., Stamm, A., Stucki, G., and Cieza, A. (2012). Individual interviews and focus groups in patients with rheumatoid arthritis: A comparison of two qualitative methods. *Quality of Life Research, 21*, 359–370.

Conlon, C., Timonen, V., Elliott-O'Dare, C., O'Keeffe, S., and Foley, G. (2020). Confused about theoretical sampling? Engaging theoretical sampling in diverse grounded theory studies. *Qualitative Health Research, 30*(6), 947–959.

Constantinou, C., Georgiou, M., and Perdikogianni, M (2017). A Comparative Method for Themes Saturation (CoMETS) in qualitative research. *Qualitative Research, 17*(5), 571–588.

Cresswell, J., and Plano-Clark, V. (2011). *Designing and conducting mixed method research* (2nd ed.). Thousand Oaks, CA: Sage.

Dodd, S., and Epstein, I. (2012). *Practice-based research in social work: A guide for reluctant researchers*. London: Routledge.

DuBois, J. (2008). *Ethics in mental health research: Principles, guidance, and cases*. Oxford: Oxford University Press.

Favourate, Y. (2020). Saturation controversy in qualitative research: Complexities and underlying assumptions, a literature review. *Cogent Social Sciences, 6*(1), 1838706.

Francis, J., Johnston, M., Robertson, C., Glidewell, L., Entwistle, V., Eccles, M., and Grimshaw, J. (2010). What is adequate sample size? Operationalising data saturation for theory-based interview studies. *Psychology & Health, 25*(10), 1229–1245.

Gaskell, G. (2000). Individual and group interviewing. In M. Bauer and G. Gaskell (Eds.), *Qualitative researching with text, image and sound* (pp. 38–56). London: Sage.

Gibson, K. (2022). Bridging the digital divide: Reflections on using WhatsApp messenger interviews in youth research. *Qualitative Research in Psychology, 19*(3), 611–631.

Gibson, S., Boden, Z., Benson, O., and Brand, S. (2014). The impact of participating in suicide research online. *Suicide and Life-Threatening Behavior, 44*(4), 372–383.

Glaser B., and Strauss A. (1967). *The discovery of grounded theory: Strategies for qualitative research*. New York, NY: Aldine.

Green, J., and Thorogood, N. (2009). *Qualitative methods for health research* (2nd ed.). Thousand Oaks, CA: Sage.

Guest, G. (2015). Sampling and selecting participants in field research. In H. Bernard and C. Gravlee (Eds.), *Handbook of methods in cultural anthropology* (2nd ed.) (pp. 215–250). Lanham, MD: Rowman and Littlefield.

Guest, G., Bunce, A., and Johnson, L. (2006). How many interviews are enough? An experiment with data saturation and variability. *Field Methods, 18*(1), 59–82.

Guest, G., Namey, E., and Chen, M. (2020). A simple method to assess and report thematic saturation in qualitative research. *PLoS One, 15*(5), e0232076.

Guest, G., Namey, E., and McKenna, K. (2017). How many focus groups are enough? Building an evidence base for nonprobability sample sizes. *Field Methods, 29*(1), 3–22.

Hagaman, A., and Wutich, A. (2017). How many interviews are enough to identify metathemes in multi-sited and cross-cultural research? Another perspective on Guest, Bunce, and Johnson's (2006) landmark study. *Field Methods, 29*, 23–41.

Hancock, M., Amankwaa, L., Revell, M., and Mueller, D. (2016). Focus group data saturation: A new approach to data analysis. *The Qualitative Report, 21*(11), 2121–2130.

Hennink, M., Kaiser, B., and Weber, M. (2017). Code saturation versus meaning saturation: How many interviews are enough? *Qualitative Health Research, 27*(4), 591–608.

Jager, J., Putnick, D., and Bornstein, M. H. II. (2017). More than just convenient: The scientific merits of homogeneous convenience samples. *Monographs of the Society for Research in Child Development, 82*(2), 13–30.

Kirchberger, I., Coenen, M., Hierl, F., Dieterle, C., Seissler, J., Stucki, G., and Cieza, A. (2009). Validation of the international classification of functioning, disability and health (ICF) core set for diabetes mellitus from the patient perspective using focus groups. *Diabetic Medicine, 26*, 700–707.

Kristensen, G., and Ravn, M. (2015). The voices heard and the voices silenced: Recruitment processes in qualitative interview studies. *Qualitative Research*, 15(6), 722–737.

LaDonna, K., Artino, A., and Balmer, D. (2021). Beyond the guise of saturation: Rigor and qualitative interview data. Editorial. *Journal of Graduate Medical Education*, 13(5), 607–611.

Lester, J. N., and O'Reilly, M. (2021). Introduction to special issue quality in qualitative approaches: Celebrating heterogeneity. *Qualitative Research in Psychology*, 18(3), 295–304.

Littlewood, D., Harris, K., Gooding, P., Pratt, D., Haddock, G., and Peters, S. (2019). Using my demons to make good: The short- and long-term impact of participating in suicide-related research. *Archives of Suicide Research*, 25(2), 315–339.

Low, J. (2019). A pragmatic definition of the concept of theoretical saturation. *Sociological Focus*, 52(2), 131–139.

Mack, N., Woodsong, C. Macqueen, K., Guest, G., and Namey, E. (2005). *Qualitative research methods: A data collector's field guide*. North Carolina: Family Health International.

Malterud, K., Siersma, V., and Guassora, A (2016). Sample size in qualitative interview studies: Guided by information power. *Qualitative Health Research*, 26(13), 1753–1760.

Mason, M. (2010). Sample size and saturation in PhD studies using qualitative interviews. *Forum qualitative Sozialforschung/Forum: Qualitative Social Research*, 11(3).

McCormick, L., Crawford, M., Anderson, R., Gittelsohn, J., Kingsley, B., and Upson, D. (1999). Recruiting adolescents into qualitative tobacco research studies: Experiences and lessons learned. *Journal of School Health*, 69(3), 95–99.

Monshat, K., Vella-Brodrick, D., Burns, J., and Herrman, H. (2011). Mental health promotion in the Internet age: A consultation with Australian young people to inform the design of an online mindfulness training programme. *Health Promotion International*, 27(2), 177–186.

Morse, J. (2015). Data were saturated... *Qualitative Health Research*, 25(5), 147–149.

Moser, A., and Korstjens, I. (2018). Practical guidance to qualitative research. Part 3: Sampling, data collection and analysis. *European Journal of General Practice*, 24(1), 9–18.

Nakkeeran, N. (2016). Is sampling a misnomer in qualitative research? *Sociological Bulletin*, 65(1), 40–49.

Onwuegbuzie, A., and Leech, N. (2007). Validity and qualitative research: An oxymoron? *Quality & Quantity*, 41, 233–249.

Oppong, S. (2013). The problem of sampling in qualitative research. *Asian Journal of Management Sciences & Education*, 2(2), 202–210.

O'Reilly, M., and Parker, N. (2013). Unsatisfactory saturation': A critical exploration of the notion of saturated sample sizes in qualitative research. *Qualitative Research*, 13(2), 190–197.

Palinkas, L., Horwitz, S., Green, C., Wisdom, J., Duan, N., and Hoagwood, K. (2015). Purposeful sampling for qualitative data collection and analysis in mixed method implementation research. *Administration and Policy in Mental Health & Mental Health*, 42(5), 533–544.

Polacsek, M., Boardman, G., and McCann, T. (2017). Paying patient and caregiver research participants: Putting theory into practice. *Journal of Advanced Nursing*, 73(4), 847–856.

Ritchie, J., Lewis, J., McNaughton Nicholls, C., and Ormston, R. (2014). *Qualitative research practice: A guide for social science students and researchers* (2nd ed.). Thousand Oaks, CA: Sage.

Saunders, B., Sim, J., Kingstone, T., Baker, S. Waterfield, J., Bartlam, B., Burroughs, H., and Jinks, C. (2018). Saturation in qualitative research: Exploring its conceptualization and operationalization. *Quality & Quantity*, 52(4), 1893–1907.

Sim, J., Saunders, B., Waterfield, J., and Kingstone, T. (2018). Can sample size in qualitative research be determined a priori? *International Journal of Social Research Methodology*, 21(5), 619–634.

CHAPTER 11

Sensitivity, vulnerability, and barriers to participation

Learning objectives

This chapter enables the reader to:

- Critically assess the meaning of "sensitive research" in relation to health research.
- Evaluate debates about participation.
- Critically evaluate the concept of vulnerability.
- Address the challenges of language, particularly in relation to the term vulnerability and "seldom-heard" and "hard-to-reach" populations.
- Recognise the ways in which some populations may be considered vulnerable by virtue of certain demographic factors.

Introduction

As has been acknowledged in previous chapters, qualitative health research undertaken by practitioners in healthcare settings can involve populations considered vulnerable, "seldom-heard" and "hard-to-reach", as well as topics that are sensitive in nature, for example in relation to mental ill-health, stigma, life threatening conditions, or child safeguarding. Indeed, healthcare practitioners can be motivated to undertake research based on ethical complexities encountered in their direct practice (see, for example, Dodd and Epstein, 2012).

Extending the discussion, this chapter considers issues of power and vulnerability in more detail than in Chapters 8 and 9, in relation to participation. We consider how participation can be promoted by you as a researcher and power shared with participants in a meaningful, rather than tokenistic, way, and what it means to undertake research on sensitive topics and/or with vulnerable populations. As part of the chapter, we also critically consider the concept of vulnerability as applied to research participants.

Levels of participation

To what level research participants are engaged in research connects to the ethical principle of justice – that is, an opportunity to contribute to and benefit from research and not be discriminated against in research based on specific characteristics. Certain groups in society have historically been excluded from research or subjected to victimisation or exploitation, raising questions about the right to informed participation and the pertinence of power. Given different power differentials in research, for participation to be meaningful, inequalities of power need to be recognised and effective ways of working managed (Beresford, 2021). Researchers also need to create pathways where participants can experience freedom and some control in the research (Gibson, 2022). We encourage you to return to Chapter 9 at this point and remind yourself of the challenge of power in relation to role identity, particularly in the context of dual roles where there may be a risk of misuse (inadvertent or deliberate) of power in the research relationship. We return to the issue of power here because of its strong connection to the challenge of participation, especially in relation to vulnerability.

A principal way in which power is realised within research is in terms of how the concept of knowledge is used, with knowledge-making considered to be the domain of adult experts (Kellett, 2014). However, as Kellett has argued, through a process of consultation, other groups, like children and vulnerable adults, can generate knowledge and have a more active role in the project. Researchers thus hold a responsibility to facilitate the active participation of those whose voices are not typically heard, and we return to some of these concepts later in the chapter.

The idea of "promotion of participation and inclusion" is frequently used in the literature and is argued to involve three main phases: listening to participants, consulting with participants, and involving participants in decision-making (Kellett, 2014). There have been various models proposed in the literature for this, some focused specifically on children as one of the unrepresented groups in society, and others more on participation generally. One example is Hart's (1992) ladder of children's participation, where Hart suggested there are different layers of participation that researchers can facilitate, from the lower rungs of manipulation and tokenism to those that are increasingly empowering, such as being informed, to being consulted and informed, to the highest rung of child-initiated shared decision making. While the ladder of participation was a helpful starting point for reflection, it is a hierarchical way of thinking about participation with the powerful bestowing rights on the powerless (John, 1996) and lacks adequate acknowledgement of cultural context (Treseder, 1997). This is not dissimilar to Arnstein's (1969) ladder as a popular model of representing involvement, like participation. Arnstein's ladder also visually represents rungs of a ladder, with the lower levels of involvement referring to non-participation and tokenism, moving up towards "degrees of citizen power" which links to partnership and ownership. Yet another well-known, but more generalised model is Shier's (2001) model of participation whereby the lower levels consider avenues for listening to participants up to higher levels of sharing responsibility and power with the researcher.

> **Key point!**
>
> Hierarchical and layered models of participation have been subject to critique as they are typically based on an individual task which is assigned a single level of participation. This fails to adequately engage with how decision-making power shifts within a research project and within the different tasks associated with the project.
>
> (Kirby and Gibbs, 2006)

Kellett (2014) argued that meaningful participation of populations who are not always heard (like children and young people) is best understood by attending to their personal experiences. She contended that participation is an "act of doing" and requires participants to be actively involved and express themselves freely. Lundy (2007) influentially conceptualised children's (and young people's) voice in terms of four interrelated elements which, though not initially focused on research, are relevant to it:

1. **Space** – children being afforded opportunities to form and express their views in a safe, inclusive environment.
2. **Voice** – children being given a platform to express their views. This includes a recognition of the possibility of them expressing these views in multiple ways.
3. **Audience** – others listening to these views. This is to say that children's views are communicated to persons identified and recognised by the children as having the power to consider their views meaningfully.
4. **Influence** – the receptiveness of others to children's views, that is, these views being taken seriously along with requisite action. This includes ensuring that the views are heard by persons with adequate power to bring about change and a recognition that children should be adequately informed about how their views were heard and influenced the process of decision-making.

Notably, the voices of vulnerable groups are starting to be heard in policy and practice, but research has further to go to ensure this becomes a norm (Kellett, 2014). Kellett further argued that agency is central to voice, as the fulfilment of participation and voice relies on agency to change or influence areas that impact them in their lives, and it is especially disempowering when those with power fail to listen and act on their views. You may or may not be including groups in your research that might be in some way disadvantaged, marginalised, or positioned as vulnerable, but promoting participation in equal and fair ways is central in health research, and giving voice to those who may not routinely be heard has benefits. Via the activity in Box 11.1, we encourage you to think about how you are giving voice and promoting inclusion in your research project

VULNERABILITY AND BARRIERS TO PARTICIPATION

> **Box 11.1**
> **Reflective activity on promoting participation**
>
> From your reading in this chapter thus far, and the section related to power and your professional identity and role in Chapter 9, we invite you to think about what active steps you are taking to promote participation, be receptive to different voices, value inclusion, and encourage agency in your own research project.
>
> In your research diary, write down some of the ways in which you might accomplish this and think about the strategies you might use to reduce issues relating to power in your work. Try to make a bullet point list of the practical ways you can attend to these issues and what challenges you might face in implementation.

Doing research involving sensitive topics

Certain kinds of qualitative projects increase the potential for risk of harm to participants more than others, such as through sensitive research. It is typically understood that some research topics are sensitive in nature. With the contemporary social concern with "cancel culture", a term which refers to the public boycotting or ostracisation of individuals, groups, or organisations for actions or statements deemed unacceptable or offensive, this has added some controversy to our understanding of what "sensitive" means for researchers (Mallon, Borgstrom, and Murphy, 2021). While the idea of what constitutes a sensitive area of research varies according to perspective and is therefore potentially complex, it is nonetheless acknowledged that the more sensitive the project, the greater the risk of possible emotional or psychological harm to the researcher and/or the participants.

> **Key point!**
>
> Harm or damage may be physical, emotional, psychological, social, political, economic, or professional, and sensitive research may lead to distress or discomfort for the researcher or the participants, or both.
>
> (Butler, Copnell, and Hall, 2019)

Sensitive topics are definable as those which involve the exploration of acutely personal experiences of participants, which are potentially laden with emotional aspects of their lives, with the likelihood of inducing short-term psychological distress as they recount their narratives (Silverio, Sheen, Bramante et al., 2022). Sensitivity can also relate to the demographic profile of the participants, in that the participants are typically vulnerable or disadvantaged (Liamputtong, 2007). Defining sensitive research requires attention, as sensitive phenomena can relate to specific culturally shaped assumptions and may reference the private worlds of participants that could generate emotional responses and may also be sensitive politically or because of societal stigma (McCosker, Barnard, and Gerber, 2001).

> **Key point!**
>
> Research exploring sensitive topics has predominantly been undertaken using qualitative approaches and methods.
>
> (Mallon and Elliott, 2021).

Although it is challenging to define exactly what constitutes a sensitive research topic (Mallon and Elliott, 2021), this is generally understood to apply in scenarios where the topic being investigated or the research situation/environment poses some kind of threat to those involved (Lee, 1993). Assumptions should not be made about what harms may be present nor about who needs protecting as issues need to be managed carefully but also effectively (Mallon et al., 2021). The very concept of sensitivity in research can elicit strong feelings in relation to a project, and yet the concept of sensitivity is subjective, as what might be considered sensitive by one researcher or participant may not be to others, and thus any judgements you might make about how sensitive your research is will to some extent be determined by your own values and ideas (Farquhar and Das, 1998). Owing to the personal nature of such judgements, we invite you to think about how your own values and ideas influence your working definition of what constitutes a sensitive topic for qualitative health research by working through the reflective activity in Box 11.2.

> **Box 11.2**
>
> **Reflective activity on sensitive topics**
>
> Inevitably, your own thoughts, feelings, and experiences will shape and influence what you view as a sensitive topic for health research and will influence your reflections on where the boundaries sit between what is sensitive and not sensitive. In your research diary, we encourage you to do the following:
>
> - Make a list of as many topics in health as you can think of that you think are sensitive.
> - Group these into clusters of "extremely sensitive", "moderately sensitive", and "mildly sensitive".
> - Add a list of topics that you think are not sensitive at all or only in a very limited way.
> - Go through each of the four clusters you have and see if you can provide a rationale for your ranking.
> - Identify some of the challenges to this task and note them, also noting where there are caveats that might influence the decision (for example, perhaps more "sensitive" for some people than others).
> - Finally, from your clustering and reasons for such categorisations, we encourage you to attempt your own definition of what constitutes a sensitive research topic.

Recruiting "vulnerable" populations

Historical events in health and social science research where there was mistreatment of certain groups have led to calls for greater protections of populations positioned as vulnerable, disadvantaged, or marginalised, as it was thought they were at greater risk of mistreatment (Hunter, 2008). Any poor treatment of vulnerable groups is unacceptable, and protectionism can play a valuable role, but homogenising vulnerability has consequently led to exclusion and disempowerment in some cases (Drewett and O'Reilly, 2023). The concept of vulnerability in qualitative research is contentious, with layered and multiple meanings, and is arguably context-dependent. That is, a person may be vulnerable in one situation or context but not necessarily in another, and furthermore assumed vulnerability should not lead to a participant's automatic exclusion from research, as that is contrary to the fundamental principle of justice and counter to inclusion and participation. In this way, a critical and reflective approach to thinking about vulnerability can be advantageous in ensuring ethical and inclusive practice in your research.

In the broader context of vulnerability (and in some ways tied to issues around sensitive topics), there are various terms employed in recruiting certain populations to a research project. In organising this section of the chapter, we first introduce the broad concepts: hard-to-reach, seldom-heard, hidden, socially disadvantaged, underserved, and marginalised. What anchors these concepts to each other is the underpinning challenge that some groups of participants are either challenging to identify and locate (referred to as "hard-to-reach"), may not wish to be found (referred to as hidden populations), or not recruited into research via traditional recruitment methods and thus often excluded (referred to as "seldom-heard") (Freeman, Skinner, Middleton, 2020). Following this consideration, we move to a discussion of vulnerability. In closing the chapter, we provide some examples of groups who are typically characterised by researchers as "vulnerable" in some way and conceptualised as "seldom-heard" or "hard-to-reach" and so on.

In thinking about your own qualitative project, it is worth reflecting on the characteristics of your population and how you might bring people in to hear the voices of those who might otherwise be otherwise missed.

- Hard-to-reach

The concept of hard-to-reach has been commonly used in the research literature (see Bonevski et al., 2014). There is no universally agreed meaning of the term hard-to-reach, or which populations fall within this category, but broadly speaking, the term refers to groups who are more challenging to access for research and where there are barriers like protective gatekeepers, additional ethical or safeguarding concerns, and issues related to communication (Williams, 2009). Thus, hard-to-reach populations can be difficult to identify for several reasons, tend to represent a small proportion of the general population, and are typically stigmatised in some way (Raifman, DeVost, Digitale, 2022). However, over time, there have been concerns raised about the potential pejorative association of this concept. This is because using the concept hard-to-reach risks positioning blame for the lack of inclusion in research with the population themselves, risks reifying the stigma they already experience, and occludes the challenge of trust in the research relationship (Duvnjak and Fraser, 2013; Islam, Joseph, Chaudry et al., 2021).

- **Seldom-heard**

The term "seldom-heard" is commonly used to refer to those voices that are not frequently heard through research and policy (Prinjha, Miah, Ali, and Farmer, 2020). This term is usually employed to designate those participant groups who have not always been given the opportunity to contribute their voices to research, especially in the context of health and service development (Social Care Institute for Excellence, 2008). This term is sometimes preferred over hard-to-reach as the responsibility for inclusion is shifted to the researchers rather than an implicit blaming of the vulnerable or marginalised population being researched (Teodorowski, Rodgers, Fleming et al., 2023).

- **Hidden**

A population can be considered "hidden" when there is no existing sampling frame and when participants may feel threatened by the revelation of their status (Heckathorn, 1997). As such, they may refuse to engage or provide unreliable answers as a way of managing their privacy. Furthermore, recruiting these populations can be difficult due to concerns about accessing services in traditional ways, and members may not disclose identities owing to fear of stigmatisation (Matthews and Cramer, 2008).

- **Socially disadvantaged**

Persons considered socially disadvantaged are those who may experience disadvantage at a social, cultural, or financial level, or all three, as compared to much of society (Bonevski, Randell, Paul et al., 2014). This means that there are individual, social, cultural, or environmental restrictions on persons in terms of affording them opportunities to participate (Marmot, Friel, Bell et al., 2008). In research, and particularly in health research, most of the groups included have tended to be educated, white, and male; with the most under-represented being those from underprivileged backgrounds (Heiat and Gross, 2002). This is largely because socially disadvantaged groups tend to be challenging to access, and yet these populations have a lot to offer our understanding of health and illness and should be afforded space to meaningfully contribute to research (Bonevski et al., 2014).

- **Underserved**

The concept of underserved has often been associated with health services and refers to a lack of inclusion in services despite a higher healthcare burden (Rochester, 2020). Those populations referred to as underserved are viewed as low socio-economic status, facing certain kinds of vulnerability, and being at greater risk of adverse events (Virapongse and Misky, 2018). Rochester (2020) noted that, in the context of research, underserved is preferable as a term to under-represented as it suggests a lack of inclusion that is by no means the fault of the community concerned. In healthcare research particularly, underserved groups need to be better represented to facilitate knowledge in meeting the needs of those populations (NIHR, 2020). Notably, however, the definition of underserved is context-specific, as it depends on the population, the conditions of the study, the research question, the context of the environment of those participants, and the contribution to be made from the research (Rochester, 2020).

- Marginalised

You will see as you start reading further on this issue that another commonly used term in the research literature is that of marginalised populations. Marginalised populations have been defined as individuals who have more reduced opportunities in their lives than those individuals who are studying them, and risk being constructed as victims, or helpless, or voiceless (Moree, 2018). Thus, marginalised voices need to be not only heard through research, but valued (Snow et al., 2018), and it is incumbent upon researchers to identify marginalised groups, while recognising that there may be groups who experience disadvantage and thus experience marginalisation that may not be overtly obvious to researchers and yet play a role in contributing to research (Moree, 2018). Moree observed that this recognition is especially important as it is often not the marginalised individuals or groups who tend to benefit from the outcomes of research.

Terms and concepts matter

From reading these short overviews of each of the common concepts, you should see there is some overlap, and indeed, there is some conflation of these in the literature. Given this overlap, and the fact the meanings of each are not fixed but context-dependent, a critical position on your preferred terms can be helpful in approaching a research project, which may involve people who may be referred to by these terms. We invite you to engage with the reflective activity in Box 11.3 to think about which concept or concepts are most appropriate in the context of your project.

> **Box 11.3**
>
> **Reflective activity on the use of concepts**
>
> Based on the reading in this chapter, particularly this section, what is your preferred term for your own project? Note down the reasons why you are going to use that concept in your work and start a literature search of papers that have used these concepts to refer to their research populations and the methods literature that debates the language used to describe them.

To some extent, what unites these concepts and the ideas associated with them is that these communities or populations tend to be less included in research than more dominant or privileged groups. Furthermore, there is an underpinning rhetoric of inequality associated with these groups. In health terms, health inequalities or health inequities have meant that there are disparities for some populations in accessing appropriate or high-quality healthcare, support, or information. One of the barriers to the achievement of health equity is research that recruits populations that are seldom-heard, underserved, marginalised, and/or hidden (Matsuda, Brooks, and Beeber, 2016). Thus, health inequality relates to the burden of disease aligning with relative social and economic inequality.

> **Key point!**
>
> For clarity, health inequalities are those differences in the health of individuals or groups (Kawachi, Subramanian, and Almeida-Filho, 2002) and health inequities are a specific type of inequality referring to a moral judgement determining whether the differences are fair or just.
>
> (Arcaya, Arcaya, and Subramanian, 2015)

In a UK context, the Equality Act refers to "protected characteristics", which are age, disability, marriage or civil partnership, sex and sexual orientation, race, religion, pregnancy, and gender reassignment, and seeks to protect these groups through anti-discrimination laws embedding a requirement for diversity and inclusion (Teodorowski et al., 2023). Teodorowski et al. commented that while the Act and its principles are not always directly applied in a research context, it is nonetheless important in thinking about participation and inclusion in research.

As a clinician-researcher, you can help move towards better representation in this arena. This is likely to be challenging as some populations may be fearful of or experience trepidation in accessing traditional service providers, making them more difficult to include, as they may be concerned about disclosing their identities or have anxieties about how their voices may be utilised by researchers and decline participation (Matthews and Cramer, 2008). As such, it remains challenging to include certain populations in research in a meaningful way (Ocloo and Matthews, 2016).

> **Key point!**
>
> Digital technologies and the rapid growth of online communities and interactions have provided new opportunities for reaching hidden, seldom-heard, marginalised populations.
>
> (Liu and Lu, 2018)
>
> (Note that we include a chapter on digital methods – see Chapter 15)

An affiliation with a certain group, an existing network with those close to the group, or a shared characteristic might facilitate the involvement of certain participants in the research. This is potentially because of trust, empathy, and a shared understanding of some of the issues faced. The extent to which this is necessary, helpful, or even a disadvantage has been subject to some debate (and we recommend you revisit Chapter 9 where we introduced insider and outsider status). Consider the reflective activity in Box 11.4.

> **Box 11.4**
>
> **Critically appraising the issue of insider status**
>
> There have been some perspectives proposed that research is of higher quality or should only be conducted/led by those with an insider perspective. For example, in the context of disability politics, arguments have been put forward that disabled researchers should lead disability research. Even in research involving children, children could lead a project, although this is arguably more complex as adults will inevitably have some control and always operate through adult assumptions (see Kellet, 2014 for some discussion). Opinions on these issues sit on a spectrum, and it can be helpful to think about your insider status (see again Chapter 9) in relation to the vulnerability and power issues present in your research. Think about:
>
> - To what extent do you have characteristics that are similar to your participants? (Age, socio-economic status, race and ethnicity, disability/ability, and so on).
> - To what extent do you feel disclosing anything about this to participants might be beneficial to the research?
> - To what extent might those shared characteristics present challenges to the research?
> - What might the benefits and limitations be of a researcher representing a group in this way? (e.g. a female researcher representing women, an autistic researcher representing autistic persons, a disabled researcher representing disabled persons, and so on).
> - How does disclosing things about yourself make you feel? Remember that reflexivity is valuable and can be largely private, but public dissemination where you actively reveal aspects of yourself and identity is necessarily selective. You need to be comfortable with what you write about in your reflexive writing.

Questioning the concept of vulnerability

From your reading in this chapter and the range of different concepts employed in research, you will see that what constitutes vulnerability bears considering critically, that is, in terms of who defines it and how it is defined. It is generally accepted that researchers hold an additional responsibility to protect and safeguard persons who are more vulnerable to harm in research, either by exploitation, or physically and emotionally. This is because vulnerable persons are typically believed to be less able to protect their own best interests.

However, the concept of vulnerability is complex. It has been difficult to create a definition of vulnerability or propose what constitutes a vulnerable group in research (Ruof, 2004) as vulnerability is contextual rather than absolute (Nordentoft and Kappel, 2011). In research settings, vulnerability tends to be positioned in terms of lacking the capacity to protect oneself from possible harm and navigating any potential risks by making informed choices (Shivayogi, 2013). However, this is a more complicated consideration than it may, on first impressions, appear, as vulnerability is more than a risk from harm. Some risks are worth taking and can be of benefit; not all risk leads to harm, and harm itself is a complex concept with multiple levels and various meanings (O'Reilly, Dogra, Levine, and Donoso, 2021).

Propositions have been put forward that we can think of vulnerability in terms of meeting two criteria (Nickel, 2006). Nickel argued that these are:

1. **Consent-based vulnerability** – meaning that a person is considered vulnerable if they lack the capacity to express autonomy and provide informed consent, as such persons have a reduced capacity to safeguard their own interests, making them vulnerable to coercion or exploitation.
2. **Fairness-based vulnerability** – meaning that some individuals do not have the freedoms or opportunities in life, as they may be unfairly impacted by economic disadvantage, have challenges with the native language, or communication challenges and thus are susceptible to being coerced.

In reflecting on the concept of vulnerability, one finds that those groups positioned as vulnerable are not homogeneous and some do have the social competencies to make informed decisions (even if they require support to do so) or have the opportunities as mitigations to ensure it are offered. In thinking about vulnerability in a more nuanced way, therefore, Rogers, Mackenzie, and Dodds (2012) argued that all persons are in some ways vulnerable and contextual and situational factors matter in research. They proposed three sources of vulnerability:

1. **Inherent vulnerability** – because of the innate humanness of individuals, all people are vulnerable to developing an illness, injury, trauma, psychological conditions, emotional challenges, and death.
2. **Situational vulnerability** – broadly, everyone is part of a political, economic, and social context, which varies across groups, but these aspects of society can influence vulnerability. Thus, the social, economic, and political environment can influence the extent of a person's vulnerability.
3. **Pathogenic vulnerability** – these vulnerabilities are created by processes of injustice and oppression, such as vulnerability to discrimination, prejudice, and stigma.

As a researcher, then, you need to think about whether the source of vulnerability is dispositional to the individual or external to them (Rogers and Lange, 2013). Often entire groups are labelled as vulnerable because of a shared characteristic like age or the presence of a health condition, for instance, adults diagnosed with a life-limiting condition, and broad decisions are made about the levels of protections that need to be afforded without considering the individual nuances of each person's identity and self-understanding in that group. Indeed, some participants may be offended to be constructed as vulnerable, like those of older adults who are of retirement age or those with a neurodevelopmental condition, simply by virtue of a defining characteristic.

One of the challenges of the idea of vulnerability in research is that those participants may be excluded from research because of a well-intentioned protectionist ideology. In our own work, an ethics committee would not initially provide approval to include autistic individuals with learning disabilities who were not considered to have the capacity to consent in our project (see Drewett and O'Reilly, 2023). However, when consulting with the families of some of those individuals, there was considerable discontent that their voices would be excluded because of issues of capacity, and family members actively supported the chance to allow them to participate if they assented and with appropriate communication techniques, safeguards, and carer consent in place.

Increasingly, academic researchers promote the inclusion of vulnerable people in research to provide essential insights for health services and interventions that have potential to improve the lives of populations who have historically been marginalised (Fisk, Dean, Alkire et al., 2018). We have highlighted through our discussion of concepts, however, that vulnerable populations can require greater effort and resources from researchers to engage in a project. This may be because of the sensitivity of the topic (Marsh, Browne, Taylor, and Davis, 2017) or because some lack trust in authority or the research process (Newman, O'Reilly, Lee, and Kennedy, 2017).

Author reflections and concluding remarks
From Nikki

As a researcher, I hold a social constructionist epistemological position. By this, I mean that the starting point of whatever academic endeavour I am involved in is that we, as humans, create the way that we understand the world we live in. Rather than concepts such as power or vulnerability being pre-existing entities, my perspective is that these are concepts or ideas that exist because we have come to a majority decision about and have found words to describe those agreements. So, in effect, concepts like "vulnerability" or "sensitivity" only exist as such because of agreement that they do. A potential research participant therefore is or is not vulnerable apart from the fact that we co-create the category and ascribe it to them. Having said that, I do strongly believe that there needs to be a shift in thinking among the research community away from doing research "on" or "to" participants, towards "with" and "for" narratives. In my idealised construct of the research endeavour, the initiative for research would lie with the would-be participants rather than the research team. My preference in research is to serve or respond to the requests of certain groups of individuals who approach me in my privileged position, to support them in gathering data about an area of their choosing. By turning the notion of who initiates the research on its head, the label of "vulnerability" becomes less relevant because the participants themselves self-select to invite research within their group. My hope is that all participants in research, no matter how they are positioned by themselves and others, are less vulnerable to being researched "on".

Turning to the idea of there being topics of research that may be more "sensitive", I draw upon my profession as a clinical psychologist to reflect on this. Again, I believe that sensitivity is a social construct. Yes, in most societies, certain topics are considered a little more taboo or uncomfortable to talk about, and these may be the topics that we refer to as sensitive in research. From this perspective, perhaps asking people about matters such as their finances, their political views, and sexual activity, could be considered "sensitive". I note here as an aside that I used the word "asking", assuming that the qualitative research would involve some form of interview. However, my preference for research is to follow a naturally occurring data agenda and to take interest in the conversations that people are already having in naturally occurring contexts and situations. When we factor in the idea that research using natural data can be extremely powerful, the concept of sensitivity starts to lose its grip. This is because whatever is being discussed is being talked about in the appropriate context, rather than being dragged out of any natural environment into the cold arena of a research interview. The concept of sensitivity, therefore, from my perspective, relates to different facets. First, there is the factor of whether the research participants themselves orient to the topic they are discussing as sensitive. The second facet is whether the topic is sensitive by virtue of the current socio-political climate, because others may have quite differing views. Third is the idea of the researcher's sensitivity to the participant, to their level of comfort in talking about the topic, and to the care taken about how their words are treated with respect and dignity both within the data gathering phase and in dissemination.

References
Arcaya, M. C., Arcaya, A. L., and Subramanian, S. V. (2015). Inequalities in health: Definitions, concepts, and theories. *Global Health Action*, 8, 27106.
Arnstein, S. (1969). A ladder of citizen participation. *Journal of the American Institute of Planners*, 35, 216–224.
Beresford, P. (2021). *Participatory ideology*. Bristol, UK: Policy Press.
Bonevski, B., Randell, M., Paul, C., Chapman, K., Twyman, L., Bryant, J., Brozek, I., and Hughes, C. (2014). Reaching the hard-to-reach: A systematic review of strategies for improving health and medical research with socially disadvantaged groups. *BMC Medical Research Methodology*, 14(1), 42.
Butler, A., Copnell, B., and Hall, H. (2019). Researching people who are bereaved: Managing risks to participants and researchers. *Nursing Ethics*, 26(1), 224–234.
Dodd, S., and Epstein, I. (2012). *Practice-based research in social work: A guide for reluctant researchers*. London: Routledge.
Drewett, A., and O'Reilly, M. (2023). Examining the value of using naturally occurring data to facilitate qualitative health research with "hard-to-reach" "vulnerable" groups: A research note on inpatient care. *Qualitative Research*, 23(3), 825–835.
Duvnjak, A., and Fraser, H. (2013). Targeting the "hard-to-reach": Re/producing stigma? *Critical and Radical Social Work*, 1(2), 162–182.
Farquhar, C., and Das, R. (1998). Are focus groups suitable for sensitive topics? In R. Barbour and J. Kitzinger (Eds.), *Developing focus group research: Politics, theory and practice*. Thousand Oaks, CA: Sage.
Fisk, R., Dean, A., Alkire, L., Joubert, A., Previte, J., Roberston, N., and Rosenbaum, M. (2018). Design for service inclusion: Creating inclusive service systems by 2025. *Journal of Service Management*, 29(5), 834–858.
Freeman, S., Skinner, K., Middleton, L., Xiong, B., and Fang, M. (2020). Engaging hard-to-reach, hidden, and seldom-heard populations in research. In A. Sixsmith, J. Sixsmith, A. Mihailidis, and M. Fang (Eds.), *Knowledge, innovation and impact: A guide for the engaged health researcher* (pp. 81–91). Cham, Switzerland: Springer.
Gibson, K. (2022). Bridging the digital divide: Reflections on using WhatsApp messenger interviews in youth research. *Qualitative Research in Psychology*, 19(3), 611–631.
Hart, R. (1992). *Children's participation: From tokenism to citizenship (innocenti essay no 4)*. Florence: UNICEF.
Heckathorn, D. (1997). Respondent-driven sampling: A new approach to the study of hidden populations. *Social Problems*, 44, 174–199.
Heiat, A., Gross, C., and Krumholz, H. (2002). Representation of the elderly, women, and minorities in heart failure clinical trials. *Archives of Internal Medicine*, 162(15), 1682–1688.

Hunter, D. (2008). The ESRC research ethics framework and research ethics review at UK universities: Rebuilding the tower of Babel REC by REC. *Journal of Medical Ethics*, 34(11), 815–820.

Islam, S., Joseph, O., Chaudry, A. et al. (2021). "We are not hard to reach, but we may find it hard to trust" .... Involving and engaging 'seldom listened to' community voices in clinical translational health research: A social innovation approach. *Research Involvement & Engagement*, 7, 46.

John, M. (1996) *Children in charge: The child's right to resources.* London: Jessica Kingsley.

Kawachi, I., Subramanian, S. V., and Almeida-Filho, N. (2002). A glossary for health inequalities. *Journal of Epidemiology & Community Health*, 56(9), 647–652.

Kellett, M. (2014). Chapter 1: Images of childhood and their influence on research. In A. Clark, R. Flewitt, M. Hammersley, and M. Robb (Eds.), *Understanding research with children and young people* (pp. 15–33). London: SAGE.

Kirby, P., and Gibbs, S. (2006). Facilitating participation: Adults' caring support roles within child-to-child projects in schools and after-school settings. *Children & Society*, 20(3), 209–222.

Lee, R. (1993). *Doing research on sensitive topics.* London: Sage.

Liamputtong, P. (2007). *Researching the vulnerable.* London: Sage.

Liu, C., and Lu, X. (2018). Analyzing hidden populations online: Topic, emotion, and social network of HIV-related users in the largest Chinese online community. *BMC Medical Informatics & Decision Making*, 18, 2.

Lundy, L. (2007). "Voice" is not enough: Conceptualising article 12 of the United Nations convention on the rights of the child. *British Educational Research Journal*, 33(6), 927–942.

Mallon, S., Borgstrom, E., and Murphy, S. (2021). Unpacking sensitive research: A stimulating exploration of an established concept. *International Journal of Social Research Methodology*, 24(5), 517–521.

Mallon, S., and Elliott, I. (2021). What is "sensitive" about sensitive research? The sensitive researcher's perspective. *International Journal of Social Research Methodology*, 24(5), 523–535.

Marmot, M., Friel, S., Bell, R., Houweling, T. A., and Taylor, S. (2008). Commission on social determinants of health. Closing the gap in a generation: Health equity through action on the social determinants of health. *The Lancet*, 372(9650), 1661–1669.

Marsh, C., Browne, J., Taylor, J., and Davis, D. (2017). A researcher's journey: Exploring a sensitive topic with vulnerable women. *Women & Birth*, 30(1), 63–69.

Matsuda, Y., Brooks, J., and Beeber, L. (2016). Guidelines for research recruitment of underserved populations (EERC). *Applied Nursing Research*, 32, 164–170.

Matthews, J., and Cramer, E. (2008). Using technology to enhance qualitative research with hidden populations. *Qualitative Report*, 13(2), 301–315.

McCosker, H., Barnard, A., and Gerber, R. (2001). Undertaking sensitive research: Issues and strategies for meeting the safety needs of all participants. *Forum: Qualitative Social Research*, 2(1).

Moree, D. (2018). Qualitative approaches to studying marginalised communities. *Oxford Research Encyclopedia of Education.* https://oxfordre.com/education/display/10.1093/acrefore/9780190264093.001.0001/acrefore-9780190264093-e-246

NIHR. (2020). Improving inclusion of under-served groups in clinical research: guidance from INCLUDE project. https://www.nihr.ac.uk/documents/improving-inclusion-of-under-served-groups-in-clinical-research-guidance-from-include-project/25435

Newman, D., O'Reilly, P., Lee, S., and Kennedy, C. (2017). Challenges in accessing and interviewing participants with severe mental illness. *Nurse Researcher*, 25(1), 37–42.

Nickel, P. (2006). Vulnerable populations in research: The case of the seriously ill. *Theoretical Medicine & Bioethics*, 27(3), 245–264.

Nordentoft, H., and Kappel, N. (2011). Vulnerable participants in health research: Methodological and ethical challenges. *Journal of Social Work Practice*, 25(3), 365–376.

Ocloo, J., and Matthews, R. (2016). From tokenism to empowerment: progressing patient and public involvement in healthcare improvement. *BMJ Quality & Safety, 25,* 626–632.

O'Reilly, M., Dogra, N., Levine, D., and Donoso, V. (2021). *Digital media and child and adolescent mental health: A practical guide to understanding the evidence.* London: Sage.

Prinjha, S., Miah, N., Ali, E., and Farmer, A. (2020). Including "seldom heard" views in research: Opportunities, challenges and recommendations from focus groups with British South Asian people with type 2 diabetes. *BMC Medical Research Methodology, 20*(1), 157.

Raifman, S., DeVost, M. A., Digitale, J. C., Chen, Y.-H., and Morris, M. (2022). Respondent-driven sampling: A sampling method for hard-to-reach populations and beyond. *Current Epidemiology Reports, 9,* 38–47.

Rochester, L. (2020). Improving inclusion of underserved groups in clinical research: Summary of findings from the National Institute for Health Research "INCLUDE" programme. https://www.ncl.ac.uk/mediav8/fms/files/INCLUDE%20Summary%20June%202020.pdf

Rogers, W. and Lange, M. M. (2013). Rethinking the vulnerability of minority populations in research. *American Journal of Public Health, 103*(12), 2141–2146.

Rogers, W., Mackenzie, C., and Dodds, S. (2012). Why bioethics needs a concept of vulnerability. *International Journal of Feminist Approaches to Bioethics, 5*(2), 11–38.

Ruof, M. (2004). Vulnerability, vulnerable populations, and policy. *Kennedy Institute of Ethics Journal, 14*(4), 411–425.

Social Care Institute for Excellence. (2008). *Seldom Heard: Developing inclusive participation in social care.* London: Social Care Institute for Excellence.

Shier, H. (2001). Pathways to participation: Openings, opportunities and obligations. *Children & Society, 15*(2), 107–117.

Shivayogi, P. (2013). Vulnerable population and methods for their safeguard. *Perspectives in Clinical Research, 4*(1), 53–57.

Silverio, S. A., Sheen, K. S., Bramante, A., Knighting, K., Koops, T. U., Montgomery, E., November, L., Soulsby, L. K., Stevenson, J. H., Watkins, M., Easter, A., and Sandall, J. (2022). Supporting researchers conducting qualitative research into sensitive, challenging, and difficult topics: Experiences and practical applications. *International Journal of Qualitative Methods, 21,* 1–16.

Snow, M., Tweedie, K., and Pederson, A. (2018). Heard and valued: The development of a model to meaningfully engage marginalized populations in health services planning. *BMC Health Services Research, 18*(1), 181.

Teodorowski, P., Rodgers, S., Fleming, K., Tahir, N., Ahmed, S., and Frith, L. (2023). "To me, it's ones and zeros, but in reality, that one is death": A qualitative study exploring researchers' experience of involving and engaging seldom-heard communities in big data research. *Health Expectations, 26*(2), 882–891.

Treseder, P. (1997). *Empowering children and young people.* London: Save the Children.

Williams, E. (2009). *Good practice in engaging "hard to reach" groups.* Cardiff: Cardiff Local Service Board Scrutiny Panel.

Virapongse, A., and Misky, G. (2018). Self-identified social determinants of health during transitions of care in the medically underserved: A narrative review. *Journal of General Internal Medicine, 33,* 1959–1967.

CHAPTER 12

Managing researcher safety

Learning objectives

This chapter enables the reader to:

- Appreciate the importance of researcher safety.
- Identify emotional risks to the researcher in doing qualitative health research.
- Identify physical risks to the researcher in doing qualitative health research.
- Recognise potential risks to a professional transcriptionist in transcribing data.
- Evaluate the relevance of the location of fieldwork in managing risk.
- Critically assess ways to mitigate risks in fieldwork.

Introduction

We deliberately dedicate a chapter to researcher safety to highlight how important it is to consider yourself and your own welfare in your research project. There has been some attention paid to researcher safety in the literature and by organisations, but the development of this area has been slow in comparison to academic work regarding the safety of participants. Although there was some work focusing on researchers in the field, the COVID-19 pandemic heightened a discourse about keeping researchers safe in their activities. There has been increased awareness of personal risk in the research context as we have moved into a more risk conscious society (Plackett, 2020), with growing attention paid to both possible physical and psychological harms (Dickson-Swift et al., 2008; Parker and O'Reilly, 2013; Social Research Association, 2005). There is now a greater emphasis placed on researcher safety training (Boynton, 2016; Tolich, Tumilty, Choe et al., 2020), although recognising that not all risks are readily apparent, nor can all be anticipated or known in advance (Sampson, 2019).

In this chapter, we guide you through some of the risks that you might face in doing your qualitative health research project and help you think about any possible physical or emotional harms that may arise for you. While the risks of harm are heightened during fieldwork, there are other aspects of the work that may lead to physical or emotional harm, and these should also be considered. In our other writing, we have strongly advocated the need to work closely with others to support your wellbeing as a researcher and to help undertake an appropriate risk assessment for your safety (Kiyimba and O'Reilly, in press). This chapter addresses core issues regarding researcher safety while making practical recommendations for you to translate to your own work.

Researcher safety in qualitative research

It is unsurprising that researcher safety has become more prominent as a concern for organisations, like universities and healthcare institutions, especially with the COVID-19 pandemic. Historically, in the context of research, concerns of risk were largely thought about in relation to threats to the health and safety of research participants (Dickson-Swift, James, Kippen, and Liamputtong, 2008), and this has become more prominent in qualitative research as it has become increasingly recognised that qualitative research imposes the potential for different kinds of risks and harms for participants (O'Reilly and Kiyimba, 2015).

The concept of risk is complicated and, in different ways, contested. Risk, put simply, is more than a possibility, but a degree of probability that an event will occur, and in research this is thought to be intrinsically tied to harm (Webber and Brunger, 2018). However, Webber and Brunger noted that harms are not always manageable and neither are they always undesired, and there is a challenge that researchers may be overly paternalistic in their practice in ways that override the autonomy of participants. Indeed, they argued that some level of risk-taking is necessary in research so that questions can be explored; experiencing some risk in the field can even enhance the production of knowledge.

> **Key point!**
>
> Do not inflate the level of risk when assessing it, and seek to be flexible in considering risk to avoid hindering the full contribution of participants, while being realistic about potential risks.
>
> (Bradley, 2007)

Evidently, it is essential that you conduct a risk assessment that not only considers the welfare and autonomy of the research participants (as we discussed in the Chapter 8 on ethics), but also addresses the risk of harm to you as a researcher and to those in your team. We include transcriptionists in our thinking about who is part of this team, as transcriptionists are often overlooked as people who may be exposed to distressing material (Kiyimba and O'Reilly, 2016a). The processes involved in doing a qualitative health research project will expose you and your participants to certain risks that can cause physical or psychological harm (Butler, Copnell, and Hall, 2019). It is likely that in considering how doing your qualitative health research project might impact you, you will need some support to think things through in planning and in managing situations as they arise. There remains a lack of formal guidelines or formalised processes, and yet safeguarding your own well-being during the process is essential (Dickson-Swift, 2022; Kiyimba and O'Reilly, 2016a). Before you go into more detail, it is useful to pause and reflect on this issue. Your own safety and well-being may be something you have already thought about and planned with your team and/or your supervisors/mentors, or it may be something you have not really considered yet. We encourage you to pause now and try the reflective activity in Box 12.1.

> **Box 12.1**
>
> **Reflective activity on planning for your safety as a researcher**
>
> Based on your reading so far in this chapter, we invite you to start making some reflective notes in your research diary in response to the following questions:
>
> - In what ways might there be potential for your physical well-being to be compromised when undertaking your research?
> - At what phase of the process are these risks most prominent?
> - In what ways do you believe your emotional, psychological, or spiritual safety might be compromised by your research?
> - At what phase of the process might these risks be most prominent?
> - What can you do to plan to mitigate, reduce, or ameliorate these risks?
> - Who is in your support network that you can contact on short notice if you need help?
> - What might your emergency planning strategy be?

Researcher safety and sensitive research

> **Key point!**
>
> Health research is a field that is often concerned with sensitive topics. Reflection on the impact of doing this kind of sensitive work with vulnerable persons is important to assess your own safety in the field.
>
> (Fenge, Oakley, Taylor, and Beer, 2019)

As we noted in Chapter 10, there is not a uniform definition of what sensitive research is, and therefore researchers must critically engage with the meaning of sensitivity in their own projects and maintain their reflexive position on their practices (Mallon, Borgstrom, and Murphy, 2021). In managing these reflexive positions, qualitative researchers need to be mindful of how working on sensitive topics might impact their own health and how this might overlap with their clinical work, professional commitments, and caseloads. There is literature showing that doing sensitive research can have some physical and emotional effects on researchers to varying degrees, including:

- Nausea, vomiting, stomach upset, and abdominal pain (Campbell, 2002).
- Sleep disturbance (Moran and Asquith, 2020).
- Poor concentration or attention difficulties (Fohring, 2020).
- Fatigue (Batty, 2020).
- Headaches (Gleeson, 2021).
- Feeling overwhelmed and unable to cope, or potentially experiencing burnout (Dickson-Swift, 2022).
- High levels of anxiety (Benoot and Bilsen, 2015).

If you start to feel any symptoms like these, or others during your research, you should seek support and help and pay attention to how the research is intersecting with other things in your personal life or clinical work that may be exacerbating the effects. You might need to take a break, you might need some formal mental health support like clinical supervision or counselling, or you may just need some debriefing with people in your team. We discuss this further later in the chapter. However, before we do so, we introduce the personal experience of Dr Calvin Swords in Box 12.2, who discusses the challenges experienced in managing safety in the field as a way of introducing some of the key issues we discuss in this chapter.

> **Box 12.2**
> **Dr Calvin Swords' experience**
>
> Dr Calvin Swords is a lecturer in social work in the School of Applied Social Studies at the University College Cork (UCC), Ireland. Prior to this, Calvin was a lecturer of social work in the Department of Applied Social Studies at Maynooth University. Before entering academia full-time, Calvin was a social work practitioner with experience in a range of settings. Calvin's PhD was funded by the Irish Research Council (IRC), which explored how mental health recovery is socially constructed in Irish mental health services. Calvin undertook and completed a PhD over a three-year period between 2018 and 2021, whilst continuing in social work practice in a hospital setting, working with individuals and families during the global pandemic.
>
> My PhD used a qualitative, interpretative, case study design to explore the experiences of individuals living with mental health challenges, family members, multi-disciplinary teams, and policymakers regarding the concept of mental health recovery and how it is socially constructed. Semi-structured interviews were used, with thematic analysis to iteratively construct codes and themes relevant to answering the research question. The research built on an earlier, smaller project which explored recovery with one multi-disciplinary team in practice (Swords and Houston, 2020). The data collection, transcription, and analysis were all undertaken by me as the lead researcher.

Exploring experiences of recovery with individuals and families using mental health services presented significant challenges to my own well-being during the research journey. Before even considering the emotional toll, this had at times done just this; the very nature of the PhD journey is well-documented as having a profound impact physically and emotionally on the individual. Interestingly, I commenced my PhD journey with a wealth of knowledge and experience regarding self-care and maintaining good emotional well-being (social work training, practice experience, and previous work in mental health services prior to becoming a social worker), yet it still did not fully prepare or protect me from the psychological impact that qualitative research on sensitive topics with vulnerable populations can have. This included sleepless nights, rational and irrational worries about the participants' well-being during the study, and self-criticism of my ability to ask the appropriate yet sensitive questions. There were plenty of good days and milestones met, but it is important to acknowledge the impact of the journey during the PhD.

Some strategies during the process that supported me included the following:

- Journaling and reflection on this with my supervisors in a safe and supportive environment throughout.
- Viewing timelines not as not deadlines, but as milestones.
- Physical activity, both running/walking when material/data was difficult to digest, but also participating in activities that involved meeting people – sport or other forms of socialising.
- Worrying was a big challenge for me – what was helpful was giving myself 2 × 5 minutes a day with a stopwatch where I literally just "worried", rationally and irrationally. However, I could not worry outside of these five-minute periods – this took practice.
- Supervision learning agreement which had scheduled supervision sessions – more often during times of data collection and analysis.
- Matching with supervisors with whom you have a relationship – knowing they have your best interests and understand you as an individual.
- Gatekeepers in the field with whom you have built rapport during the data collection phase.
- Several meetings were held with participants in the study to build rapport and understand their circumstances.

Emotional safety

One of the main ways you may be affected, especially if your research explores a sensitive topic and/or involves vulnerable persons, is emotionally. Indeed, it is important to attend to your emotional states and think about how you are responding emotionally to your participants and to your data. If you are dealing with difficult or sensitive topics and are frequently exposed to emotional or distressing narratives, then this might influence you and may lead you to ruminate (Silverio, Sheen, Bramante et al., 2022). This is more likely in qualitative research, as researchers remain immersed in the data through data collection, transcription, coding, analysis, and dissemination (Williamson, Gregory, Abrahams et al., 2020).

> **Key point!**
> Inexperienced researchers are likely to have a stronger emotional investment in research, and while this is not necessarily problematic, postgraduate students and doctoral researchers studying sensitive topics tend to be at greater risk of a detrimental emotional impact.
> (Orr, Durepos, Jones, and Jack, 2021)

In qualitative research, this potential for rumination is exacerbated by the nature of the work. As a qualitative researcher, you will build something of a relationship with your participants. You will need to build rapport, respect, and trust. You are likely to have some empathy in building this with your participants, and in so doing, this will likely promote an emotional connection with those participants (Coles and Mudaly, 2010).

> **Key point!**
> Remember that the emotional impact of undertaking your research is not complete when you finish your fieldwork, but it continues through the analysis and dissemination of that work.
> (Butler et al., 2019)

Problematically, in research, the academic endeavour is frequently viewed as objective, detached, and neutral where researchers are expected to distance themselves from the project. Yet, research is almost never neutral, and researchers are not passive or unaffected (Williamson et al., 2020). We argue that researcher emotional safety is critical in qualitative health research, as there are possible consequences of burnout, vicarious traumatisation, and secondary traumatic stress if this is ignored or remains unnoticed by research teams.

Emotional burnout, vicarious traumatisation, and secondary traumatic stress

When undertaking a qualitative health research project, you may experience a range of different emotional reactions. This may vary from mild upset and some recognition that you are experiencing some emotional discomfort, right through to experiencing vicarious trauma (Etherington, 2007), i.e. as part of the process of empathically engaging with the narratives of traumatic experiences (Pearlman and Saakvitne, 1995), or experience of secondary traumatic stress, i.e. a consequence of empathically hearing the traumatic experiences of others (Devilly, Wright and Varker, 2009). Be mindful to consider the possible cumulative effect of working with your participants and data, as you may reach a point of emotional saturation (Sherry, 2013). Notably, the terms vicarious trauma, secondary traumatic stress, burnout, and compassion fatigue tend to be used interchangeably by researchers, and while there is overlap, there are some differences in these terms and thus, we address each separately here.

Burnout – depending on your profession, you may be familiar with different terms for similar experiences. Job burnout is the term used to refer to a collection of behaviours, attitudes, and feelings that are characterised by chronic exhaustion and cynicism about the workplace (Demerouti, Bakker, Nachreiner, and Schaufeli, 2001). In the helping professions, burnout tends to be a more common term for compassion fatigue, which refers to a reduction in interest or concern regarding the suffering of others (Figley, 2013). Burnout and compassion fatigue, unfortunately, are common among healthcare practitioners, and even for those not involved in research in addition to clinical responsibilities there is a great need for compassionate self-care (Larson and Bush, 2006), through intentionally investing time in activities that are self-nurturing (Boyle, 2011). A couple of helpful questions to ask are "What can I do to help myself in this moment?" and "How can I be kind to myself?" (Kiyimba, 2020). Developing a day-to-day integrated mindfulness practice also has a good evidence base to demonstrate its effectiveness in managing stress and burnout (Christopher, Goerling, Rogers et al., 2016).

Vicarious trauma – refers to a change in a person that results from empathic engagement with trauma survivors (Moran and Asquith, 2020). Vicarious trauma can potentially occur if you are researching the experiences of vulnerable populations who have experienced violence, abuse, and trauma (Campbell, 2017). By exposing yourself to the impact of participants' traumatic experiences, you are engaged with the emotional context of those narratives (Coles, Astbury, Dartnall, and Limjerwala, 2014), and this may trigger something in you, especially if you have experiences of a similar or related nature yourself. In research, this kind of intensive engagement with traumatised participants can lead to pain, especially if the trauma is shared, but can also be the case even if there is an absence of a "shared traumatic reality" (Eriksen, 2017). The experience of vicarious trauma can result in a range of possible impacts on the researcher, noted by Smith et al. (2021) as being:

- Nightmares.
- Intrusive thoughts.
- Hopelessness.
- Despair.
- An altered view of themselves.
- Social withdrawal.
- Disconnection from family and friends.

Secondary traumatic stress – has some overlap with the concept of vicarious trauma and refers to the acquisition of negative emotional states arising because of extended contact with persons who have experienced adverse events (Motta, 2008). In the context of research, secondary traumatic stress has not been well researched, as it has in the field of clinical and psychotherapeutic practice, and yet there is potential for researchers to experience this in relation to their emotional safety (Williamson et al., 2020). Specifically, where researchers may be involved in collecting data from participants who have experienced trauma, the possibility is increased.

The Secondary Traumatic Stress Scale (STSS) is a short questionnaire that can quickly give an indication of a person's experiences in the symptom clusters associated with secondary traumatic stress, which are: intrusion, avoidance, and arousal (Bride, Robinson, Yegidis, and Figley, 2004). This simple self-scoring screening tool has been successfully adopted by mental health professionals to assess clinician well-being after exposure to potentially traumatic events immediately, 48 hours later, and four weeks later (Sillitoe, Kimbya, Milliken, and Bennett, 2021). This is an example of responsibility being taken up at an organisational level for staff in a particular department or area of work. Sprang, Lei, and Bush (2021) advocate for organisational-level support and argued that policies and procedures to manage secondary traumatic stress by using an STSS to identify it at an organisational level can have a direct positive benefit to the well-being of individuals within the organisation (Sprang, Miech, and Gusler, 2023). For clinician-researchers, organisational support to avoid or manage secondary traumatic stress may be initiated by senior colleagues within the clinical setting, or by the leads of the research project.

> **Key point!**
>
> When a researcher experiences burnout, vicarious trauma, or secondary traumatic stress, this may lead to compassion fatigue. Compassion fatigue is a consequence of the emotional, physical, and psychological impact of helping other people.
>
> (Figley, 2013)

We have focused on the emotional labour of doing sensitive or challenging qualitative health research in this section of the chapter and considered the possible consequences of deep and meaningful engagement with your participants' emotional experiences, and possibly traumatic narratives. Of course, it depends on your participants, their experiences, how they report them to you, the empathy you have, your own emotional state and experiences at the time of doing the work, and a range of other factors in terms of how you respond and feel when undertaking your project. Nonetheless, there are some important things to remember regarding researcher emotional well-being, and we outline these in Box 12.3.

> **Box 12.3**
>
> **Important things to remember regarding emotional well-being**
>
> In reflecting on your emotional well-being while undertaking your qualitative health research project, these are some helpful things to be mindful of:
>
> - Managing your emotional safety can be impeded by balancing the demands of the project. There may be time pressures to complete fieldwork within a certain timeframe, and this may lead the researcher to expose themselves to material of a sensitive nature, for example, regarding painful emotional experiences, in a shorter space of time than is comfortable (Williamson et al., 2020).

- Your research is likely to be emotionally demanding if it is sensitive in nature, so recognising this is essential for managing this side of the work. You can take some responsibility for your own welfare by undertaking a risk assessment during the planning stage and work with others to identify strategies to minimise and manage your emotional reactions, as the emotional impact can often go unaddressed (Orr et al., 2021).
- Self-care in research is necessary to manage the potential emotional impact on you. Being reflective about this will ensure you manage your emotional safety, and in doing so, it is necessary to be honest with yourself about the emotional impact of the work (Bowtell, Sawyer, Aroni, et al 2013).
- Vicarious trauma, secondary traumatic stress, burnout, and compassion fatigue have been identified as possible occupational risks for researchers (Eades, Hackett, Raven et al., 2020; Gleeson, 2021) and being aware of these risks is vital for your planning (Dickson-Swift, 2022) so you might recognise any effects and take steps to address them.
- In managing the emotional risks to you in your research, you might find it beneficial to seek out training regarding this (Dickson-Swift, 2022) and ensure you have avenues to access support.

Physical safety

It is necessary to think about whether there are any physical risks being taken in undertaking a project as well as the emotional risks. There are various physical risks you may be exposed to, such as the possibility of infection, injury, or violence (Parker and O'Reilly, 2013) and the characteristics of participants will be central to the likelihood of these. Problematically, there is only limited literature on physical risks in qualitative research, especially due to violence, as threats of violence and physical injuries tend to be under-reported by researchers (Bloor, Fincham, and Sampson, 2007). In planning qualitative research, physical risks tend to be more easily recognisable than emotional ones (Bowtell et al., 2013) and you can take some time to identify what these might be.

It is noted, however, in the literature that researchers often only think about the basic safety issues in terms of their physical vulnerabilities. Aside from situations where there is an obvious danger, such as in a participant's living environment (e.g. in the context of armed conflict) or their characteristics (e.g. having a history of violent offending), researchers often do not think about their physical safety (Bahn and Wetherill, 2013). Even when they do think about their safety, they may plan to use public transport during daylight hours, avoid quiet places like parks, and have steps to manage risks for infection if needed, but unanticipated events may still occur that threaten their safety. We have some experience of this ourselves, as we acknowledge in the following example.

A physical threat in our research: In a health research project, one of our team (Nikki) was investigating the psychological impact of acquiring an infectious disease. In the initial risk assessment, careful attention was given to minimising the risk of infection to the researcher. Preparations included wearing protective clothing, use of hand sanitisation practices, and protection of recording equipment from contamination. In addition, thought was given to the fact that some of the interviews were to be conducted in the community, and some in hospital settings. For those interviews in the community, owing to the risk of infection, as well as practical considerations regarding recording quality, it was deemed most advantageous to conduct interviews in participants' homes. Because of this, the organisation's lone worker policy was actioned, which meant that the researcher informed a colleague of the date, time, and location of the interviews, and arranged that the colleague would contact the police if the researcher had not checked in with the colleague at a specified time to confirm she was safe and well. Unfortunately, despite these well-laid plans, a different physical risk emerged in one of the interviews. The participant in question had hidden a taser gun under the seat where the researcher was invited to sit for the interview in the participant's home. At the start of the interview, he spoke of prior violence he had engaged in and mental instability that may pose a threat to the researcher. He advised that the researcher should access the weapon and be educated on its use, as it was possible that she may need to use it on him in self-defence if he became physically aggressive during the interview.

Due to this being a research interview rather than a clinical appointment or intervention, information about the participant's history had not been shared with the researcher prior to the interview, and this raises an interesting question about how much personal information about prospective participants in health research is necessary. For those readers who are now feeling a little alarmed, do not worry, Nikki was able to remove herself safely from the situation (Parker and O'Reilly, 2013 - *Parker is now Kiyimba). Also, it is valuable to consider that situations like this are variable and, in this instance, the meaning of providing a weapon may be thought of as arising from a place of concern on the part of the participant, for the researcher to be provided with a means of self-defence should she need this. Before outlining a few of our learning points from this experience (we recommend you read our chapter, Kiyimba and O'Reilly, in press, for more details), we encourage you to think about your own safety in research and do the activity in Box 12.4.

Box 12.4

Reflective activity on concerns for physical safety

Based on your reading of this example, we encourage you to reflect on these questions:

- How do you feel after reading our account?
- What do you think could have been done to prevent this situation from occurring?
- What lessons might you take from this in relation to managing your own physical safety in your research project?

Learning points

Reflecting on our example and the contents of this chapter, we encourage you to ask questions about how much information a researcher needs to have about a potential participant to make an informed decision about risk, and how lone worker policies might be updated to take better account of how police services operate (i.e. a police policy may be to wait 24 hours before acting on a report of a missing person). In terms of our personal learning, the following is not a comprehensive list but highlights a few of the factors that we have since considered in our own work as a research team:

- To incorporate into the research ethics review process, consideration of the researcher's physical and emotional safety, and the well-being of other research team members.
- To consider the proximal distance of the field researcher from others in the research team so that those collecting data are not physically far away or in an isolated place.
- To consider during research planning whether there may be a need for a co-researcher to attend the site of data collection if any risk is anticipated.
- To be aware that organisational lone worker policies may have been developed unilaterally without consultation with other relevant agencies, such as collaboration with local police services.
- An advantage that clinician-researchers have in data collection is a background in clinical skills for working in challenging situations. To ensure that those collecting data are suitably trained in managing their own safety when collecting data in the field, this would include:
  - ☐ risk assessment on arrival at a venue, including pets, other people, harmful substances, escape route planning, etc.
  - ☐ ability to de-escalate a situation if a participant becomes agitated or aggressive.
  - ☐ ability to discern the probable intentions of the participant.
  - ☐ awareness of safety protocols and adherence to procedures, such as emergency notification of a colleague, the importance of check-ins, and others knowing where you are.

Choosing a location for fieldwork
There are many different locations where qualitative fieldwork can take place. One area of physical safety that has received some attention in the literature relates to the geographical location and nature of the space in which data collection takes place. There are some fieldwork situations where risk is heightened considerably, such as countries at war or natural disasters, institutional settings where there may be a greater risk to physical health, like hospitals or other medical environments, or where there is an increased potential for violence, such as prisons. However, there can be a physical risk when entering the homes of your participants, which you should explore in more depth. It is common for researchers to work in the interests of their participants and help them feel more relaxed and comfortable by doing fieldwork in participants' homes, and this is where we turn our attention now.

- Fieldwork in the participant's home

There are advantages to undertaking fieldwork in the homes of your participants. For example, this environment can help provide a space that ensures participants feel comfortable, which can promote rapport. Therefore, the home setting can help to create a more equal partnership between the researcher and researched (Borbasi et al., 2002).

If you ultimately decide to undertake your data collection in your participants' homes, then you need to think about the possible risks. This is necessary as you have no control over who else will be in the home at the time of data collection, and neither will you have been able to gain information about those persons and their mental health, criminal history, or substance use status (Bahn and Weatherill, 2013). You need to be mindful of how certain geographic areas may heighten risks to personal safety and personal property (Borbasi, Chapman, and Read, 2002).

Even in cases where you are physically safe in the home environment, doing research in this location can cause you stress because of the more limited control you have and the need to quickly adapt to a changing environment and unanticipated challenges (MacDonald, 2008). For example, MacDonald noted that, in this environment, it can be difficult to negotiate space and privacy to talk to your participant, and other members of the household may interrupt you or try to join in your conversation. The home of the participant may be a busy, even chaotic space, and there is a risk that it may be a hostile or uncomfortable environment (Bushin, 2007) where you would need to be able to manage situations as they arise.

- **Fieldwork in the hospital or hospice**

The hospital environment may be an inappropriate site for conducting qualitative health research as hospital wards are characterised by a lack of privacy, making it difficult to achieve the sense of collaboration required (Borbasi et al., 2002). However, undertaking research in hospital settings or other healthcare contexts where physical care procedures are provided in a more intensive way enables the researcher to be close to the direct delivery of care, which can be beneficial in terms of the insight afforded into actual practice. You will need to ensure that your presence as a researcher does not interfere with or compromise this care, alongside other issues relating to infection control and your physical safety as a researcher in this environment. Emergency care departments, for example, are highly pressurised work environments. In other direct access care contexts, there are also risks around perceived or actual threats of physical violence. Safety planning in advance of commencing any fieldwork in this type of setting is thus critical, as well as considering triggers that would prompt action (and designating the type of action entailed).

- **Fieldwork in the mental health in-patient hospital or outpatient clinic**

Similar things can be said about undertaking research in mental health treatment settings, including both in-patient and outpatient care contexts. The researcher or research team needs to reflect carefully on what their presence will involve in these settings and how it may affect – and what it will mean for – the workings of the clinic or care unit. Working alongside a gatekeeper or link-professional is also an integral consideration in this respect.

Depending on the setting, the researcher (even if they are a professional working in the same area in which the research is based) should take time to familiarise themselves with the processes in place to manage different risks that are recognised in the context, for example, around medication management and the supervision of service users. In in-patient care settings, there are usually a range of procedures in place that are instituted to manage the risks that service users may pose to themselves via self-injurious behaviour, which are important to be aware of.

The researcher should make efforts to ensure they are unobtrusive in their presence and take care to consider how this can create additional risks around well-being and physical safety that need to be considered, including ways their presence may, unwittingly, hinder the provision of care or treatment. Establishing informed consent from any service users or professionals who participate in the research is, again, significant with this. In planning and reflecting on their involvement with a mental health care setting, researchers should begin from an understanding that these are places of care for individuals who are, sometimes, acutely unwell.

- Voluntary/charity and community settings

Some researchers recruit in the community, and some with the support of the voluntary or charity sector. There are many different places where research can take place in the community, including (not an exhaustive list):

- Faith organisations.
- Homeless shelters.
- Community support groups (e.g. alcohol support groups, art groups).
- Aid organisations.
- Libraries.
- Temporary medical units.
- Recreational grounds.
- Community cafes/centres.
- Village halls.

Part of the assessment around risk to your safety will relate to the location of the data collection and the extent to which you are supported by any community group, leader, or organisation. You may have the responsibility for finding a venue for data collection, but you may be provided with space by the supportive community partners or professionals. This leads to issues regarding who else has access to that space, who else is likely to enter the space, and the possible unpredictability of the space.

Consider also that some community or charity settings may be in areas where there are considerable risks to safety, such as following a natural disaster or regions impacted by war and conflict. Such settings carry clear issues relating to safety and security that need to be managed and mitigated if you are going to carry out your fieldwork in those places. It is important to navigate the security challenges, attend to power issues, and be reflective so that you might challenge any stories that perpetuate harm and insecurity (Gordon, 2021). Gordon argued that it can be helpful to undertake a conflict analysis to identify, assess, prioritise, and avoid threats, to create a security plan which needs to be constantly revisited.

We have offered up a discussion of these four settings as common examples of places where researchers interact with their participants and may need to consider their safety, rather than as an exhaustive list. As a summary, then, we offer some summative practical tips in Box 12.5.

> **Box 12.5**
>
> **Important things to remember about physical well-being**
>
> In reflecting on your physical well-being while undertaking qualitative health research, there are some things you need to be mindful of:
>
> - Managing your physical safety is an ongoing consideration, and you need to think through all aspects of this before you begin engaging with others in PPIE activities, working with your team, and undertaking fieldwork.
> - Make sure you are mindful of the environment for fieldwork. If you are entering the homes of your participants, you may not know all the occupants and you have little control over who comes into the space (Bloor et al., 2010).
> - Do not overlook physical safety risks. Develop a written safety protocol and take active steps to safeguard your personal safety during all parts of the project (Dickson-Swift, 2022).
> - Take care to consider the physical toll of undertaking the research, in quite practical terms, for example, sitting for several hours undertaking ethnographic observations or interviews.
> - Risks to your physical safety as a researcher are not limited to contact with participants or the subjects of the research but also include other aspects of the research environment, which should be considered.

Transcriptionist safety

We have previously argued that transcriptionists are often not afforded the necessary attention in relation to safety in qualitative research (Kiyimba and O'Reilly, 2016a, 2016b). However, as human beings, transcriptionists will also experience emotional reactions to the data. As such, their emotional well-being should be considered when undertaking qualitative health research. Indeed, some have suggested that researchers have a duty of care toward their transcriptionists to minimise or ameliorate any potential emotional harm (Hennessy, Dennehy, Doherty, and O'Donoghue, 2022). Hennessy et al. argued that reference to "the researcher" means the "research team" and this includes the transcriptionist.

> **Key point!**
>
> Often researchers contract transcription services to external companies, so the researcher needs to be aware of the kind of material they are exposing the transcriptionist to and put processes in place to manage any impact.
>
> (Dickson-Swift, 2022)

It is certainly possible that transcriptionists can become emotionally affected by the accounts they hear in research interviews or other recordings (Tilley, 2003), and in some cases they may feel distress or feelings of helplessness (Kiyimba and O'Reilly,

MANAGING RESEARCHER SAFETY

2016a; Wilkes, Cummings, and Haigh, 2015). We have argued, therefore, that there needs to be more attention paid to the risks of secondary traumatic stress or vicarious traumatisation for the transcriptionist (Kiyimba and O'Reilly, 2016b). As we noted earlier in the chapter, these consequences are possible for researchers working with sensitive and emotionally challenging data, and researchers can be left feeling burnt out, and transcriptionists are not immune to this either.

> **Key point!**
>
> Transcriptionists may be working on multiple projects in a given timeframe, in succession or in parallel, and this can increase the potential for long-term emotional impact.
>
> (Hennessy et al., 2022)

There are steps you can take as a qualitative researcher to help your transcriptionist manage any emotional impact. We have made some suggestions, and we outline those practical steps in Box 12.6 (Kiyimba and O'Reilly, 2016b).

> **Box 12.6**
> **Practical steps to help support the transcriptionist (Kiyimba and O'Reilly, 2016b)**
>
> There are some practical steps you can take to help support the transcriptionist working on your project during three key stages in the research (see Kiyimba and O'Reilly, 2016b):
>
> 1. **Prior to the transcription task** – you can brief the transcriptionist about the nature of the data, the characteristics of the participants, the topic of conversation, and anything that came up that was especially upsetting or difficult to hear. Provide a simple protocol for them in terms of what they can do and who they can contact should they find themselves adversely affected. As a researcher, you are likely to be one person on that list due to the confidentiality and protection of participants in of the data collection process, but charitable organisation helplines or other sources may also be included. In the section relating to researcher safety on the ethics application, a short piece about the emotional well-being of the transcriptionist should be included.
> 2. **During the transcription task** – make yourself available to the transcriptionist if they need to talk. Provide them with contact details so that if they find themselves negatively affected during the task, they can take a break and talk to you about how they are feeling.
> 3. **Post the transcription task** – have regular check-in or debrief meetings with the transcriptionist as they hand over batches of transcription to check on their welfare and give them an opportunity to share their experiences. You can remind the transcriptionist of other sources of support should they find they want to make use of them. Additionally, researchers could be more active in reporting and publishing their experiences and encouraging a culture of sharing (see also Parker and O'Reilly, 2013) so that these issues are discussed more often in research teams.

In thinking about the emotional welfare of the transcriptionist, we recognise that some of our readers may be experienced health researchers who have developed coping techniques and may even have become desensitised to the emotional impact of the research on them. In these cases, we encourage researchers to be reflective and consider how transcriptionists, and less experienced researchers in the team, may experience working with data (Kiyimba and O'Reilly, 2016b). We note that it is unusual for researchers to work completely individually and in isolation, as it is normative for them to have collaborators, co-investigators, mentors, supervisors, stakeholder groups, or other team members supporting the project. In supporting transcriptionists with their emotional well-being, a team approach can be hugely helpful, provided that individual is treated as a team member.

In our own research interviewing professional transcriptionists, we found that they mostly felt that they had limited or inadequate formal support for the intensity of the emotional work they conducted (Kiyimba and O'Reilly, 2016a). Indeed, transcriptionists taking part in the study felt it was challenging to manage the impact of exposure to distressing material. Moreover, we found that there was considerable heterogeneity among transcriptionists as a professional group, with many working privately on short-term contracts. This is particularly problematic as there tend to be no official safeguarding protocols for this working group, especially on short contracts, and they may not have had any training or preparation to deal with the issues arising from the work. Thus, in closing this section of our chapter, we encourage you to consider how you might support your transcriptionist and highlight some useful things to remember for this task in Box 12.7.

Box 12.7

Important things to remember about transcriptionists (and their safety)

In reflecting on the role of the transcriptionist, there are some things to be mindful of:

- Remember that transcriptionists are often invisible workers, and researchers do not always think about them in terms of coming to emotional harm.
- It is essential for you to consider the welfare of the transcriptionist working on your project if you employ one to undertake the work. Transcriptionist safety should not be overlooked (McCosker, Barnard, and Gerber, 2001).
- Transcription is not merely a mundane task (Lapadat and Lindsay, 1999). Because of the labour and depth involved, the transcriptionist will be affected by the process of the task (Gregory, Russell, and Phillips, 1997; Kiyimba and O'Reilly, 2016a).
- Be mindful that your transcriptionist will likely listen to the data multiple times to capture the words accurately and is therefore more likely to be emotionally affected (Gregory et al., 1997; Kiyimba and O'Reilly, 2016a; Lalor, Begley, and Devane, 2006).
- The transcription work can become emotionally overwhelming, and this may influence the decisions of transcriptionists to leave the profession or refuse certain kinds of transcription work (Wilkes et al., 2015).
- Appreciate that your transcriptionist may be working in isolation and may have no or limited access to support (Kiyimba and O'Reilly, 2016a). You may need to take some

> responsibility to provide your transcriptionist with the opportunity to debrief, and you should also prepare them in advance that there may be emotional effects (Etherington, 2007). This is important, as transcriptionists are rarely given any formal supervision or support (Etherington, 2007).

Managing researcher safety in practice
As we draw this chapter to a close, we synthesise recommendations from the wider literature and reiterate some of the practical strategies we have proposed in our own work. While having some sense of what the issues are is helpful, having practical management strategies in research practice is vital. Researchers need to be well-equipped to competently address challenges that arise in their work and engage with their networks when undertaking sensitive or difficult topics of research (Silverio et al., 2022). This is due to "researcher vulnerability", a concept introduced by Tang, Cheung, Zhou, and Leung (2020) referring to the necessity of having strategies and protocols in place for protecting researchers, especially in unpredictable situations. In our previous writing, we have proposed some practical ways of developing these strategies, having operational management techniques, and planning with safety in mind, and we proposed these in five clusters (Kiyimba and O'Reilly, in press), which we reconsider and redevelop here in the context of health research more specifically:

1. Preparatory thinking and planning.
2. Developing policy.
3. Prevention.
4. Managing risk in-situ.
5. Actions post event or incident.

Preparatory thinking and planning
We have proposed that researcher safety needs to be thought about and considered from the outset of the project and should be reflected in the preparatory thinking and planning stage (Kiyimba and O'Reilly, in press; O'Reilly and Kiyimba, 2015). Researchers need to be mindful of what risks may occur during their work, specifically emotional and physical ones, but also considering any reputational risk or other kinds of possible risks that may arise in relation to the topic, the participants, the location of fieldwork, and so forth. Some of these risks are quite specific to health and illness and healthcare environments, and others are more general to qualitative research. We outline our recommendations that we made in our previous work (Kiyimba and O'Reilly, in press) which were based on the wider literature, our own experiences, and our research in Table 12.1 and here in this chapter we apply them to health research more specifically.

Developing policies
It is considered good practice for organisations to have a clear policy directive that accounts for researcher safety and for these policies to ensure that they are operational

Table 12.1 Planning recommendations for researcher safety (originally discussed in Kiyimba and O'Reilly, in press in relation to research generally)

Action	Description
Raise awareness	It is important when planning to read about researcher safety and be aware of what risks you might face in preparing and doing your health research project. A planning risk assessment can help raise this awareness for you and your team, as this actively encourages reflection on what is possible. Ethics applications should include explicit questions about possible risks to the research team, and there should be space for you to specify how you have mitigated and considered those risks. For example, there may be obvious risks of infection when working with certain participants (e.g. going onto a ward with patients who are infectious) or in specific health environments (e.g. visiting prisoners in relation to their health). The risk assessment should be examined by health research experts who can ask appropriate questions and critically examine the safety protocol. Thus, we advise you to partner with or seek advice from experts in your topic area.
Training	Training is core business for researchers and is often mandated. Indeed, healthcare practitioners generally engage with continuing professional development and regularly attend training courses. We have recommended that researchers engage in safety training that addresses assessment procedures, risk management techniques, basic de-escalation or self-defence techniques, and the theory and practice of lone working and encourage you to look at various training options available to you. Training in relation to safety, as well as other ethics and integrity issues, should be a part of a researcher's professional development (see Winfield, 2022), and for many clinical practitioners will align with their health and safety training for their clinical practice.
Risk assessment and management	Many clinical practitioners undertake risk assessments as part of their practice, and some of those skills will be beneficial in the context of research. Thus, you may already have skills in this practice. For research, preferably, the risk assessment should be a formal written record and be part of your ethics application for an audit trail. The risk assessment should provide you with a view of possible physical, emotional, situational, and temporal risks and could provide information links to sources of support and institutional policy. The risk assessment form and procedure should be reviewed regularly by the institution and/or researcher, and action plans should be made available.

and map against other relevant institutional policies. We outline our recommendations, based on the wider literature, our own experiences, and our research and frame these in relation to health research in Table 12.2.

Preventing harm

In the context of researcher safety, steps need to be taken to prevent harm to the researcher (and the team and organisation they represent) emotionally, physically, and

Table 12.2 Developing a researcher safety policy (originally discussed in Kiyimba and O'Reilly, in press)

Action	Description
Have a policy in place	It is useful for you to check if your organisation has a policy in place in relation to researcher safety, or to see what safety protocols ther are for clinical practice which might help you in the research context. Policies are useful in organisations as they provide protocols for engaging in research, and most healthcare organisations and universities will have policies related to their research code of conduct. Policies should be reviewed regularly, and any policy that considers researcher safety may overlap with other relevant policies like those for lone workers, health and safety, and ethics. Policies on researcher safety need to be developed with safety at the centre and should be written in consultation with experts in the field and contextualised in relation to the discipline of health. Any conflicts with other policies (either within the organisation or a partner organisation) need to be identified, and persons with responsibility should be appointed, so it is worth you seeking out these individuals if you have questions. In so doing, organisations should aim for an institutional culture that is supportive of the well-being of researchers and navigates any barriers there may be in accessing support (see Smith et al., 2021).
Policies need to be operational and functional	Policies need to be checked to ensure they are substantial enough to protect researchers from harm, and contextual factors specific to health research should be accounted for. There need to be procedures related to the policy that can be followed and implemented by researchers, and we recommend you take steps to protect yourself from harm. Policies need to be accessible and easy to find for those who need them and so it is worth checking if this is the case in your own organisation.
Policies need to align with those of other agencies	Risk assessments and policies often signpost to other organisations or agencies for further information or support. Professionals developing organisational policy can consult with other relevant agencies about best practices and obtain advice. Any policy developed, though unique to the organisation, should be compatible with those of other comparable organisations.

reputationally. In the planning stages of the project and in carrying out a risk assessment, researchers ideally ought to do as much as possible to identify and mitigate the possible risks of undertaking the research project. We have made some recommendations for this in practice in relation to research generally (Kiyimba and O'Reilly, in press) which are outlined in Table 12.3 and here we contextualise those proposals in terms of health research more specifically.

In addition to this, the literature advises that a trauma-informed approach to research is useful in avoiding the re-traumatisation of research participants, but also to reduce the likelihood of vicarious trauma for the researcher (Campbell, Goodman-Williams, and Javorka, 2019). A trauma-informed approach is relevant as this means that the practice accounts for any possible or actual trauma experience (Knight, 2019). Such an approach necessitates institutions to understand how trauma may impact a person, and the risks associated with this trauma (Orr et al., 2021).

Table 12.3 Preventing harm (originally discussed in Kiyimba and O'Reilly, in press)

Action	Description
Avoid personal spaces for field work	Earlier in the chapter, we discussed possible locations for data collection and identified some of the plausible risks associated with them. Although a participant might feel more comfortable talking in their own home, from experience, we recommend, where possible, to avoid personal spaces for data collection. There may be risks such as the presence of animals, access to weapons, or house guests who may be a threat to you. There are alternatives, such as library rooms, community centres, and organisational spaces. Of course, you may be collecting data as part of your working role which may involve visiting people at home and consequently be unavoidable. Nonetheless, discussions about the research aspect of the work with your supervisors, managers, and other relevant stakeholders are needed even where it forms part of your day-to-day practice so that policies and plans can account for the research aspect of the task.
Avoid lone working	Lone worker policies were created for a range of professional groups because many practitioners needed to visit their clients at home. In research, we advise you to be mindful of the risks you may be taking and the organisational infrastructure to protect you in going into personal or even some professional spaces alone. We have previously advised researchers not to visit participants alone in private spaces, and where possible, to have a second researcher accompany them through fieldwork.

Table 12.4 Managing risk (originally discussed in Kiyimba and O'Reilly, in press)

Action	Description
Be calm	If you face risk or danger within the field, try to stay calm. Regulate your breathing, and keep calm and steady. Remain grounded in the environment by paying attention to your five senses. Allow your mind to focus on the situation to find a solution. Your clinical skills may come in useful, as it is possible you have faced difficult situations as part of your practice. It might be necessary to use those clinical skills in this context and draw upon your clinical training to manage the situation.
De-escalation	It is often the case that organisations recommend the termination of data collection (like the interview) as quickly as possible and removing oneself from the situation (Ritchie, Lewis, Elam et al., 2014), but be mindful that this action may provoke alarm and aggression, and de-escalation may be more appropriate (Bashir, 2018). You will need to use your own judgement about what is sensible and appropriate depending on the specifics of your situation and again draw on your practitioner skills if helpful to do so. In de-escalating a situation, think about your posture and body language and speak in a tone of voice that is calm and slow. Try to keep your facial expression neutral or pleasant and move the conversation onto safer topics. As good practice, it may be useful to complete some training in de-escalation techniques if you have not done so previously.
Disengage	When possible and as quickly as you can, disengage from the risky situation. It is always useful to have planned exit routes and think about where you are seated in relation to the participants. Indicate as soon as you can your indication to leave and offer a timeframe to do so.

MANAGING RESEARCHER SAFETY

Managing risk in the moment

Not all risks can be prevented or predicted, and so it is important that researchers are equipped with skills and techniques for managing challenges that occur during fieldwork or at any other point in the process. We outline our recommendations, based on the wider literature, our own experiences, and our research in Table 12.4.

In the planning stages, it is useful to have a "buddy system" in place (Silverio et al., 2022). Silverio et al. pointed out that this is useful in the sense of having a pre-planned telephone chain of contact, that is, a nominated point of contact, and a second buddy should be available in case the primary buddy is away from the phone or experiencing illness.

Post incident

In the previous section, we made some suggestions for how to manage an event while it is occurring, and it is also helpful to consider post-incident management factors as there are likely to be additional steps to take afterward. Our recommendations are provided in Table 12.5.

Table 12.5 Post-incident recommendations (originally discussed in Kiyimba and O'Reilly, in press)

Action	*Description*
Inform those who need to know	There will likely be several people who need to understand the incident. You may be part of a research team, and your colleagues need to know what happened. Additionally, you may need to tell senior members of the team, representatives of the organisation, the ethics board, your supervisor if you have one, and any other relevant party. Speak with your safety contact person and take the opportunity to debrief as you may be emotionally affected. If the research is related to your organisation or your work, then you will need to speak to your line manager.
Assess if other formal parties need to know	If the incident was serious, criminal in nature, or has serious implications for the safety of others, you may need to contact external organisations or agencies, such as social services, general practitioners, or the police. You will need to review your research participation confidentiality breach clause in your information sheet and other documents, and you may need to seek advice from others in your organisation to support you.
Debriefing	Debriefing is an important process as it establishes facts, identifies support needs, and determines who needs to be informed. Try to have a clearly written narrative of what happened to share with those you need to.
Make changes	You may decide to review your research processes and procedures and make changes to promote safety. Consultation and discussion with others in the team and other experts can help in making those changes. The data collection process may need to be changed, or the topic may need to be altered slightly. New gatekeepers may be needed.

In bringing this chapter to a close, we invite you to reflect on the lessons you have learnt and the thoughts you now have about your safety. Consider the reflective activity in Box 12.8.

> **Box 12.8**
>
> **Reflecting on your own safety**
>
> Based on the topic of this chapter, we invite you to take a few moments to reflect on your own role as a clinician-researcher.
>
> - What topics have been covered that you had not previously thought much about?
> - How will this new knowledge change the way that you and your research and/or clinical team operate?
> - What additional information, training, or supervision arrangements might you need to negotiate for yourself and your research team?
> - Consider whether sharing your own experiences in managing researcher safety might helpfully add to the information and literature available to others.

Author reflections and concluding remarks
From Nikki

To conclude this chapter, I will offer a few reflections on the topic of researcher safety. It is interesting for me, as the person who was a doctoral student at the time of the physical safety example earlier in the chapter, to reflect on how that experience has shaped the way that I have subsequently engaged in research, and the way that I now support my students, research assistants, and transcriptionist colleagues. At the time of writing this book, more than a decade has passed since that incident, and I have learnt a lot more about how important the emotional and physical safety of the whole research team is. As a student, apart from a university supervisor, most of my experiences were of being quite independent, collecting, transcribing, and analysing all the data myself. What I have come to value greatly as a clinician-researcher are the wonderful, supportive, interesting, and collaborative relationships that emerge through being part of a research team. Often, as the lead researcher, it is my role to take responsibility for the welfare of the research assistants and colleagues involved in interviewing participants. I am much more conscious of ensuring regular contact with each of them, as apart from the potential emotional toll, it can feel quite isolating working on an aspect of a project alone. I know I have not always been great at doing this – my own work pressures, deadlines, and responsibilities at times have distracted me away from this. But with hindsight, I now know that maintaining the welfare of the beautiful humans in the research team needs to be a top priority.

Also, it truly is a joy – the most vibrant, interesting, and productive times are when we meet together either in pairs or small groups to look at data, to debrief from a block of interviews, or to touch base regularly about what is coming up in the data during the transcription process. I am extremely grateful to the transcriptionist involved in the "we're alone in the house" project (Parker and O'Reilly, 2013) who showed me just how much she cared for my well-being and how my reciprocation of care about her well-being was just as important as getting my project completed. More recently, I am very grateful to the wonderful interviewers, transcriptionists, and research assistants I have been working with on the international phase of the LOSST LIFFE project (see Thorne and O'Reilly, 2022 for UK model). These research colleagues have been amazing partners in learning about how to support one another through the emotional challenges of listening to the narratives of front-line workers responding to suicide. I have ever more deepening respect for those participants for sharing their pain and courage, and for each person in my research team for their genuine passion to serve our participants by providing a place for them to be heard, and for their willingness to engage in this emotionally challenging work.

References

Bahn, S., and Weatherill, P. (2013). Qualitative social research: A risky business when it comes to collecting "sensitive" data. *Qualitative Research*, 13, 19–35.

Bashir, N. (2018). Doing research in peoples' homes: Fieldwork, ethics and safety – on the practical challenges of researching and representing life on the margins. *Qualitative Research*, 18(6), 638–653.

Batty, E. (2020). Sorry to say goodbye: The dilemmas of letting go in longitudinal research. *Qualitative Research*, 20(6), 784–799.

Benoot, C., and Bilsen, J. (2015). An auto-ethnographic study of the disembodied experience of a novice researcher doing qualitative cancer research. *Qualitative Health Research*, 26(4), 482–489.

Bloor, M., Fincham, B., and Sampson, H. (2007). *QUALITI (NCRM) Commissioned inquiry into the risk and well-being of researchers in qualitative research*. Cardiff: ESRC.

Bloor, M., Fincham, B., and Sampson, H. (2010). Unprepared for the worst: Risks of harm for qualitative researchers. *Methodological Innovations*, 5(1), 45–55.

Borbasi, S., Chapman, Y., and Read, K. (2002). Perceptions of the researcher: In-depth interviewing in the home. *Contemporary Nurse*, 14(1), 24–37.

Bowtell, E., Sawyer, S., Aroni, R., Green, J., and Duncan, R. (2013). "Should I send a condolence card?" Promoting emotional safety in qualitative health research through reflexivity and ethical mindfulness. *Qualitative Inquiry*, 19(9), 65.

Boyle, D. (2011). Countering compassion fatigue: A requisite nursing agenda. *The Online Journal of Issues in Nursing*, 16(1), 1–13.

Boynton, P. (2016). *The research companion: A practical guide for those in the social sciences, health and development*. London: Routledge.

Bradley, M. (2007). Silenced for their own protection: How the IRB marginalizes those it feigns to protect. *ACME: An International Journal for Critical Geographies*, 6(3), 339–349.

Bride, B., Robinson, M., Yegidis, B., and Figley, C. (2004). Development and validation of the secondary traumatic stress scale. *Research on Social Work Practice*, 14(1), 27–35.

Bushin, N. (2007). Interviewing children in their homes: Putting ethical principles into practice and developing flexible techniques. *Children's Geographies*, 5(3), 235–251.

Butler, A., Copnell, B., and Hall, H. (2019). Researching people who are bereaved: Managing risks to participants and researchers. *Nursing Ethics*, 26(1), 224–234.

Campbell, R. (2002). *Emotionally Involved: The impact of researching rape*. New York, NY: Routledge.

Campbell, R. (2017). Qualitative fieldwork within the criminal justice system. *Qualitative Psychology*, 4(3), 315–325.

Campbell, R., Goodman-Williams, R., and Javorka, M. (2019). A trauma-informed approach to sexual violence research ethics and open science. *Journal of Interpersonal Violence*, 34(23–24), 4765–4793.

Christopher, M., Goerling, R., Rogers, B. S., Hunsinger, M., Baron, G., Bergman, A., and Zava, D. (2016). A pilot study evaluating the effectiveness of a mindfulness-based intervention on cortisol awakening response and health outcomes among law enforcement officers. *Journal of Police & Criminal Psychology*, 31(1), 15–28.

Coles, J., Astbury, J., Dartnall, E., and Limjerwala, S. (2014). A qualitative exploration of researcher trauma and researchers' responses to investigating sexual violence. *Violence against Women*, 20(1), 95–117.

Coles, J., and Mudaly, N. (2010). Staying safe: Strategies for qualitative child abuse researchers. *Child Abuse Review*, 19(1), 56–69.

Demerouti, E., Bakker, A., Nachreiner, F., and Schaufeli, W. (2001). The job demands-resources model of burnout. *Journal of Applied Psychology*, 86(3), 499–512.

Devilly, G., Wright, R., and Varker, T. (2009). Vicarious trauma, secondary traumatic stress or simply burnout? Effect of trauma therapy on mental health professionals. *Australasian Psychiatry*, 43(4), 373–385.

Dickson-Swift, V. (2022). Undertaking qualitative research on trauma: Impacts on researchers and guidelines for risk management. *Qualitative Research in Organizations & Management*, 18(4), 469–486.

Dickson-Swift, V., James, E., Kippen, S., and Liamputtong, P. (2008). Risk to researchers in qualitative research on sensitive topics: Issues and strategies. *Qualitative Health Research*, 18(1), 133–144.

Eades, A.-M., Hackett, M., Raven, M., Liu, H., and Cass, A. (2020). The impact of vicarious trauma on indigenous health researchers. *Public Health Research & Practice*, 31(3), 1–6.

Eriksen, C. (2017). Research ethics, trauma and self-care: Reflections on disaster geographies. *Australian Geographer*, 48(2), 273–278.

Etherington, K. (2007). Working with traumatic stories: From transcriber to witness. *International Journal of Social Research Methodology*, 10(2), 85–97.

Fenge, L., Oakley, L., Taylor, B., and Beer, S (2019). The impact of sensitive research on the researcher: Preparedness and positionality. *International Journal of Qualitative Methods*, 18, 1–18.

Figley, C. (2013). *Compassion fatigue: Coping with secondary traumatic stress disorder in those who treat the traumatized*. New York, NY: Routledge.

Fohring, S. (2020). The risks and rewards of researching victims of crime. *Methodological Innovations*, 13(2), 1–11.

Gleeson, J. (2021). Troubling/trouble in the academy: Posttraumatic stress disorder and sexual abuse research. *Higher Education*, 1, 1–15.

Gordon, E. (2021). The researcher and the researched: Navigating the challenges of research in conflict-affected environments. *International Studies Review*, 23(1), 59–88.

Gregory, D., Russell, C., and Phillips, L. (1997). Beyond textual perfection: Transcribers as vulnerable persons. *Qualitative Health Research*, 7(2), 294–300.

Hennessy, M., Dennehy, R., Doherty, J., and O'Donoghue, K. (2022). Outsourcing transcription: Extending ethical considerations in qualitative research. *Qualitative Health Research*, 32(7), 1197–1204.

Kiyimba, N. (2020). *Trauma-informed mindfulness: A practitioner's guide to one-to-one work*. Chester: Chester University Press.

Kiyimba, N., and O'Reilly, M. (2016a). An exploration of the possibility for secondary traumatic stress amongst transcriptionists: A grounded theory approach. *Qualitative Research in Psychology*, 13(1), 92–108.

Kiyimba, N., and O'Reilly, M. (2016b). The risk of secondary traumatic stress in the qualitative transcription process: A research note. *Qualitative Research*, 16(4), 468–476.

Kiyimba, N., and O'Reilly, M. (in press). Lone worker policies: What to do in risky situations when theory and practice fail to align. In K. Hughes, A. Tarrant, J. Hughes, and G. Sykes (Eds.), *Tales of the unexpected: Learning from doing social sciences research* (Title subject to change). London; Sage

Knight, C. (2019). Trauma informed practice and care: Implications for field instruction. *Clinical Social Work Journal*, 47(1), 79–89.

Lalor, J., Begley, C., and Devane, D. (2006). Exploring painful experiences: Impact of emotional narratives on members of a qualitative research team. *Journal of Advanced Nursing*, 56(6), 607–616.

Lapadat, J., and Lindsay, A. (1999). Transcription in research and practice: From standardization of technique to interpretive positioning. *Qualitative Inquiry*, 5(1), 64–86.

Larson, D., and Bush, N. (2006). Stress management for oncology nurses: Finding a healing balance. In R. Carroll-Johnson, L. Gorman., and N. Bush (Eds.). *Psychosocial nursing along the cancer continuum* (pp. 587–601). Pittsburgh, PA: Oncology Nursing Society.

MacDonald, K. (2008). Dealing with chaos and complexity: The reality of interviewing children and families in their own homes. *Journal of Clinical Nursing*, 17(23), 3123–3130.

Mallon, S., Borgstrom, E., and Murphy, S. (2021). Unpacking sensitive research: A stimulating exploration of an established concept. *International Journal of Social Research Methodology*, 24(5), 517–521.

McCosker, H., Barnard, A., and Gerber, R. (2001). Undertaking sensitive research: Issues and strategies for meeting the safety needs of all participants. *Forum: Qualitative Social Research*, 2(1).

Moran, R., and Asquith, N. (2020). Understanding the vicarious trauma and emotional labour of criminological research. *Methodological Innovations*, 13(2), 1–11.

Motta, R. (2008). Secondary trauma. *International Journal of Emergency Mental Health*, 10(4), 291–298.

O'Reilly, M., and Kiyimba, N. (2015). *Advanced qualitative research: A guide to contemporary theoretical debates*. London: Sage.

Orr, E., Durepos, P., Jones, V., and Jack, S. M. (2021). Risk of secondary distress for graduate students conducting qualitative research on sensitive subjects: A scoping review of Canadian dissertations and theses. *Global Qualitative Nursing Research*.

Parker, N., and O'Reilly, M. (2013) "We are alone in the house": A case study addressing researcher safety and risk. *Qualitative Research in Psychology*, 10(4), 341–354.

Pearlman, L., and Saakvitne, K. (1995). *Trauma and the therapist: Counter-transference and traumatisation in psychotherapy with incest survivors*. London: Norton.

Plackett, B. (2020). The British department trying to reset workers' attitudes toward health and safety: The health and safety executive, charged with safety research and regulation, hopes COVID-19 will bring needed change. *Chemical & Engineering News*, 98(41). https://cen.acs.org/safety/British-department-trying-reset-workersattitudes/98/i41

Ritchie, J., Lewis, J., Elam, G., Tennant, R., and Rahim, N. (2014). Designing and selecting samples. In J. Ritchie, J. Lewis, C. McNaughton-Nicholls, and R. Ormston (Eds.), *Qualitative research practice: A guide for social science students and researchers* (pp. 111–146). London: Sage.

Sampson, H. (2019). "Fluid fields" and the dynamics of risk in social research. *Qualitative Research*, 19(2), 131–147.

Sherry, E. (2013). The vulnerable researcher: Facing the challenges of sensitive research. *Qualitative Research Journal*, 13(3), 278–288.

Sillitoe, K., Kimbya, N., Milliken, J., and Bennett, P. (2021). Peer assessment after clinical exposure (PACE): An evaluation of structured peer support for staff in emergency care. *British Journal of Nursing*, 30(19), 1132–1139.

Silverio, S. A., Sheen, K. S., Bramante, A., Knighting, K., Koops, T. U., Montgomery, E., November, L., Soulsby, L. K., Stevenson, J. H., Watkins, M., Easter, A., and Sandall, J. (2022). Supporting researchers conducting qualitative research into sensitive, challenging, and difficult topics: Experiences and practical applications. *International Journal of Qualitative Methods, 21*, 1–16.

Smith, E., Pooley, J. A., Holmes, L., Gebbie, K., and Gershon, R. (2021). Vicarious trauma: Exploring the experiences of qualitative researchers who study traumatized populations. *Disaster Medicine & Public Health Preparedness, 17*, e69.

Social Research Association. (2005). Staying safe: A code of practice for the safety of social researchers. www.the-sra.org.uk

Sprang, G., Lei, F., and Bush, H. (2021). Can organizational efforts lead to less secondary traumatic stress? A longitudinal investigation of change. *American Journal of Orthopsychiatry, 91*(4), 443–453.

Sprang, G., Miech, E., and Gusler, S. (2023). The role of secondary traumatic stress breakthrough champions in reducing worker trauma and improving organizational health using a configurational analysis approach. *Implementation Research & Practice, 4*.

Swords, C., and Houston, S. (2020). Exploring the concept of recovery in Irish mental health services: A case study of perspectives within an inter-professional team. *Irish Journal of Applied Social Studies, 20*(1), 31–46.

Tang, X., Cheung, M., Zhou, S., and Leung, P. (2020). The vulnerable researcher phenomenon. *Open Journal of Philosophy, 10*(4), 511–527.

Thorne, B., and O'Reilly, M. (2022). Operationalizing strategic objectives of suicide prevention policy: Police-led LOSST LIFFE model. *Death Studies, 46*(9), 2077–2084.

Tilley, S. (2003). Transcription work: Learning through co-participation in research practices. *Qualitative Studies in Education, 16*(6), 835–851.

Tolich, M., Tumilty, E., Choe, L., Hohmann-Marriott, B., and Fahey, N. (2020). Researcher emotional safety as ethics in practice: Why professional supervision should augment PhD candidates' academic supervision. In R. Iphofen (Ed.), *Handbook of research ethics and scientific integrity* (pp. 589–602). Cham, Switzerland: Springer.

Webber, V., and Brunger, F. (2018). Assessing risk to researchers: Using the case of sexuality research to inform Research Ethics Board guidelines. *Forum Qualitative Social Research, 19*(3).

Wilkes, L., Cummings, J., and Haigh, C. (2015). Transcriptionist saturation: Knowing too much about sensitive health and social data. *Journal of Advanced Nursing, 71*(2), 295–303.

Williamson, E., Gregory, A., Abrahams, H., Aghtaie, N., Walker, S.-J., and Hester, M. (2020). Secondary trauma: Emotional safety in sensitive research. *Journal of Academic Ethics, 18*, 55–70.

Winfield, T. (2022). Vulnerable research: Competencies for trauma and justice-informed ethnography. *Journal of Contemporary Ethnography, 51*(2), 135–170.

CHAPTER 13

Methods of data collection

> **Learning objectives**
>
> This chapter enables the reader to:
>
> - Differentiate between naturally occurring and researcher-generated data.
> - Identify the value of different methods of qualitative data collection.
> - Recognise the value of visual, audio, and text-based methods of data collection.
> - Critically assess the benefits and challenges of different kinds of methods.
> - Appreciate the value and challenges of using secondary data sources.

Introduction

There are many methods of data collection in qualitative research. The most common ways to collect data are via interviews and focus groups, and we have thus dedicated a whole chapter to these two methods in the next chapter. In this chapter, we introduce you to the two types of research data: data that occur naturally and are used for research purposes, and data that are generated specifically for research. As we progress through the chapter, we also introduce you to the common qualitative data collection methods other than interviews and focus groups: case studies, diaries, observations, use of documents, and World Café methods. We additionally provide some information about participatory techniques and using secondary data.

Naturally occurring and researcher-generated data

Collecting data for qualitative research has generally been conceptualised into two broad types: (1) researcher-generated data and (2) naturally occurring data.

> **Key point!**
>
> Researcher-generated data are produced by a researcher for the purpose of a project. These data would not exist if it were not for the activities of the researcher.
>
> (Kiyimba, Lester, and O'Reilly, 2019)

> **Key point!**
>
> Naturally occurring data denotes the capturing and recording of activities that occur naturally for the purpose of research. These activities would continue to occur without the active involvement of the researcher.
>
> (Potter, 2002)

A preference for either naturally occurring data collection or researcher-generated data collection methods can be strong for some researchers, and some qualitative approaches involve one or the other. However, other methodological approaches allow for either type or even a combination of both. In thinking through which type of data collection is most suitable for your project, you should consider the theoretical, epistemological, and ontological framework of your research, as your methods of data collection need to be congruent with them.

You should be mindful that whilst we are differentiating naturally occurring data from researcher-generated data, there are some scholars who argue that the distinction between the two is not at all clear-cut and can be overstated (Silverman, 2010). Arguably, all data collected for research purposes are to some extent "generated", and when recording naturally occurring activities, the researcher will have some influence, even if it is minimal (Kiyimba et al., 2019). Arguably, then, as Peräkylä (2005) noted, "the difference between researcher-instigated data and naturally occurring data should … be understood as a continuum rather than as a dichotomy" (p. 870). Before we provide more detail, we note some things for you to be aware of in planning and undertaking your own research in Box 13.1.

> **Box 13.1**
>
> **Important things to remember about your data collection method**
>
> There are some things to reflect on when choosing what kind of data to collect for your own project:
>
> - Consider your ontological and epistemological assumptions as a researcher and ensure that the method you choose is congruent with them.
> - Think through the practical challenges that you might face in collecting your data and whether these will influence your choices.

METHODS OF DATA COLLECTION

- Ensure that you have completed the necessary ethical applications and have in place required consents before starting your data collection.
- Be mindful that your qualitative approach and type of analysis need to link to the type of data collection you choose to undertake.
- Consider the resources you will need and whether these impact your ability to collect your data in the way you prefer.
- Carefully plan how much data will be sufficient for your project. Collecting too much data to manage and analyse within a prescribed timeframe or other project parameters may be an inappropriate imposition on your participants. Likewise, collecting too little data may not provide you with adequate material to justify your analytic claims.

Naturally occurring data

In understanding naturally occurring data, it can be helpful first to think about what is meant by naturally occurring activities. Naturally occurring activities or events (including text-based activities) refer to those interactions in everyday or institutional settings, with a range of reasons and goals (Kiyimba et al., 2019). Kiyimba et al. noted that naturally occurring activities or texts become data when they are selected by a researcher with the intention of using them for analytic purposes to address a research question. The collection of naturally occurring data is, therefore, consistent with the ontological and epistemological position that reality is situated and co-created through interactions where shared meanings are negotiated and navigated.

The concept "naturally occurring" is used as opposed to "natural" as it is recognised that, because of ethical obligations and the presence of a recording device, the events captured may be subtly influenced, although it is also acknowledged that the presence of a recording device is usually forgotten quickly (Speer and Hutchby, 2003). Nonetheless, the events and activities are naturally occurring in the sense that these are events and activities that would still occur even without the presence of the researcher (Potter, 2004). Consequently, the event or activity continues regardless of the research project and only counts as data if there is an active research process engaged (Potter, 2002). Naturally occurring data are contrasted with researcher-generated data, which are those data produced with active input from a researcher and would not exist if it were not for the researcher (Kiyimba et al., 2019).

Key point!

Much qualitative research involves researcher-generated data as the researcher actively engages their participants in learning about their lives through methods like interviews, focus groups, and diaries where the researcher is a co-interlocutor in the process.

(Potter, 2002)

The collection of naturally occurring data is especially advantageous in qualitative health research where the researcher can observe what is actually happening, rather

Table 13.1 Benefits of collecting naturally occurring data (Kiyimba et al., 2019)

Benefit	Description
Person-centred approach to collecting data.	The collection of naturally occurring data helps in understanding the social and institutional lives of people and can thus be considered a person-centred approach. Collecting naturally occurring data enables the researcher/analyst to explore people's activities in their natural environments, allowing them to explore, describe, and interpret those activities in a real-world context.
Data are context rich.	Qualitative research is typically described as contextually rich (Denzin and Lincoln, 2011), but naturally occurring data also captures the context in which the healthcare interactions arise. The collection of naturally occurring data is situated, local, and contextually focused, providing real-world insights into healthcare and health-related activities.
The collection of naturally occurring data is typically emic.	Emic perspectives have a goal to understand the world through the eyes of the participants, and thus researchers collecting naturally occurring data centre their interpretations on the activities of participants.
Practical advantages to collecting naturally occurring data in relation to time and expenses.	When collecting data through researcher-generated methods like interviews, researchers often have to pay for out-of-pocket expenses for participants, but capturing data via naturally occurring activities does not usually require this. Researcher-generated data also places an additional burden on participants to commit time to participate in research. In contrast, they elect to participate in their naturally occurring activities, and so no additional time burden is created.
Ethical advantages to collecting naturally occurring data in relation to risk and safeguarding.	In addressing ethical issues, the researcher must consider the benefits of the research against any possible risks to participants. In collecting naturally occurring data, there are ethical concerns to be addressed, but some elements, such as safeguarding of participants, are likely accounted for as part of the natural clinical practice and will not be the responsibility of the researcher.
Naturally occurring data provide transparency of context.	Naturally occurring data have the advantage of transparency. Instead of relying on retrospective accounts, capturing this data affords insight into the actual lives and worlds of health and illness. These data retain the original context and arguably the authenticity of the original event or activity.
Benefits to the researcher–participant relationship.	In the collection of naturally occurring data, the researcher is likely to have minimal direct contact with the participants (notwithstanding ethical discussions), and thus they are less likely to influence the interaction. This will likely minimise the potential for social desirability and reduce the need to reflect on the intersubjective nature of the relationship between researcher and participant.

(Continued)

METHODS OF DATA COLLECTION

Table 13.1 (Continued)

Benefit	Description
There is integrity within the collection of naturally occurring data.	The process of acquiring naturally occurring data has some quality indicators built in, such as transparency, trustworthiness, and credibility, as the data reflect natural and real-world interactions. This provides field validity in relation to healthcare practices, which are arguably more meaningful to those working in the field.
Collecting naturally occurring data can provide a mechanism to support practice change.	The collection of naturally occurring data supports the researcher in developing recommendations for practice that are based on an understanding of real-world interactions and healthcare practices. These data enable an illumination of best practices or where things could be improved. This means that actual examples can be used in training those new to a profession by supervisors in supervision, and/or provide a basis for team dialogue.

than what is reportedly happening in different clinical settings. Healthcare comprises naturally occurring institutional and non-institutional activities which can be captured as data. Researchers recording or capturing naturally occurring activities in the field can advance our knowledge of real-world practices and professional communications. Using naturally occurring data provides a source of evidence regarding how professionals and patients/clients experience, understand, and navigate their institutional interactions, with information generated that can be translated into improved care, practices, or processes (Kiyimba et al., 2019). Kiyimba et al. also noted that naturally occurring data are particularly valuable because of the potential to generate theories of care and practices grounded in actual healthcare work rather than from abstract conceptualisations or retrospective accounts. We outline some of these benefits in Table 13.1 originally discussed by Kiyimba et al. (2019).

Researcher-generated data

As we have noted, researcher-generated data are those intentionally created for the purposes of research to address a specific research question. This is to say that the researcher has a role in creating a situation whereby those data can be collected. There are many methods for researcher-generated data, but the most common are interviews and focus groups, whereby participants are invited to attend a location and talk with the researcher about a specific topic area or issue (see Chapter 13). Researchers who collect researcher-generated data tend to operate from epistemological and ontological positions based on a standpoint that researchers can access people's thoughts and perspectives, their versions of reality, by asking them questions (Kiyimba et al., 2019).

There are a range of benefits and advantages to collecting researcher-generated data as described by Kiyimba et al. (2019) and we outline these in Table 13.2.

There are many different methods of data collection available to the qualitative health researcher, and we consider the more common ones in turn (notwithstanding interviews and focus groups, which we discuss in the next chapter).

Table 13.2 Benefits of researcher-generated data (Kiyimba et al., 2019)

Benefit	Description
Immediacy to the production of data.	In terms of time commitment, there can be an advantage in some researcher-generated methods, as they can be set up quickly and the time spent with the participant(s) is often (but not always) a single unit of time – such as a one-hour interview.
Authenticity in data.	Where consistent with an epistemological position, some researchers argue that researcher-generated data have authenticity as it is argued that these data reflect what people think.
Versions of the "truth" become accessible.	Advocates of researcher-generated data argue that these methods support access to participants' versions of the truth and therefore afford valuable knowledge about people's perspectives and experiences.
Allows a focus on a topic or issue.	Researchers are active in setting the agenda or schedule of questions, which creates opportunities for those researchers to focus on specific topics or experiences.
Allows flexibility.	Researcher-generated methods of data collection enable the researcher to interact flexibly with participants according to what they wish to focus on.

Observations

There are a range of different ways of undertaking observations, most of which are researcher-generated, although it is possible to employ an observation method in a naturally occurring way. Observation is a method that has an obvious affinity with the tasks and sensibilities of clinical practitioners as they are typically trained in observing their patients/clients, and systematically recording data about their health and illness, behaviour, or other factors (Mays and Pope, 1995). In the context of research, this can involve systematic observation of both verbal and non-verbal aspects of social behaviour or practices and recording these in detail via field notes. Opting for an observation method means that the researcher can capture more than just the verbal dialogue of participants and move beyond privileging the spoken word to capture the ordinary connections to material artefacts (Aagaarda and Matthiesen, 2015), in other words, the way people interact with material objects within the physical space.

If you are using an observation method, you will play a role in that task. Creswell (2016) argued that there are four types of observer role:

1. **Complete participant** – when you are engaged with those you are observing.
2. **Participant as observer** – when you participate in the activity, and work to gather views as an insider of the group (these can also be ethnographic observations when associated with that methodology).
3. **Non-participant** – when you are an outsider from your participant group, and you observe, but not from a distance.
4. **Complete observer** – a more covert form of observation where you observe without attracting attention and without interacting with the subjects of the research.

METHODS OF DATA COLLECTION

There are some practical steps if you decide to use observations. Creswell (2016) outlined various things you need to consider, which we note in Box 13.2.

Box 13.2

Practical steps to consider when undertaking an observation (Creswell, 2016)

There are many practical things to consider if you opt to gather data via observational means, as outlined by Creswell (2016):

- Select a setting (or settings) where you want to observe your participants and make notes about the physical setting, the interactions, and the activities.
- Develop a protocol for the recording of information.
- Consider what events or situations to capture.
- Decide which role you want to adopt as an observer.
- Recognise the influence of your own behaviours as you observe others.
- Start your observation with broad objectives and narrow down the information sought that is more specific to your research question.
- Take detailed, descriptive, and reflective field notes.
- You will need to be patient and adjust to any obstacles that arise during the process.
- At the start of the observation, you may feel overwhelmed by the task and worry that you cannot capture everything you are observing and experiencing. Try to be patient and focus on the activities observed or the phenomenon of interest.

Using observations gives you access to considerable, rich, and detailed information for analysis. Your field notes are the principal means through which you capture this detail, including the sensory information, so that you can translate or interpret this in the process of analysis. Some have argued that the data collection method of observation provides richer insight into people's lives and social practices by enabling a more holistic understanding of the research subjects and their relationships (see, for example, Aagaarda and Matthiesen, 2015).

Case studies

Case studies are one of the common qualitative research approaches (Yazan, 2015). However, they are arguably a much underused and undervalued approach to collecting data, with considerable practical utility for engaged research that can meaningfully inform organisational change, policy, and practice at a local level (Flyvberg, 2001). This undervaluing may be due to misunderstandings about what constitutes a case study and how this method of data collection might inform professional practice or evidence-based decision-making (Baxter and Jack, 2008). Yet, case study methods allow researchers to explore individuals or organisations and offer the opportunity for discovery about complex interventions, relationships, communities, and programmes (Yin, 2003). For Yin, case studies can be well-utilised when the researcher is addressing "how" or "why" type questions and is interested in exploring phenomena. Indeed, in different respects, a case study is more of a design frame than a method specifically (Thomas, 2011). Simply stated, a researcher may choose a single case study design or a multiple case study design. A multiple case study design affords a way for researchers to explore differences or similarities across cases, whereas a single case might be used to represent an extreme or unusual case either at a single point in time or longitudinally across numerous points over time (Yin, 2003).

Beyond this simple differentiation, there are three main schools of thought regarding the process of engaging in case study research. By "case", this could mean an event, a group, an organisation, or a patient/client/service user. Usually, in practice, the term refers to an individual person. Yazan (2015) provided an overview of the nuances of different case study approaches, which can be used to inform your decisions regarding which approach (or combination of approaches) is most appropriate for your health-related research project. In terms of the different functions of the case study, George and Bennett (2005) have proposed six different types, these are outlined in Table 13.3.

These different approaches to case study research provide different frameworks for the researcher. Consequently, in choosing your approach, it is worth thinking about the goals of the research and the goals of the case study, as this will determine what kind of case study you conduct. Whilst there are functions of case study and different ways of conducting the research, this approach to data collection has a commitment to studying complex processes in different real-life situations and relationships (Simons, 2009). Regardless of the type or function of case study you elect to pursue, it is still relevant to engage in the inquiry in a reflexive way to provide a quality piece of work. Reflecting on your own epistemic position and that of your research participants as coming from different worldviews, the layers of interpretation that occur in the endeavour of analysis must be accounted for overtly. As Merriam (1998, p. 22) emphasised:

> The researcher brings a construction of reality to the research situation, which interacts with other people's constructions or interpretations of the phenomenon being studied. The final product of this type of study is yet another interpretation by the researcher of others' views filtered through his or her own.

Table 13.3 Types of case study and their functions (George and Bennett, 2005)

Case study type	Description of the function
Atheoretical or configurative idiographic	Illustrative case studies that do not aim to contribute to the development of theory.
Disciplined configurative	Case studies where established theories are drawn upon to explain the case.
Heuristic	Case studies in which new causal pathways are identified, and attention is paid to outlier cases.
Theory testing	Case studies designed to assess the scope and validity of a single theory or competing theories.
Plausibility probes	Case studies designed to determine if additional research is warranted and feasible.
Building block	Case studies of specific types or subtypes, or of a specific phenomenon to identify common patterns.

Although we have mentioned previously that there are three main approaches to case study research (Yazan, 2015), as an example, we offer one of these here, which illustrates the practical steps to take (as proposed in Yin's (2003) model). These steps are outlined in Box 13.3.

Box 13.3

Conducting a case study (Yin, 2003)

There are several steps you need to take in conducting a case study:

1. **Your question should guide your case study** – how and why prefaced research questions are typically most appropriate for case studies. Your question will need to be informed by relevant scholarly literature. You will need some development of theory for your research at this stage.
2. **Work through the literature** – initially use the literature to focus your interest on key topics and do not be too concerned with your questions at this point. Once you have narrowed your focus, identify some key studies of relevance, and explore the questions in those studies and areas identified for future research. Endeavour also to explore additional literature to reinforce the relevance and importance of your questions and find ways to refine them.
3. **Address the propositions of the case study** – each proposition of the case study directs attention to what needs to be examined within the scope of the study. By stating propositions, the research can move in the right direction, so these propositions need to reflect theoretical issues and guide the researcher toward appropriate evidence in the field.
4. **Identify the units of analysis** – these are related to the fundamental problem of defining your case, as each case study requires a focus. For example, in each situation, an individual person can be the case being studied, and thus becomes the single unit of analysis per case. Alternatively, the unit of analysis might be an event or entity.
5. **A general definition of the case needs to be established** – this clarification is referred to as bounding the case, which is needed to determine the scope of the data collection and differentiate the subject of the case study from data external to the case.
6. **Assess the logic linking the data to the propositions** – data needs to be linked to propositions, and you need to be aware of how the choices you make might affect the case study for later analysis.
7. **Address the criteria for interpreting the findings** – this is particularly important if your case study is quantitative, and you are completing some form of statistical analysis. However, for qualitative research, this is still important and needs to be connected to the broader theoretical framework.

Diaries as data

Collecting data in the form of diary entries, also known as journaling, is a valuable method in health research. Using diaries creates an opportunity for the researcher to collect information over a protracted period, providing insights into the lives and experiences of the participants (Day and Thatcher, 2009). Broadly speaking, there are two ways to collect data using diaries:

1. **The solicited diary** – the most common diary method. With this approach, participants produce diarised accounts of their lives at the request of the researcher, and require the participant and researcher to agree on what events or experiences will be covered, the content of the entries, who those entries will be shared with, and the format for doing so (Mackrill, 2008). They require a time commitment from participants, as you are likely to ask them to write in the diary (or record entries in a digital diary) at regular intervals, usually requesting a reasonable level of detail.
2. **Non-solicited diary** – which is less well-utilised in research. These are diaries written unprompted by researchers (Mackrill, 2008). People write diaries for many different reasons, to document their feelings, to detail events, and for therapeutic purposes (Pennebaker, 1997). These diaries are personal accounts of people's lives, they can be difficult to access, and they are likely to contain information that may not be pertinent to the research project (Mackrill, 2008).

The solicited or researcher-generated diary is more commonly used in health research as the focus of the entries can be guided by the research agenda (Hayman et al., 2012). Entries in these diaries provide valuable insights into the topic of the project and are related to the wider research questions. The researcher may elect to encourage a more structured approach to entries in terms of quite precise guidance or may encourage an unstructured approach, giving the participant more freedom in what to write about (Willig, 2008). Whatever way you structure your diary approach, it can be helpful to run a short training session for your participants and provide them with a clear information package about expectations and requirements (Day and Thatcher, 2009). For instance, it may be useful to provide them with a template or an example entry, so they have a clear understanding of what you are requesting.

Using a diary method has several advantages. This approach to data collection means that the data tend to have good fidelity. This is because the participants are encouraged to write in their diary at the point of a situation or event, or very soon afterward, and this can counter or eliminate memory errors, increasing data accuracy (Cucu-Oancea, 2013). Cucu-Oancea also noted that because of the way in which data are recorded as a text-based or audio personal record in a personal space, this is an especially useful method for obtaining information from populations who are typically more difficult to recruit, with diaries providing a mechanism for self-expression, and the participant has a sense of control over what they reveal (Mackrill, 2008). Relatedly, diary methods can provide access to information that can be otherwise difficult to obtain, whilst also generating data that are temporally ordered (Willig, 2008).

> **Key point!**
>
> Diary methods can have the advantage of being a cathartic experience for participants. Participants in diary studies have reported that completing a diary has a therapeutic effect, helping them to make sense of experiences and process emotions.
>
> (Day and Thatcher, 2009)

METHODS OF DATA COLLECTION

Like all methods of data collection, the use of diaries also entails various challenges that need to be navigated. Of particular concern is that the use of diaries is heavily reliant on the participant's memory and a participant being motivated to complete their entries at appropriate time points and with sufficient detail (Day and Thatcher, 2009). Day and Thatcher argued, therefore, that prior agreements will be necessary in consultation with the participants to avoid disruption to their daily activities and enhance compliance.

> **Key point!**
>
> A useful mechanism for supporting data collection is to send text message reminders to participants at appropriate points in the project – with their prior agreement to do so.
> (Day and Thatcher, 2009)

Documents as data

> Documents do not stand alone. They do not construct systems or domains of documentary reality as individual, separate activities. Documents refer – however tangentially or at one remove – to other realities and domains.
> *(Atkinson and Coffey, 1997, p. 55)*

The large array of documents produced in many contexts and for different purposes is a rich and useful source of research data. In the area of health especially, there are large numbers of different documents that can be "mined" for interesting in-depth information, which can reveal insights about organisations, individuals, and health conditions, as well as the processes involved in and effectiveness of care delivery (Epstein, 2009). Documents are "standardised artefacts" that occur in specific formats (e.g. reports, certificates, case reports, letters, expert opinions, magazine/newspaper articles, to name a few), with some functioning as official documents, others as private documents, and some as public documents (Wolff, 2004). Documents are not simply sources of information but a form of social activity or element of the social world and thus are a record of social realities (Drew, 2006).

Documents are mostly comprised of texts, but may also contain images, diagrams, and other elements. Largely, documents are naturally occurring data as they are produced in the real world for natural purposes. In this way, then, using documents as data is a way of capitalising on the use of data that already exist (O'Leary, 2014) especially as organisations will often produce documents that are designed for public consumption (Atkinson and Coffey, 1997). Of course, some documents are private and require individual permissions to access. For example, a healthcare service may have a brochure and copies of their policies on their website, but patient records and clinical notes associated with treatment will be private and secure.

When using documents for research, it is likely that you will undertake some kind of textual analysis, which will require reflection and refinement, whereby you will need to consider the issue of subjectivity and bias (O'Leary, 2014). O'Leary advised that researchers need to locate and acquire any documents they intend to use and assess their credibility, addressing questions about the author, audience, circumstances of production, style, goals, background, and document type to fully assess the data produced. In interrogating the data, you can explore the communication practices through the text as a way of engaging with the processes through which organisations constitute a shared social reality and the knowledge relating to it (Bloomfield and Vurdabakis, 1994). You will need to attend to how the document is constructed as well as the textual organisation (Atkinson and Coffey, 1997).

World Café methods
The World Café approach was developed in the 1990s by Brown and Isaacs initially as a change-management tool (Schieffer et al., 2004) and thus the literature we draw upon in this section is a blend of scholarly work, whereby the approach has been used in business and management for driving change, as well as adaptations and applications of the method in a research context. In our discussion of the World Café method, we are contextualising its value as a research data collection tool, albeit recognising that its use extends beyond research.

As the name suggests, the method uses a café-style approach, whereby different groups of people sit around a table or tables, usually with refreshments, and engage in a focused task or topic of conversation for each table. This conversational process encourages groups to engage in constructive dialogue and fosters collaborative learning (Fouché and Light, 2010). Fouché and Light characterised the World Café approach as founded on two assumptions:

1. Knowledge and wisdom required for research are already present and accessible if the right people are engaged in meaningful dialogue.
2. Intelligence emerges from collaborative discussions in creative ways.

With the World Café approach, each table has a host who remains with the table and guides the focal point of discussion as the groups move around the room. Each table discusses a certain topic or addresses a question, and the host uses text, symbols, or sketches to facilitate dialogue (e.g. using paper tablecloths to draw/write on) and share their ideas with the whole group at the end of each discussion (Löhr, Weinhardt, and Sieber, 2020). Through these different discussions and materials, the researcher can identify patterns and collective knowledge (Brown and Isaacs, 2005). At the end of the café, the insights, ideas, discussions, and additional materials are "harvested" and explored with all those in the room to capture the collective knowledge of the group (Biondo et al., 2019).

The World Café approach is a practical and creative way to bring together different stakeholders to discuss a topic, engage with project-related activities, and meet the broader goals of a research project. The approach provides a mechanism for the generation of ideas in a way that accounts for the collective wisdom of all the different stakeholders and groups (Brown and Isaacs, 2005). The service user/patient group is actively engaged in this method of data collection and contributes to the overall discussions (Terry, Raithby, and Cutter, 2015). Therefore, in bringing together your stakeholders and other interested parties to the World Café, it is useful to centre your approach around a dialogic effort and participatory discussion (Jorgenson and Steier, 2013).

Although there are some similarities with focus groups, whereby a moderator guides small group discussions with participants to address a research question (Morgan, 2018), the World Café can have groups of any size to engage in dialogue whilst remaining connected to the larger group conversation (Fouché and Light, 2010). Fouché and Light noted that these small, intimate group conversations thus link to previous ones and build up a café dialogue towards solutions, ideas, and following research agendas, thus "creating actionable knowledge". The approach should be utilised in a flexible way, as its principles need to be balanced with local circumstances and environments (Steier, Brown, Mesquita, and de Silva, 2015).

> **Key point!**
>
> World Café approaches are advantageous when you have large groups of participants from different backgrounds brought together to collaboratively discuss a specific topic where you want diversity in views.
>
> (World Café, 2015)

The World Café method requires conversations that build and develop as people move between different groups whereby ideas become cross-pollinated and new connections about the guiding questions are forged (Schieffer, Isaacs, and Gyllenpalm, 2004). There are different roles required for the World Café method as delineated by Schieffer et al. (2004) and these are listed in Table 13.4.

The hosts of the café are influential actors in its process, as they support dialogue that encourages participants to use an appreciative position to engage in social enquiry (Fouché and Light, 2010). In essence, the hosts and others involved in the project *are* the café event. This solution-focused dialogic style of the World Café approach is indicative of its transformative potential. Indeed, the founding theorists Brown and Isaacs recognised the transformative intent of the World Café method, seeing it as an approach for meaning-making through its inductive approach to knowledge creation (Lorenzetti, Azulai, and Walsh, 2016). The World Café method facilitates discussions of difficult problems through meaningful conversations to influence social change (Carson, 2011). In this way, it can function as a tool to change organisational cultures by empowering those who work for them and promoting more "democratic intraorganizational relationships" (Lorenzetti et al., 2016, p. 204). This is because this approach allows participants from different social positions and roles to collaborate and engage in reflective knowledge building, making social transformation possible through the personal contribution of each participant and directly addressing the power dynamics between them (Tan and Brown, 2005). The World Café method is arguably egalitarian in style in the sense that it recognises the rights of all participants, seeking to empower them to contribute to a worthwhile dialogue on an issue they consider significant (Lorenzetti et al., 2016).

Table 13.4 World Café roles (Schieffer et al., 2004)

Role	Description
Café convenor	The convenor is the lead of the project insofar as they initiate the organisation of the café and typically issue invitations for attendance.
Café host	The café host is usually the project manager who oversees the process. They host the café and steer the agenda, chair the event, ensuring conversational coherence but not control.
Table host	In a World Café, there is usually one host per table, and the table host stays with the allocated table throughout the event, welcomes new arrivals, explains the tasks or focus, and facilitates conversation at the table. In this way, table hosts are facilitators but also an equal member of the conversation and contribute to the dialogue.
Member or participant	These are stakeholders who have been invited to the café event and travel between the tables to cross-pollinate ideas and contribute to conversations.
Design team	This usually includes the host and is the group responsible for the design and implementation of the World Café method.

If you decide to organise a World Café, then you will need to consider practical ways in which the event will be undertaken. This includes considering who you are inviting, the reason for the invitation, ways in which your smaller groups will be organised, the types of questions and tasks set for each table, that you have sufficient materials to encourage dialogue, that there are enough moderators (one at each table), and that an agenda and format are set for the day. Often the World Café starts with a welcome lunch, followed closely followed by a keynote presentation that sets the goals of the day and the topic of focus, with introductions and establishing a common understanding of the project (Biondo, King, Minhas et al., 2019). Schieffer et al. (2004) posited seven procedures as important for a successful World Café:

1. Ensure that the context is clarified.
2. Foster a welcoming environment.
3. Address the questions pertinent to your project.
4. Facilitate dialogue so everyone's contribution is elicited and valued.
5. Encourage cross-pollination of ideas and links between diverse views.
6. Create space for the whole room to listen and collaboration to identify patterns and insights to develop deeper questions.
7. Harvest the collective discoveries and share findings.

Participatory techniques

During data collection, you might choose to utilise participatory techniques to help the participants you are working with to engage. It is common to use participatory techniques with populations who might find it difficult to verbally articulate themselves, may find it anxiety-provoking to talk to a researcher, or may have some vulnerability whereby the participatory technique supports members of these groups to tell their story. There are a wide range available including story games, vignettes, mapping, drawing, photographs, or videos. Underpinning the use of participatory techniques to support your data collection is the belief that these techniques facilitate the researcher in treating the participants as experts in their own experiences and opinions (Thomas and O'Kane, 1998). Whilst there are many techniques, we review some common ones to help you see how these might be useful for certain populations and in some forms of data collection. Before we get into specifics, we invite you to reflect on the possible value and possible limitations of using these participatory techniques as part of the data collection specifically for your own research project in Box 13.4.

> **Box 13.4**
>
> **Reflections on the benefits and limitations of participatory techniques**
>
> In the context of your own project, consider these questions:
>
> - Are you recruiting a population that may find it difficult to engage with your data collection method? Might they need support to build rapport and engagement, or might they need help to articulate their stories?
> - Might you need to invite the participants to have a support person or advocate with them?
> - What kind of participatory technique are you considering using, and what are the benefits of that technique?
> - What additional reading might you need to engage in regarding that technique to use it competently?
> - Who else can you consult to help you reflect on and discuss the value or limitations of that technique?

Vignettes

Succinctly described, vignettes are stories based on fictional accounts that can appear as text or be verbally told by the researcher. To put it another way, they are short stories about a hypothetical person or people to help participants identify their own beliefs and experiences. Notably, though, they can be based on real-world cases rather than fictional or hypothetical ones (Sampson and Johannessen, 2020). With vignettes, participants are asked to reflect on a scenario. These scenarios vary in form and content and usually relate to an event which is central to the topic being explored or investigated (Sampson and Johannessen, 2020).

Vignettes are a useful participatory technique and have been deployed by researchers in the health and social sciences for a long time. Typically, vignettes are used to support data collection methods like interviews, focus groups, and World Cafés but can be used in diverse ways to support the researcher. Vignettes are a helpful way of exploring social issues and problems, particularly those of a sensitive nature, as, for example, they provide a means for participants to share their perceptions about dealing with adversity indirectly and to reflect on possible solutions (Tremblay, Turcotte, Touati et al., 2022). This is because vignettes can be less personal and provide a non-threatening way of exploring something sensitive (Schwappach et al., 2013), allowing for some distance between the participant and researcher and for the participant to comfortably disclose anything of personal significance (Kandemir and Budd, 2018).

Using vignettes with participants provides an opportunity for reflexive learning and to consider responses to difficult situations (Tremblay et al., 2022). As such, they can be used to encourage participants to be open about their own related experiences, reduce the likelihood of idealised responses, facilitate trust and rapport, and increase credibility (Sampson and Johannessen, 2020). Vignette techniques are a flexible method and can be introduced to participants at any point during data collection, which may be early on or much later in the process (Barter and Renold, 2000). In this way, the researcher establishes the content and format of the vignette and selects a delivery approach, ensuring the content reflects the project by consulting experts in the field, such as clinicians in health research (Tremblay et al., 2022).

If you choose to use vignettes to support your data collection, you should be mindful of some of the limitations of this participatory technique. For instance, the use of vignettes in health research has been critiqued because the decision-making explored through the vignette does not fully reflect decisions navigated in real-world situations (Thalén, Heimann Mählenbock Almkvist et al., 2017). Indeed, it may be argued that vignettes are overly simplistic when compared to real-world health situations (Murphy, Hughes, Read et al., 2021).

Drawing and art

Another common participatory method is to ask participants to draw pictures or create some form of art. Drawing is something most people learn from a young age, and participants will vary in talent and skill at producing something creatively. By using drawing as a participatory method, you may want to have a range of artistic materials available to your participants, depending on their age, preferences, and the nature of the project. You may use different materials, like paints, coloured pens, glitter, glue, feathers, buttons, card, paper, and so on.

An advantage of using drawing or art as a participatory technique is that whilst the participants are engaging with the creative task, a narrative can unfold between them and the researcher. The communication can evolve around the drawing, or the drawing can be used to help relax and occupy the participant whilst they talk about something difficult or complex (Treacher, 2006). In this way, communication can be facilitated, as the activity positions the participant as the expert (Horstman et al., 2008). Thus, the drawing or piece of artwork can help to bridge any communication barriers between researcher and participant and provide a focus for reflections on the content or motivations behind the art (Søndergaard and Reventlow, 2019). Søndergaard and Reventlow argued that the strength of using this technique is that it can help thoughts and feelings to materialise whilst fostering a sense of community between researcher and participant as the participants visually express their feelings and experiences. Moreover, the drawings afford a basis for verbal elaboration as they relate to their drawing and provide explanations (Driessnack and Furukawa, 2012).

If you choose to use drawings or art to support your data collection, it is helpful to explore with your participant group what their views are about using this method. Some participants will enjoy the experience, but others may have previously had negative experiences with such activities or be hindered by beliefs about their lack of creativity or ability. For some populations, like children and young people, drawing is something they regularly engage with in their education and at home, but it is still important not to make assumptions. When working with participants as they sit with their artwork, it can be helpful to be cognisant of the context in which the work is created and what kind of instructions you provide them for the activity (Søndergaard and Reventlow, 2019). What is especially helpful about this participatory technique, in relation to that context, is that the drawings are less reliant on language and participants communicate with you through the visual. This can be useful in many ways as the drawings allow participants to express themselves through the art.

In some of our own research in various majority world countries (Brazil, South Africa, Turkey, Pakistan, and Kenya), we have used drawings as a participatory technique to encourage children to communicate things about their lives. Children were asked to represent noteworthy events in their lives using drawings and bring those drawings to focus groups as a focal point for dialogue (see Haffejee, Vostanis, O'Reilly et al., 2022, for some examples). The project was conducted during the COVID-19 pandemic, the topic was potentially sensitive, and the children arguably vulnerable. Whilst the project was facilitated by local partners and professionals working with children, trust needed to be built. The research team (led by a clinical academic psychiatrist, Professor Vostanis, whose voice is represented in Chapter 15) engaged partners from all countries. It was felt that the use of drawing would help retain engagement with the project whilst supporting children to select the topics to talk about in the focus groups by bringing drawings as a focal point (see O'Reilly, Haffejee, Eruyar et al., 2024, for further discussion regarding the methods used).

PhotoVoice and photography

PhotoVoice is a participatory technique used to generate dialogue about a specific topic or area using photographs taken by participants (Wang and Burris, 1997). One way in which PhotoVoice can be used is through a digital diary, whereby participants take photographs and insert them alongside their reflections on the images in the form of a diary (Volpe, 2019). Volpe commented that this method can reduce the potential for participants to feel out of place as they are possibly well versed in using photographs and narration through digital media, like social media platforms, and are likely experienced in using a phone to take photographs. Whatever their experience with technology, the taking and sharing of photographs for research can be a helpful means of centring the conversation and deployed as a foundation for participants to tell their stories (Nardon, Hari, and Aarma, 2021).

In some ways, like art and drawing, due to the creativity of the participatory technique, the use of photographs can be a valuable means of promoting engagement, supporting participants in telling their stories, and collecting additional data to supplement the verbal information from the interview or focus group (or other means). Using photographs affords the participants choice over what they share and what pictures they take. These pictures can then be used to generate discussion in a way that further engages them in dialogue about the photograph and about the events or situations those images represent (Strack, Magill, and McDonagh, 2004).

The use of photographs can also provide a mechanism for visual storytelling where participants create a series of photographs, for example, centred around a particular health condition, and then narrate the impact of the condition or, for instance, discuss different things they do to manage associated symptoms (Drew, Duncan, and Sawyer, 2010). This supports participants in making sense of their experiences and generating personalised meanings of their worlds as they talk about their pictures with the researcher (Bruce, Ungar, and Waschbusch, 2009). Moreover, on this basis, the researcher can ask open questions, draw the participant's attention to the image to probe about specific details, and request clarification where helpful (Mandleco, 2013).

Whilst it was previously the case that researchers would provide participants with disposable cameras and print pictures, it is now more common for participants to use the camera on their mobile phones and send the images digitally to the researchers using email or an app like WhatsApp™. Of course, you might recognise that not all your participants will have access to a mobile phone or have the funds for the data required to send those images to you, and so this will need to be accounted for if you use photographs as a participatory technique. The mobile phone camera has, all the same, served to expand the opportunities available to researchers for using photographic methods (Volpe, 2019). Indeed, more specifically, digital technology has allowed the use of PhotoVoice to be more readily available. Whichever means is used, this must be declared and discussed through the ethics approval process of your project.

Key point!

If you use photographs or PhotoVoice as a participatory technique, you need to take care with privacy issues as the photographs may include images of persons who have not given consent.

(Volpe, 2019)

Secondary data analysis

In recent years, growing attention has been paid to the value of analysing secondary data to generate knowledge. A key discussion regarding this, however, relates to how primary and secondary data are conceptualised, which is not as straightforward as it first appears. In simple terms, primary data are those collected by the initial research team, with primary data analysis considered the first analytic process by a research team. Secondary data, on the other hand, are those data that already exist, with secondary data analysis being the re-analysis of data collected by another researcher (O'Reilly and Kiyimba, 2015). We have previously highlighted some inconsistencies in the way the terms primary and secondary data, and primary and secondary data analysis, have been used, as these terms do not fully account for the differentiation between naturally occurring and researcher-generated data (O'Reilly and Kiyimba, 2015). We have argued that publicly available data that may have previously been referred to as secondary data (such as newspapers, documentaries, websites, social media videos, and so on) would be better referenced as naturally occurring data, thus making the analysis of those materials primary data analysis (Kiyimba et al., 2019).

In discussing secondary data, we specifically refer to researcher-generated data that has already been subject to primary analysis by a research team that collected those data. Following this, it becomes available to a second research team who engages in secondary data analysis. Recordings of naturally occurring activities, whereby the recordings are collected for the purpose of an initial research project, may also be subject to secondary data analysis. In qualitative research, there have been relatively few researchers engaged in secondary data analysis of primary data already collected by another research team (Alexander et al., 2020). This is perhaps surprising, given that the analysis of data already collected is arguably cost-effective, convenient, and a credible method for generating further knowledge (Heron, 1989). Furthermore, the second research team, who were not involved in the recruitment of participants and the initial development of a project, may view the data with greater detachment, which may be an advantage or disadvantage (Szasbo and Strang, 1997).

> **Key point!**
>
> Secondary data analysis relies on data sharing. Data sharing may be accomplished directly, where there are existing relationships between researchers, or it may be accomplished indirectly through a data repository.
>
> (Alexander, Jones, Bennett et al., 2020)

Part of the challenge in accessing data for secondary analysis is that because qualitative research is typically driven by relatively broad research questions, researchers may use that data for analysis over an extended period. This can therefore blur the boundaries between primary use and secondary analysis of one's own data (Hammersley, 2010). In our own work, we have differentiated four types of analysis to try to create working definitions representing the way in which data are used by different researchers (O'Reilly and Kiyimba, 2015). We proposed:

1. **Primary analysis** – the analysis of primary data collected by a researcher to address the initial research question. These data may be naturally occurring or researcher-generated.
2. **Re-use or re-analysis** – the analysis of that primary data set collected by the same researcher, but to address a new research question.
3. **Secondary analysis** – the analysis of data collected by a different researcher for the purpose of answering a new and different research question.
4. **Simultaneous analysis** – the analysis of the same data set by different researchers concurrently. These different researchers may be part of the same research team or independent of each other.

Although in the modern environment of funding, where researchers are encouraged to archive their data so that it is accessible to other researchers for secondary analysis, we note several challenges. First, there is the challenge of context. We have argued that the challenge of context is threefold (O'Reilly and Kiyimba, 2015): (i) researchers not involved in the initial project have limited information about the situated nature of the data collected, including the political and cultural setting; (ii) data are collected for the purpose of addressing a specific question and may not be a good fit with the purpose of the secondary analysis; and (iii) epistemology informs methodology and method, and the researcher acting as a secondary analyst may not have all relevant theoretical information pertinent to this. With this issue, there are risks of potential misrepresentation because of selective interpretation (Corti and Thompson, 2004).

Second is the challenge of ethics. On one hand, it is arguably ethically useful to engage in secondary analysis of existing data as this prevents the need to recruit more participants (Heaton, 1998). On the other hand, this is challenging if the primary researchers did not account for the possibility of secondary analysis when seeking institutional ethical approval for the study and designing participant consent procedures. This challenge is especially problematic if the topic is sensitive or the participant group is vulnerable because of the emphasis on managing data and safeguarding (O'Reilly and Kiyimba, 2015). In this respect, the process of informed consent is crucial in managing the ethical challenges, and whilst there is greater guidance now regarding secondary analysis and archiving, this is not always followed or understood by research teams, which can create problems with data sharing at later points in the project (Alexander et al., 2020).

Third, there are matters related to quality. Of particular concern in this is the quality requirement of transparency. Limited transparency is possible for the secondary research team as they may not have sufficient information to report details that were pertinent in the project data collection processes. There are also challenges with reflexivity for the secondary analysis, as the researcher analysing the data was not present during the earlier phases of the project. Indeed, in qualitative research, the intersubjective relationship between the participant and researcher is important to consider to support reflexive insights (Heaton, 1998).

Author reflections and concluding remarks
From Philip

Helping to write this chapter was a useful reminder to me of the diverse range of approaches available for gathering data beyond interviews and focus groups. This perhaps seems like a strange thing to say as an active researcher with training involving instruction relating to different methods. Yet, in practice, I have found it can be easy to retreat to what is familiar and to use the same (or similar) methods to those that one has used previously. Of course, making use of unfamiliar methods is far from easy, and care must be taken to ensure sensible and ethical application.

Based on this experience, my advice for fledgling clinician-researchers would be to keep an open mind about which methods to use and not overlook those that one knows less about. Familiarity with other methods can be built by reading literature relating to those methods and, where possible, by pursuing opportunities to be involved in projects with more experienced researchers.

Indeed, completing my own research training and PhD, one of the most valuable experiences I had was assisting with a large-scale evaluation study that looked at the embedding of a new way of working across an entire local authority children's services provision. A key component of this research was the observation of social workers as they went about their work, in their offices and the community – something I had no experience with in research up to that point. Working alongside my doctoral supervisor, who was an advocate for research that gets close to the actual "doing" of social work practice, I learnt a great deal, both in observing and hearing from him about the process involved, as well as in experiencing it firsthand as a member of the research team.

References

Aagaarda, J., and Matthiesen, N. (2015). Methods of materiality: Participant observation and qualitative research in psychology. *Qualitative Research in Psychology*, 13(1), 33–46.

Alexander, S., Jones, K., Bennett, N., Budden, A., Cox, M., Crossas, M., Game, E., Geary, J., Hardy, R., Johnson, J., Karcher, S., Motzer, N., Pittman, J., Randell, H., Silva, J., Da Silva, P., Strasser, C., Strawhacker, C., Stuhl, A., and Weber, N. (2020). Qualitative data sharing and synthesis for sustainability science. *Nature Sustainability*, 3, 81–88.

Atkinson, P., and Coffey, A. (1997). Analysing documentary realities. In D. Silverman (Ed.), *Qualitative research: Theory, method and practice* (pp. 45–62). London: SAGE.

Barter, C., and Renold, E. (2000). "I wanna tell you a story": Exploring the application of vignettes in qualitative research with children and young people. *International Journal of Social Research Methodology*, 3(4), 307–323.

Baxter, P., and Jack, S. (2008). Qualitative case study methodology: Study design and implementation for novice researchers. *The Qualitative Report*, 13(4), 544–559.

Biondo, P. D., King, S., Minhas, B., Fassbender, K., and Simon, J. (2019). How to increase public participation in advance care planning: Findings from a World Café to elicit community group perspectives. *BMC Public Health*, 19, 679.

Bloomfield, B., and Vurdabakis, T. (1994). Re-presenting technology: IT consultancy reports as textual reality constructions. *Sociology*, 28(2), 455–478.

Brown, J., and Isaacs, D. (2005). *The World Café: Shaping our futures through conversations that matter*. San Francisco, CA: Berrett-Koehler.

Bruce, B., Ungar, M., and Waschbusch, D. (2009). Perceptions of risk among children with and without attention deficit/hyperactivity disorder. *International Journal of Injury Control and Safety Promotion*, 16(4), 189–196.

Carson, L. (2011). Designing a public conversation using the World Café method. *Social Alternatives*, 30, 10–14.

Corti, L., and Thompson, P. (2004). Secondary analysis of archived data. In C. Seale, G. Gobo, J. Gubrium, and D. Silverman (Eds.), *Qualitative research practice* (pp. 327–343). London: Sage.

Creswell, J. (2016). *Essential skills for the qualitative researcher*. Thousand Oaks, CA: Sage.

Cucu-Oancea, O. (2013). Using diaries – a real challenge for the social scientist. *Procedia – Social and Behavioral Sciences*, 92, 231–238.

Day, M., and Thatcher, J. (2009). "I'm really embarrassed that you're going to read this…": Reflections on using diaries in qualitative research. *Qualitative Research, in Psychology*, 6(4), 249–259.

Denzin, N., and Lincoln, Y. (Eds.). (2011). *The Sage handbook of qualitative research* (4th ed.). Thousand Oaks, CA: Sage.

Driessnack, M., and Furukawa, R. (2012). Arts-based data collection techniques used in child research. *Journal for Specialists in Pediatric Nursing, 17*, 3–9.

Drew, P. (2006). When documents "speak": Documents, language and interaction. In P. Drew, G. Raymond, and D. Weinberg (Eds.), *Talk and interaction in social research methods* (pp. 63–80). London: Sage.

Drew, S., Duncan, R., and Sawyer, S. (2010). Visual storytelling: A beneficial but challenging method for health research with young people. *Qualitative Health Research, 20*(12), 1677–1688.

Epstein, I. (2009). *Clinical data-mining: Integrating practice and research.* Oxford: Oxford University Press.

Flyvbjerg, B. (2001). *Making social science matter: Why social inquiry fails and how it can succeed again.* Cambridge: Cambridge University Press.

Fouché, C., and Light, G. (2010). An invitation to dialogue: The world café in social work research. *Qualitative Social Work, 10*(1), 28–48.

George, A., and Bennett, A. (2005). *Case studies and theory development in the social sciences.* Cambridge, MA: MIT Press.

Haffejee, S., Vostanis, P., O'Reilly, M., Law, E., Eruyar, S., Fleury, J., Hassan, S., and Getanda, E. (2022). Disruptions, adjustments, and hopes: The impact of the COVID-19 pandemic on child well-being in five Majority World Countries. *Children & Society, 37*(1), 8–28.

Hammersley, M. (2010). Can we re-use qualitative data via secondary analysis? Notes on some terminological and substantive issues. *Sociological Research Online, 15*(1), 5. https://doi.org/10.5153/sro.2076.

Hayman, B., Wilkes, L., and Jackson, D. (2012). Journaling: Identification of challenges and reflection on strategies. *Nurse Researcher, 19*(3), 27–31.

Heron, D. (1989). Secondary data analysis: Research method for the clinical nurse specialist. *Clinical Nurse Specialist, 3*(2), 66–99.

Heaton, J. (1998). Secondary analysis of qualitative data. *Social Research Update, 22.* http://sru.soc.surrey.ac.uk/SRU22.html

Horstman, M., Aldiss, S., Richardson, A., and Gibson, F. (2008). Methodological issues when using the draw and write technique with children aged 6–12 years. *Qualitative Health Research, 18*(7), 1001–1011.

Jorgenson, J., and Steier, F. (2013). Frames, framing, and designed conversational processes: Lessons from the World Café. *Journal of Applied Behavioral Science, 49*(3), 388–405.

Kandemir, K., and Budd, R. (2018). Using vignettes to explore reality and values with young people. *Forum: Qualitative Social Research, 19*(2), 23. https://doi.org/10.17169/fqs-19.2.2914.

Kiyimba, N., Lester, J., and O'Reilly, M. (2019). *Using naturally occurring data in health research: A practical guide.* Cham, Switzerland: Springer.

Löhr, K., Weinhardt, M., and Sieber, S. (2020). The world café as a participatory method for collecting qualitative data. *International Journal of Qualitative Methods, 19*, 1–15.

Lorenzetti, L., Azulai, A., and Walsh, C. (2016). Addressing power in conversation: Enhancing the transformative learning capacities of the World Café. *Journal of Transformative Education, 14*(3), 200–219.

Mackrill, T. (2008). Solicited diary studies of psychotherapy in qualitative research – pros and cons. *European Journal of Psychotherapy & Counselling, 10*(1), 5–18.

Mandleco, B. (2013). Research with children as participants: Photo elicitation. *Journal for Specialists in Pediatric Nursing, 18*, 78–82.

Mays, N., and Pope, C. (1995). Qualitative research: Observational methods in health care settings. *British Medical Journal, 311*, 182–184.

Merriam, S. (1998). *Qualitative research and case study applications in education.* San Francisco, CA: Jossey-Bass.

Morgan, D. (2018). *Basic and advanced focus groups.* London: Sage.

Murphy, J., Hughes, J., Read, S., and Ashby, S. (2021). Evidence and practice: A review of vignettes in qualitative research. *Nurse Researcher, 29*(3), 8–14.

Nardon, L., Hari, A., and Aarma, K. (2021). Reflective interviewing – increasing social impact through research. *International Journal of Qualitative Methods*, 20, 1–12.

O'Leary, Z. (2014). *The essential guide to doing your research project* (2nd ed.). London: Sage.

O'Reilly, M., Haffejee, S., Eruyar, S., Sykes, G., and Vostanis, P. (2024). Benefits and challenges of engaging Majority World children in interdisciplinary, multi-qualitative-method, mental health research. *International Journal of Social Research Methodology*, 27(2), 219–233.

O'Reilly, M., and Kiyimba, N. (2015). *Advanced qualitative research: A guide to contemporary theoretical debates*. London: Sage.

Pennebaker, J. (1997). Writing about emotional experiences as a therapeutic process. *Psychological Science*, 8(3), 162–166.

Peräkylä, A. (2005). Analyzing talk and text. In N. Denzin and Y. Lincoln (Eds.), *The Sage handbook of qualitative research* (3rd ed., pp. 869–886). London: Sage.

Potter, J. (2002). Two kinds of natural. *Discourse Studies*, 4(4), 539–542.

Potter, J. (2004). Discourse analysis as a way of analysing naturally occurring talk. In D. Silverman (Ed.), *Qualitative research: Theory, method and practice* (2nd ed., pp. 200–221). London: Sage.

Sampson, H., and Johannessen, I. A. (2020). Turning on the tap: The benefits of using "real-life" vignettes in qualitative research interviews. *Qualitative Research*, 20(1), 56–72.

Schieffer, A., Isaacs, D., and Gyllenpalm, B. (2004). World café methods: Part one. *World Business Academy Transformation*, 18(8).

Schwappach, D., Frank, O., and Davis, R. (2013). A vignette study to examine health care professionals' attitudes towards patient involvement in error prevention. *Journal of Evaluation in Clinical Practice*, 19(5), 840–848.

Silverman, D. (2010). *Doing qualitative research* (4th ed.). London: Sage.

Simons, H. (2009). *Case study research in practice*. London: Sage.

Søndergaard, E., and Reventlow, S. (2019). Drawing as a facilitating approach when conducting research among children. *International Journal of Qualitative Methods*, 18. https://doi.org/10.1177/1609406918822558.

Speer, S., and Hutchby, I. (2003). From ethics to analytics: Aspects of participants' orientations to the presence and relevance of recording devices. *Sociology*, 37(2), 315–337.

Steier, F., Brown, J., and Mesquita de Silva, F. (2015). The World Café in action research settings. In H. Bradbury (Ed.), *The Sage handbook of action research* (pp. 211–219). London: Sage.

Strack, R., Magill, C., and McDonagh, K. (2004). Engaging youth through photovoice. *Health Promotion Practice*, 5(1), 49–58.

Szasbo, V., and Strang, V. (1997). Secondary analysis of qualitative data. *Advances in Nursing Science*, 20(2), 66–74.

Tan, S., and Brown, J. (2005). The World Café in Singapore: Creating a learning culture through dialogue. *Journal of Applied Behavioral Science*, 41(1), 83–90.

Terry, J., Raithby, M., Cutter, J., and Murphy, F. (2015). A menu for learning: A World Café approach for user involvement and inter-professional learning on mental health. *Social Work Education*, 34(4), 437–458.

Thalén, L., Heimann Mählenbock, K., Almkvist, O., Eriksdotter, M., Sundström, E., and Tallberg, I.-M. (2017). Do adapted vignettes improve medical decision-making capacity for individuals with Alzheimer's disease? *Scandinavian Journal of Psychology*, 58(6), 497–503.

Thomas, G. (2011). A typology for the case study in social science following a review of definition, discourse, and structure. *Qualitative Inquiry*, 17(6), 511–521.

Thomas, N., and O'Kane, C. (1998). The ethics of participatory research with children. *Children & Society*, 12, 336–348.

Treacher, A. (2006). Children's imaginings and narratives: Inhabiting complexity. *Feminist Review*, 82(1), 96–113.

Tremblay, D., Turcotte, A., Touati, N., Poder, T., Kilpatrick, K., Bilodeau, K., Roy, M., Richard, P., Lessard, S., and Giordano, E. (2022). Development and use of research vignettes to collect qualitative data from healthcare professionals: A scoping review. *BMJ Open*, 12, e057095.

Volpe, C. (2019). Digital diaries: New uses of PhotoVoice in participatory research with young people. *Children's Geographies, 17*(3), 361–370.
Wang, C., and Burris, M. (1997). Photovoice: Concept, methodology, and use for participatory needs assessment. *Health Education & Behavior, 24*(3), 369–387.
Willig, C. (2008). *Introducing qualitative research in psychology* (2nd ed.). Milton Keynes: Open University Press.
Wolff, S. (2004). Analysis of documents and records. In U. Flick, E. von Kardoff, and I. Steinke (Eds.), *A companion to qualitative research* (pp. 284–289). London: Sage.
World Café. (2015). A quick reference guide for hosting a world café. http://www.theworldcafe.com/wp-content/uploads/2015/07/Cafe-To-Go-Revised.pdf
Yazan, B. (2015). Three approaches to case study methods in education: Yin, Merriam, and Stake. *The Qualitative Report, 20*(2), 134–152.
Yin, R. (2003). *Case study research: Design and methods* (3rd ed.). Thousand Oaks, CA: Sage.

CHAPTER 14

Interviews and focus groups

Learning objectives

This chapter enables the reader to:

- Identify different methods of interviewing.
- Critically assess the value of different types of interviews.
- Recognise the complexity of interviews as a method of data collection.
- Appreciate the practical decisions involved in interviewing.
- Identify different modalities of interviewing.
- Critically assess the value of focus groups.
- Design a schedule of questions for an interview or focus group.
- Appraise the mechanisms of conducting focus groups.
- Evaluate the benefits and challenges of interviews.
- Evaluate the benefits and challenges of focus groups.

Introduction

Interviews and focus groups are arguably the most commonly deployed methods of data collection in qualitative health research. It is this commonality that was the basis for our decision to devote an entire chapter to these two methods. Through this chapter, we introduce a range of different kinds of interviews and address the different modalities through which interviewing and focus groups can be accomplished. The interview method (and, for that matter, the focus group method) relies heavily on the effective delivery of the question–answer sequences, which are informed by the approach taken by the researcher (Roulston, 2021). We therefore focus some of our chapter on how to design interview and focus group questions and consider the style and nature of questioning as tied to methodological design. We close our chapter with some critical consideration of the disadvantages and critical issues in doing interview-based and focus group research.

A simple heuristic

When you read qualitative research methods textbooks, a simple heuristic is often deployed to differentiate three broad ways of conducting an interview:

- **Structured** – usually associated with quantitative research as the question design and order of asking is rigidly applied.
- **Semi-structured** – a common way of delivering an interview with a loose guide of questions in clusters to shape the direction of the interview.
- **Unstructured** – qualitative interviews with fewer questions that are participant-led.

This heuristic is a helpful way to categorise different formats of designing interview schedules and is widely adopted by researchers, especially students new to qualitative research. Most often, for qualitative research, your interviewing approach to formulating and delivering questions is likely to either be semi-structured or unstructured. Semi-structured formats tend to be favoured by many researchers as they afford the interviewer flexibility in how they ask their questions and the order they do, as well as space for them to actively listen to participants and respond accordingly (O'Reilly and Dogra, 2016). Having an interview schedule that is designed to be asked in a semi-structured way means that the interviewer can adapt the interview to suit the individual in front of them whilst remaining faithful to the research agenda (Flewitt, 2014). The unstructured interview format is more appropriate for some researchers as this gives most of the control over the direction and content of the conversation to the interviewee (Corbin and Morse, 2003).

In selecting one of these formats for asking interview questions, you need to think about how the aim of your project will guide the interview's nature, content, style, and substance, based on the appreciation that interviewing in practice is more complex than initially evident in this heuristic. This is to say, whilst you may favour a semi-structured style or an unstructured style, ultimately the design and approach of your interview need to be strongly anchored to the theoretical foundation and overarching research methodology.

> **Key point!**
>
> Researchers sometimes do not properly appreciate the relationship between the method of data collection employed and the underpinning theoretical framework, and consequently the interview is treated as a generic research tool.
>
> (Wimpenny and Gass, 2000)

The qualitative interview is not a generic research tool. In deciding on semi-structured or unstructured styles of questioning, researchers need to be more specific in relation to the purpose of their research and their theoretical frameworks regarding how we can learn about the social world so that the interview is tied to a methodology (Roulston, 2021). Before we go into specifics about the different approaches to interviewing, we encourage you to think about your knowledge on this topic first by completing the reflective activity in Box 14.1.

Box 14.1

Reflecting on your interview knowledge

If you are contemplating using interviews for your own research project, consider what you know about this method of data collection. Make some notes in your research diary to answer the following questions:

- What reading, if any, have you engaged in beyond the simple heuristic of interviewing approaches?
- What kind of reading might you need to develop your understanding beyond this heuristic?
- What are your initial thoughts about how the interview approach needs to be anchored to your methodology and epistemology?

Types of interview

> The very virtue of qualitative interviews is their openness.
>
> *(Kvale, 1996, p. 84)*

In this chapter, we provide you with a simple overview of the most common interview approaches and encourage you to do more reading for depth on the approach that you choose to utilise for your own project. We remind you that the approach to interviewing you adopt needs to be congruent with your design, methodology, and epistemology, and should enable you to address the aims of your research. In other words, the notion of semi-structured and unstructured will help you to ascertain the level of flexibility you have in your question delivery and order in which you ask them, but the type of interview you do should be related to a theory and methodology. Thus, the appropriateness and choice of interviewing approach are related to those factors and need to be explained as such when you write up your research project.

Narrative interviews

The narrative interview, usually anchored to narrative methodology, is an alternative approach to interviewing in the sense that it is not a conventional question–answer style of seeking information from participants. The unique feature of a narrative interview is that instead of using questions as a foundation for talking with participants, it is guided by thematic concerns, prompting the participant to respond via a "storied" account of their experience. Thus, by engaging with a narrative interview approach, the data elicited become enriched by plots, subplots, and characters (McKenzie and Payne-Gifford,

2023). Storytelling is a useful way of generating an understanding of participants' lives, experiences, and events, as the story will consist of characters, scenes, places, or contexts which are organised along a timeline (Anderson and Kirkpatrick, 2015). As Anderson and Kirkpatrick noted, these narratives can be biographical accounts and provide a whole life story of an individual.

A narrative interview affords the participant the freedom to provide an account of their experience in a way that is meaningful to them (McKenzie and Payne-Gifford, 2023). By eliciting stories from participants, it enables a participant-centred way of privileging the meanings conveyed by them (Anderson and Kirkpatrick, 2015). A specific way interviewers can help encourage the participant to tell their story as a narrative is to not just list events but link meanings across time to give the plot of their narrative. In guiding the participant through their story, a structure should not be imposed. Instead, the participant is encouraged to use their own personal language to narrate their experiences (Bauer, 1996).

> **Key point!**
>
> A narrative interview approach can help the researcher shift the balance of power in favour of the participant, centralising their perspectives by putting them at the centre of their own story.
>
> (McKenzie and Payne-Gifford, 2023)

If you are new to narrative interviews, it may feel intimidating to undertake an interview with minimal questions. However, this approach is premised on an appreciation that the researcher should allow accounts of experience to unfold through a more conversational style, with the participant leading the direction of that conversation. Narrative researchers have offered some guidance to help, and we summarise practical steps involved in Box 14.2.

> **Box 14.2**
>
> **Practical steps in narrative interviewing (Anderson and Kirkpatrick, 2015)**
>
> Anderson and Kirkpatrick developed practical guidance for narrative interviewers, suggesting that it can be helpful to divide the interview into four sections:
>
> 1. **Introductions** – as with any form of interview, it is useful to introduce the interview and yourself as researcher, whilst explaining the process and going through the core ethical parameters again with the participants. It is important that participants are informed that it is their story, in their own words, with their own examples that are at the centre of the conversation.
> 2. **The narrative** – the interviewee should be guided to begin their story, with regular non-verbal encouragement and acknowledgement of the words they use. Interviewers

should not interrupt the flow of the story, and interviewees should be encouraged to continue with the different parts of the story.
3. **Questions** – some semi-structured or unstructured style questions can be utilised based on the story told by the participant. Whilst questions are generally not required in a narrative interview, occasional questions or clarification-seeking probes can encourage the interviewee to continue with their story, help fill in gaps, and be used to pursue additional information in areas of pertinence to the research aims.
4. **Conclusions** – this is a short, concluding part of the interview where the interviewee is given an opportunity to ask questions, is reminded of any next steps, and thanked for their participation.

Reflective interviews

Reflective interviews require the interviewee to actively reflect during the interview process and for the interviewer to be reflexive in situ and post-interview. Interviewees can be encouraged to reflect on something specific, such as a segment of video material that you may have recorded, or to reflect on a past event, experience, or feeling. Indeed, with reflective interviews, you may ask your participant to prepare something beforehand as a focal point for reflection, such as a story, a photograph, or a drawing. In this way, there are a range of tools that can facilitate reflection (as noted by Nardon, Hari, and Aarma, 2021):

- Participants reflect on their life stories.
- Participants draw on metaphors to help make sense of their reflections.
- Participants reflect on photographs as the focus of a conversation.

> **Key point!**
>
> Reflective interviews are a forum to facilitate reflection in a way that helps the interviewer and interviewee make sense of the interviewee's feelings and experiences in a collaborative way.
>
> (Cunliffe and Scaratti, 2017)

With a reflective interview, it is essential that the participant is given time to think and engage in a process of critical thinking by examining their experiences and learning from them (Nardon et al., 2021). This way, there is collaboration between the interviewer and interviewee as they reflect and learn together. The collaborative style of reflective interviewing creates a space for both parties to think, which can help foster trust in the relationship between interviewee and interviewer (Nardon et al., 2021). The relationship between interviewer and interviewee is central to the way the interview is shaped and so this relationship needs to be open and trusting (Johnston, 2016) and the interviewer actively empathic (Wolgemuth and Donohue, 2006).

Reflective interviewing can have a solution-focused style in the way reflective activities are approached. Through open dialogue between interviewer and interviewee, the reflective interview process allows both parties to work together and provides a platform for a solution-focused approach (Nardon et al., 2021). Nardon et al. argued that interviewees should be encouraged to reflect on micro and macro-level problems and solutions to empower them to talk through their reflections. We offer some practical advice in Box 14.3.

Box 14.3

Practical advice for undertaking reflective interviews

There are some practical things to think about if you choose to do reflective interviews:

- Before you start your interview, help your participant to understand the aim of the interview and, particularly, the focus on the reflective aspects of the questions and the relationship dynamic between interviewer and interviewee (Nardon et al., 2021).
- During the interview, as the interviewer, you should actively seek to create several spaces for the interviewee to pause and reflect (Nardon et al., 2021). In so doing, the interviewee needs to be encouraged to articulate what they are thinking and feeling whilst also asking them to evaluate their assumptions and biases (Kayes, 2002).
- Reflective activities can be used to support the reflective account, such as videos, photographs, and narratives, to anchor the reflective conversation in the interview (Nardon et al., 2021).
- Once the interview is finished, you are likely to have additional questions, feelings, or thoughts to share with the participants, and participants will need time to process the experience of being interviewed. Therefore, reconnecting later can be a helpful exercise with the use of reflective interviews (Nardon et al., 2021).

Researcher reflexivity is central to reflective interviewing (Roulston, 2010). During the interview, the interviewer should keep reflexive notes and acknowledge their feelings, reactions, and thoughts as private reflective journaling. Once the interview is complete, reflexivity occurs when the interviewer considers how they shaped and influenced the process and critically reflects on the dynamic relationship as well as their role in the development of the interview.

Empathy interviews

Empathy interviewing is an approach with empathy at the heart of the method. Notably, there is only limited methodological literature on empathy interviewing, and therefore we offer you a simple introduction to the approach here. The central idea underpinning empathy interviewing is that humans, as social beings, need to actively work to understand the experiences and feelings of other people, deeply listening to their stories and perspectives (Nelsestuen and Smith, 2020). In this way, the empathy interview is a participant-centred conversation with the goal of gathering perceptions or experiences about the focal point of the research from the participant's point of view (Lochmiller,

2023). This kind of interview is also a dyadic conversation that relies on open questions, which encourage storytelling about a person's experiences and probe the lived experiences of participants (Nelsestuen and Smith, 2020).

In empathy interviewing, empathy is the interviewer's ability to understand the interviewee's experience, that is, to put themselves in their shoes, even when this experience is (perhaps considerably) different from their own (Lochmiller, 2023). This affords a way to gain insights into participants' thoughts and feelings with a focus on storytelling and dialogue rather than using a simple question–answer format (Nelsestuen and Smith, 2020).

> **Key point!**
>
> As an empathic research interviewer, you will need to consider how you feel and how you are reacting to what your participant is saying to you.
>
> (Nelsestuen and Smith, 2020)

Empathy interviews are typically guided around a certain concern or problem, with improvement to solve the challenge at the centre. Talking with participants using an empathy style allows the interviewer to gain an understanding of the challenges faced and consider how change may impact the individual's experiences (Lochmiller, 2023). Lochmiller noted that the process of encouraging participants to empathise helps them to identify any issues that may need addressing and work on ways to solve those problems. To achieve this in practice, the empathy interview needs to be conducted with awareness of potential power dynamics between interviewer and interviewee (Nelsestuen and Smith, 2020). Although the literature on empathy interviewing is limited, Lochmiller (2023) and Nelsestuen and Smith (2020) have offered some practical guidance, and we summarise this in Box 14.4.

> **Box 14.4**
>
> **Practical steps in empathy interviewing**
>
> There are several practical concerns to be mindful of when conducting empathy interviews:
>
> - In a traditional semi-structured interview, the goal is to explore the participant's perspective on a phenomenon. Contrastingly, in empathy interviewing, the goal is to obtain a deep exploration of how the experience was lived in the way that it was (Lochmiller, 2023).
> - When preparing for your empathy interview, you will need to plan and identify points of interest as well as explore the interviewee's experiences via a learning conversation after the interview so that you can identify areas for development (Lochmiller, 2023).
> - Ideally, an empathy interview should be conducted with only one participant at a time, not in a group, and questions should be iteratively developed with that participant's experiences in mind as the interview unfolds (Lochmiller, 2023).

- The questions you are asking should be tailored to the individual and to the context, so the questions should be personalised as well as focused on equity and equality (Nelsestuen and Smith, 2020).
- When you design your interview schedule, you need to be clear about the purpose of the interview, listen in depth to the participant, and consider the power dynamics at play (Nelsestuen and Smith, 2020).
- Use some questions to ascertain details about what has contributed to the interviewee's experience or their perspective on the matter discussed (Lochmiller, 2023).
- You will need to think about how to best structure your conversation with participants so that you can better understand their unique experiences and use this to expand on positive narratives (Lochmiller, 2023).
- Avoid asking leading questions (Lochmiller, 2023).
- Avoid having too many questions for an empathy interview, with guidance suggesting about four to eight open, story-based questions, with prompts and encouragements (Nelsestuen and Smith, 2020).
- Try to stay neutral in your questions and allow the interviewee space to express their perspective (Nelsestuen and Smith, 2020).
- It can be advantageous to take notes during the interview (Nelsestuen and Smith, 2020).

Ethnographic interviews

Ethnographic interviewing is an approach founded in ethnography and thus a method of data collection with the goal to study the culture and social ways of living of a certain population or community. From the reading you have engaged regarding ethnography so far in this book, you may have noticed that this is a methodological approach most associated with participant observation, and yet the ethnographic interview can also be a highly valuable method (Weeks, 2020). Ethnographic interviews are typically conducted only within a wider ethnographic inquiry whereby ethnographers generate data about the culture of a group so that what the participant says in their interview is interpreted in relation to the time, place, and wider context of their lives (Walford, 2018).

In ethnographic interviews, the interviewer seeks to explore the meanings that individuals give to their own cultural worlds through discourse (Roulston, 2021). It has been argued that there are different modes, referred to as declarative, non-declarative, and public modes, with different levels of those cultures manifesting in an ethnographic interview (Lizardo, 2017).

Key point!

The focus in an ethnographic interview is to encourage participants to describe events and concerns to provide insight into their cultural worlds.

(Roulston, 2021)

Arguably, interviewing has value as part of an ethnographic approach because this method of data collection enables the researcher to learn about how people understand and make sense of their everyday experience (Weeks, 2020). By undertaking an ethnographic interview, the researcher can build a relationship with participants via conversations which may or may not be recorded and yet all contribute to the ethnography (Rinaldo and Guhin, 2022). Specifically, then, in the interview itself, the ethnographic interviewer prompts the participant to describe their culture as well as help provide explanations of any terms routinely used by members of the culture (Roulston, 2021).

> **Key point!**
>
> There are some tensions about what constitutes an ethnographic interview. Thus, the ethnographic interviewer must balance the challenge of ethnographic traditions from cultural anthropology and qualitative sociology to understand how people use language to make sense of their culture.
>
> (Roulston, 2010)

The ethnographic interview is an opportunity for the researcher to engage with and question members of a community or group in ways that may reveal the roots of a cultural tradition or mindset through shared and individual experiences, memories, and emotions (Finesurrey, 2019). This emphasis on culture and symbolic meaning means that the ethnographic interviewer attempts to immerse themself in their participants' worlds (Roulston, 2010), and recognises that that interview is co-constructed, that is, knowledge is produced by both the participant and the researcher (Finesurrey, 2019). We offer some practical advice in conducting your ethnographic interview in Box 14.5.

> **Box 14.5**
>
> **Practical steps in ethnographic interviewing**
>
> There is guidance on how to conduct an ethnographic interview, and we outline some key aspects of the approach here:
>
> - There needs to be careful consideration of the population you are recruiting as it is their cultural world that is the focus (Walford, 2018).
> - The participants you recruit for ethnographic interviews will be involved because of their belonging to a specific group or their position within an organisation or community (Walford, 2018).
> - Ethnographic interviewers need to be directly linked to participants' lives through the wider ethnography, and there should be a longer-term engagement with those participants (Troman, Gordon, Jeffrey, and Walford, 2006).

- The ethnographic interviewer must approach the interviews from a position of curiosity and avoid a "static" or "flat" understanding of the culture they are investigating.
- As with other approaches to interviewing, the ethnographic interviewer should reflect on how the interview discourse serves to produce a "reality" that is co-constructed in the interview encounter.
- In attempting to immerse themselves in the culture of the participants or subjects of their research, the ethnographic interviewer should ensure they keep detailed field notes regarding interviews, as well as interview recordings and transcripts.

Naturally occurring interviews

The idea of the naturally occurring interview is likely to be less familiar to you than other approaches as this kind of interview has arguably received less attention. Naturally occurring data is central here, as we discussed in Chapter 13. Before we consider the naturally occurring interview, we remind you that naturally occurring data are typically audio or video recordings of naturally occurring events or activities, or they are naturally occurring text material that is selected by a researcher to use as data for a project (Kiyimba, Lester, and O'Reilly, 2019).

As it involves naturally occurring data, this type of interview does not rely on the researcher's actions (O'Reilly and Dogra, 2016). In other words, these are recordings of interviews that occur naturally in institutions or other contexts which are captured for the purpose of research. Consider these examples:

- When police officers interview a suspect or witness as part of the organisational business.
- When a social worker interviews members of a family regarding child protection concerns.
- When a panel of employers interviews a candidate who has applied for employment.
- When a reporter interviews a government representative about a national health concern.
- When a Human Resources representative interviews a worker over a case of misconduct in the workplace.
- When an assessor interviews an individual about their health and capacity to work.
- When a celebrity is interviewed for a magazine about their struggles with mental health.

Recording interviews or utilising text-based interviews that occur naturally as part of some institutional business provides the researcher with data that constitutes a naturally occurring interview. The use of naturally occurring interviews for research ensures a commitment to exploring how people use language and attribute meaning to their experiences, to produce a holistic understanding of a phenomenon (Kiyimba et al., 2019). There are some practical issues you need to consider if you want to record interviews that are naturally occurring, even if they are in the public domain. We outline some steps in Box 14.6.

> **Box 14.6**
>
> **Practical steps in managing naturally occurring interviews**
>
> We offer some guidance on how to record interviews that occur naturally in the public and private domains, and we outline them here:
>
> - Engage in background work to identify the acceptability of what you are proposing to do.
> - Be clear about the possible benefits of the research widely, but also to the organisation (if there is one).
> - Be mindful of the ethical parameters of recording interviews, even in relation to those already in the public domain (see also our guidance about online methods).
> - If you are recording institutional interviews, you will need to build a good relationship with the gatekeepers and the participants to reassure them that you are not seeking to judge their work or criticise it.
> - People are more likely to feel accountable if their work is being recorded and explored, and so having partners will help you manage this.
> - Careful conversations about confidentiality and informed consent with the participants and with the research team are useful to ensure participants are protected in terms of their privacy and agency (see Chapter 8 for our disscussion on this in relation to ethics).

Transformative or interventionist interviews

In the context of health research, some interviews are conceptualised as transformative or interventionist. Transformative or interventionist approaches to interviews are broadly defined as those that intend to bring about change and are based on principles of social justice or empowerment. They can draw from ideas linked to various theoretical approaches, for example, related to feminist theory, critical theory, psychoanalysis, or hermeneutics (Roulston, 2010) and are informed by a concern for social justice (Farias, Rudman, Magalhães, and Gastaldo, 2017).

> **Key point!**
>
> Transformative or interventionist interviews assume that the relationship between interviewer and interviewee is less asymmetrical than in other interview forms, with an aim to hold a transformative dialogue.
>
> (Roulston, 2010)

The focus on social justice means transformative or interventionist interviews have a slightly different goal compared to other forms of qualitative interviews. An underpinning idea behind these interviews is a process of change or learning. As such, transformative learning theory proposes that learning needs to involve a process of the revision of the "mental models" of action and consequence, which consequently leads to a change in the interpretation of action and experience (Mezirow, 1990). There are a range of transformative or interventionist interview approaches, and three of the most common are therapeutic interviews, dialogic interviews, and emancipatory interviews (Nardon et al., 2021; Roulston, 2010). Arguably, because of their epistemological foundations, feminist interviews and psychoanalytically informed interviews can also be represented as transformative.

We acknowledge there are researchers who argue that some of the interview approaches we have already discussed could be conducted in a transformative way if social justice and power are centralised within them, and thus the boundaries are not always easy to identify. For example, Nardon et al. (2021) argued that when participants are encouraged to actively reflect in a reflective interview, this can help them work toward changes in the way they relate to others and thus, potentially, contribute to personal or social change. As such, there is a connection between reflection and transformative learning, and reflective interviewing can be conducted as a form of transformative intervention.

Therapeutic interviews

It is recognised in the research literature that qualitative interviews of any nature may have a therapeutic effect for the participants (Lakeman, McAndrew, MacGabhann et al., 2013) and we return to this in Chapter 17. Some qualitative research, in exploring private aspects of participants' lives, creates a space where they are invited to self-disclose through an interview that is therapeutic in nature (Birch and Miller, 2000).

> **Key point!**
>
> Research interviews that are therapeutic support participants to make use of meaning-making spaces as they reflect and think through their personal experiences via a conversational exchange with the interviewer.
>
> (Birch and Miller, 2000)

A function of a therapeutic interview is to help the participant reflect on aspects of the self and how their experiences have shaped who they are and their beliefs, and thus the interview conversation can help to bring about some changes in the ways they view themselves (Birch and Miller, 2000) and be experienced as cathartic (Rossetto, 2014). For the therapeutic interview, a therapeutic experience for the participant may or may not be identified as the goal of the research from the outset, but may help the participants reach a more in-depth understanding of their personal experiences (Birch and Miller, 2000).

However, in setting this type of experience as a goal, therapeutic interviews can be a useful qualitative approach for those with counselling or psychotherapy training, who may actively aim to engage in an interview process that is transformative (Nelson, Onwuegbuzie, Wines, and Frels, 2013). Nelson et al. emphasised that researchers with clinical skills undertaking therapy interviews need to be mindful to seek guidance, as they will need to change their mindset from positioning themselves as having expertise in psychological treatment to instead viewing participants as experts in their own experiences.

> **Key point!**
>
> In the therapeutic interview, the well-being of the participants is a central concern, and this is enabled through the interviewer–interviewee relationship.
>
> (Birch and Miller, 2000)

When conducting therapeutic interviews for research, skills gained from clinical practice need to be translated carefully for transformative interviews (Archard and O'Reilly, 2022; Nelson et al., 2013). As Nelson et al. argued, skills like empathic responding, self-awareness on the part of the interviewer, and reflexive thinking can be central in considering how the interview process might impact the participants and in managing the process of data collection so that the experience can be therapeutic for the interviewee. As with the other interview methods reported here, we encourage you to study this approach carefully before using it. This is particularly important as a clinician-researcher, as separating the two roles is especially relevant for this approach.

Emancipatory interviews

Emancipatory interviews have a central tenet to recognise the social and political freedoms and rights of participant groups (Brinkmann, 2007; Wolgemuth and Donohue, 2006). Framed by an emancipatory framework, there is an explicit interventionist intent in emancipatory interviewing (Nardon et al., 2021). Consequently, it is through the interview that social change is promoted by encouraging the participants to question their beliefs and assumptions, with possible challenges to their previously held perspectives (Wolgemuth and Donohue, 2006). Wolgemuth and Donohue argued that to achieve this, the emancipatory interviewer should have a predetermined research agenda through which they guide their participants towards transformation. They noted that care must be taken in this approach for the researcher to be honest in reflecting on what informs their own worldview, as a risk in this approach is that it can seem quite "expert driven", with caution in reflecting on whether one's belief in "emancipation" is not merely a cultural artefact.

> **Key point!**
>
> The emancipatory paradigm, as the name implies, is about the facilitation of a politics of the possible by confronting social oppression at whatever level it occurs.
>
> (Oliver, 1992, p. 110)

With emancipatory interviewing, the researcher is innovative in the interviewing approach. Thus, participants can explore their health in the context of their identity, across spaces, temporality, and different life stages, with interviewers obtaining interesting insights about the interconnections of health and identity that are both emancipatory and supportive of social justice (Boutain, Evans-Agnew, Liu, and Rosemberg, 2018). Aligned with this standpoint, emancipatory research is not designed to empower people per se, but rather, if people make their decision to be empowered then research should facilitate that, and researchers need to utilise their knowledge and skills in the service of their participants so they can utilise them in ways that benefit them (Oliver, 1992).

A focal point in emancipatory interviews is both parties questioning and justifying their opinions and views by using actively confronting questions that can critically challenge their beliefs and/or defend their positions (Brinkmann, 2007). More specifically in health research, emancipatory interviews are designed in a way that supports the exploration of how "identity privileging and marginalizing informs health" as the emancipatory focus broadens participants' descriptions about their health identities (Boutain et al., 2018, p. 305).

Dialogic interviews

Interviewing through a dialogic lens means that interviewers encourage participant perspective-taking as a means of transformation (Way, Kanak Zwier, and Tracy, 2015). Thus, the dialogic interview is interventionist as it focuses on the intersubjective knowledge co-created between the two parties (Tanggaard, 2009). Congruent with this stance, the aim of a dialogic interview is not to discover an objective truth, but rather to examine the social creation of truth by the interviewee in dialogue (Nardon et al., 2021). These social truths or accounts that are provided by interviewees are viewed as embedded in certain contexts, in the sense that interviewees and interviewers explore how the social relationship resonates with the interviewee's background (Tanggaard, 2009).

> **Key point!**
>
> Dialogic interviews are dialogic social events, and interviewers and interviewees utilise repertoires of culturally and socially embedded discourses.
>
> (Tanggaard, 2009)

Through the dialogic interview, situated knowledge is identified. This allows a re-evaluation of the commonly accepted understanding of phenomena, reflecting participants' experiences embedded within a historical, cultural, social, and political space (Cunliffe and Scaratti, 2017). Within the interview, then, utterances are seen as discursively created phenomena where the interview is conceptualised as a shared dialogic event that will reveal conflicts embedded in social lives, blurring the boundaries between (personal) subjective meanings and objective (social) realities (Tanggaard,

2009). Tanggaard also argued that for the interviewee to co-construct meaning, their own and others' discourses must be engaged. The interviewer, therefore, must provide space for questioning, change, and transformation, so that the participants can engage whilst suspending their assumptions about the world and opening themselves to new viewpoints (Way et al., 2015). Way et al. (2015) offered three practical strategies for a dialogic interview, and we outline these in Box 14.7.

> **Box 14.7**
> **Strategies for undertaking dialogic interviews (Way et al., 2015)**
>
> Way et al. (2015) offered three strategies to conduct dialogic interviewing:
>
> 1. **Probing questions** – questions designed to encourage participants to reflect, explain, and modify statements they made in the interview. These can be valuable when participants express uncertainty.
> 2. **Member reflections** – most beneficial once some initial analyses of the interview data have been undertaken and often helpful for promoting self-reflexivity.
> 3. **Counterfactual prompting** – this requires participants to imagine the world in different ways from their originally expressed view. This might be accomplished by talking through other ways of being in the world or encouraging participants to think about new ideas or perspectives.

Feminist interviews

The feminist standpoint emphasises the need for research to provide a foundation for the empowerment of research participants as a way of promoting social change and an egalitarian relationship between female interviewees and their female interviewers (Roulston, 2010). To promote empowerment, rapport is needed, which is created by minimising the power hierarchy and fostering genuine trust between the two parties (Oakley, 1981). Oakley argued that empowering participants through feminist interviewing allows researchers to hear voices that are typically unheard, allows participants to take leading roles, provides a platform for equal sharing of opinions and ideas, reduces the power hierarchy, and ultimately minimises any exploitation of the participant whereby a researcher uses their account of their experience or views and offers little in the way of reciprocity. In her more recent work, Oakley (2016) emphasised that there are complex conditions shaping research relationships, greater than initially observed in her early work, a relationship that is political and social, and this cannot necessarily easily be positioned in a feminist paradigm of research. Thus, within the feminist paradigm, there are a range of feminist theories that are linked by a common commitment to equality and resistance to the oppression of women.

Nonetheless, the relationship between researcher and researched and the power dynamic between them are central to empowerment and to feminist-informed work. Indeed, those utilising feminist methodologies work in ways that are reflexive and relational (Devault and Gross, 2012). More specifically, feminist interviewers actively reflect on the power differential between themselves and their participants, and the reflexive style of questioning promotes the empowerment of the participant whilst scrutinising the power dynamics as they unfold interactionally (Del Busso, 2007).

Psychoanalytic interviews (the free association narrative interview method)

The free association narrative interview method (FANIM), acknowledged previously in Chapter 6, is arguably the most well-known approach to research interviewing that makes explicit use of principles drawn from clinical psychoanalysis, as a broad body of ideas and practices concerned with the unconscious (Archard, 2020a). Developed by Hollway and Jefferson (2013), FANIM has some similarities with other articulations of a psychoanalytically inspired interview approach (see, for example, Cartwright, 2004; Holmes, 2017). It is a based on a theorisation of the research participant as a "defended psychosocial subject" and Hollway and Jefferson elaborated this via a combination of ideas from the Kleinian tradition of psychoanalytic psychology.

Central to the method, as its title suggests, is the psychoanalytic idea of free association. In clinical psychoanalysis, the patient giving voice to whatever comes to mind, i.e. by free associating, affords a means of insight into the unconscious. In a narrative research interview, the participant is encouraged to talk freely. Thereafter, in the analysis of the interview material, the researcher considers the "associative" ordering (or sequencing) of a participant's account, as well as other, more subtle aspects of the communication, which may not be picked up if the data is coded in a way that fragments the account. To give a simple example from research one of us (Philip) undertook, examining how child welfare professionals experience and account for the suffering of parents, child protection professionals who were interviewed often spoke about children's difficulties and experience when asked about parents' problems (Archard, 2020b). This suggested a difficulty in being able to hold in mind both the (suffering) parent and child.

In different ways, a FANIM-based approach assumes conversance with different psychoanalytic concepts, and training or experience in psychotherapy can be valuable to use this approach in an ethical way (see, for example, Archard, 2020a). The method, and indeed the idea of doing research interviews using principles drawn from psychoanalytic therapy, is complex (see, for example, Holmes, 2017). Hollway and Jefferson's work regarding FANIM has been criticised as an expert-driven application of psychoanalytic ideas, where the researcher occupies a much more powerful position than the participant in making sense of the interview material. Whilst there are ways in which the method may be adapted to be more "democratic" in application (see Hoggett et al., 2010), there should be careful reflection on how well qualified the researcher is to share insights regarding assumed unconscious processes with a participant and the extent to which the participant consents to a research interview that parallels psychotherapy (Archard, 2020a; Archard and O'Reilly, 2022).

Phenomenological interviews

If you are engaging with a phenomenological design for your qualitative research, then for coherence, ideally, your interviewing should be phenomenological in style. Phenomenological interviewing is an approach that requires depth and engages with participants' lived experiences (Adams and van Manen, 2008). Phenomenological interviews are designed to generate in-depth descriptions of human experience, and the interview format tends to be unstructured to follow the way participants describe their own subjective experience. Follow-up interviews are also often used to promote depth (Roulston, 2010).

Of course, it is a skill to obtain descriptions of people's life worlds, and thus the interview should be structured through phenomenological theory (Kvale and Brinkmann, 2009). With this, the researcher needs to appreciate differences in phenomenological theories (see Chapter 3 where we discussed theory). Broadly, there are two related styles of phenomenological interviewing: those which focus on the lived experiences of participants, and the hermeneutic style which focuses on the meanings ascribed to those lived experiences (Adams and van Manen, 2008). Acknowledging this means you are less likely to get waylaid by the complexities in the polarisation of descriptive and interpretive orientations of phenomenology, as such debates can distract from the practical application of phenomenological interviewing (Bevan, 2014). It is the experience of the participants' life-worlds that is under investigation (Giorgi, 1997) and thus, at the heart of the phenomenological interview is a concern with reporting the person's experiences as they experience them (Bevan, 2014).

> **Key point!**
>
> Phenomenological interviewers need to be flexible in the examination of lived experiences so that data are obtained in a phenomenological manner and are appropriate for analysis.
>
> (Bevan, 2014)

Practically speaking, the theoretical orientation does have implications for how you conduct your phenomenological interview. For example, in Husserl's theoretical position on phenomenology, the phenomenological interviewer will need to bracket off parts of the self throughout the interviewing process so that their preconceptions and presuppositions about the world do not influence the participant's narratives of the phenomenon (Wimpenny and Gass, 2000). Husserl (1970) argued that through bracketing, the researcher sets aside what they already know about a phenomenon. Practically, this requires researchers to be consciously aware of their own life-world and how that might be taken for granted (Merleau-Ponty, 1962). As such, by undertaking a "phenomenological reduction" the interviewer endeavours to remain faithful to the lived experiences of participants or phenomenological attitude referred to as epoché, a "critical-position-taking attitude", whereby the interviewer accepts that they should take nothing for granted (Bevan, 2014).

Some problems with interviews
You need to be as certain as you can that interviews are the appropriate method to meet the goals of your project and answer your research questions. The method of data collection needs to be congruent with your methodology, theory, and goals of the work.

Table 14.1 Criticisms of interviewing (Roulston, 2021)

Criticism	Description
Challenge of validity	It has been suggested that the data produced through interviews can be biased and thus have limited validity. This argument stems from the idea that self-reported information simply reflects the beliefs of a person rather than the social reality.
Skewed perceptions	It is argued that interview data will be, in some way, skewed by participants' perceptions of what they think they do rather than what they actually do in certain situations. Thus, recollection can vary over time.
Rigour	There are criticisms of the rigour of the analysis of interview data. This relates to concerns about the role of theory in the development of an interview schedule and approach.
Culture	Concerns have been expressed about how appropriate interviews are for use with individuals and communities of different cultures, with arguments proposed that they need to be developed for use with population groups outside of the minority world.
Research relationship	There are concerns expressed about the treatment of participants in terms of the researcher imposing their belief system on the research.

In making this decision, a critical stance is needed regarding the use of interviews. Just because they are popular and widely used is not reason enough. You will still need a robust rationale for using them, and to do that, you need to understand criticisms and disadvantages of interviewing as a research method. Roulston (2021) has identified five criticisms of the use of interviewing in qualitative research, which we outline in Table 14.1.

In providing a rationale for your decision to use interviews, it can be helpful to contextualise them as a form of interaction. Remember, this will be tied to your epistemology and your understanding of "truth", "objectivity", and "subjectivity". Often interviews are treated as an unproblematic medium for the transmission of information, and yet, interviews themselves are a type of social interaction between two or more parties (Wooffitt and Widdicombe, 2006). As such, the relationship between interviewer and interviewee, and the talk from both parties, will shape the nature and direction of the interview and any outcomes (O'Reilly and Kiyimba, 2015). This means that it is important not to erase the researcher's role in the production of the data (Potter, 2002). For example, the way that questions are asked may "subtly coach the participant in a relevant social science agenda" (Potter and Hepburn, 2012, p. 20), thus towards circularity.

Additionally, try to tease out if possible whether the participant is speaking on their own behalf or on behalf of others in their "category". This is referred to as "footing" (Goffman, 1981) and applies to whether the interviewer is treating the interviewee as a conduit to report on their own experiences or as a representative of the experiences of others in their population. Furthermore, it is often the case that people orient not just in their everyday and institutional talk to the matters of stake and interest (Edwards and Potter, 1992), but also in a research interview context. People have an "interest" of some kind in the way that what they say is perceived, or what judgements may be made about them from what they have said. One factor to bear in mind is that of "demand characteristics", whereby participants have been found to try to be "good" participants and design their responses to support the hypothesis of the research (Orne, 1962). This is a feature that has been found to be further exaggerated when participants reported that they viewed the researcher favourably (Nichols and Maner, 2008). Recognise then, that the interviewee is not merely reporting on what they know but framing what they say to be relevant to the context of the research interview. The interviewee thus shapes what they say and how they say it, not just in response to the questions, but in response to the person of the interviewer and their perception of the project overall.

In response to some of these concerns, Potter and Hepburn (2012) have offered some helpful guidance on ensuring greater transparency and reflexivity when reporting the interview in the dissemination of research, which are:

- Greater transparency during the set-up phase of the interview.
- Acknowledging how the interviewer played an active role in the interview.
- Demonstrating the way that the interview was interactionally produced.
- Connecting analytic comments with specific aspects of the interview elements.

Focus groups and group interviews

We now turn our attention to focus groups as our emphasis has been on interviews. Focus groups are a beneficial method of data collection that is well suited to qualitative health research. There are different kinds of focus groups, which have been conceptualised as high and low moderation focus groups (Morgan, 2018). As Morgan noted, high moderation groups have a lot in common with group interviews as they comprise serial interactions between the moderator and individual focus group participants, whereas low moderation groups are closer to generating socially constructed collective meaning that develops through a shared dialogue.

We open this section with a reflective activity to encourage you to consider your current level of knowledge now that you have read all about the complexity of interview design and the different approaches to interviewing – see Box 14.8.

Box 14.8
Reflective activity: reflecting on knowledge

Before you continue with this section on focus groups and group interviews, we invite you to reflect on your knowledge and knowledge gaps. In your research diary, write your answers to these questions:

- From reading about different interview approaches, what additional learning do you think you need to consolidate your knowledge about them?

- Many of the interview approaches (not all) can be adapted for a group interview or potentially for a focus group project. What reading would you need to do to be able to translate and adapt (if appropriate) those approaches for group interviews or focus groups?
- Consider what information you need to decide whether to engage in individual or group data collection. Who do you need to speak to so you can make that decision, or what material do you need to familiarise yourself with?
- What might the practical benefits and limitations be of engaging in a group interview or focus group for your research?

Table 14.2 Focus groups and group interviews

Group interview	*Focus group*
A group interview maintains the question–answer structure from most types of interview design and is generally guided by the research agenda (O'Reilly and Dogra, 2016).	Focus groups tend to be less structured, with only general guidance from a moderator to maintain the research focus (O'Reilly and Dogra, 2016).
In a group interview, the interviewer plays an active role in directing the conversation and asking questions (O'Reilly and Dogra, 2016).	In a focus group, the moderator remains in the background as much as possible. The dialogue is participant-directed (O'Reilly and Dogra, 2016).
In the group interview, participants may be given the opportunity to comment on or add to the contributions of others, but this will be directed by the questions and the interviewer.	In focus groups, there are opportunities for participants to respond to and comment on each other's contributions, and, where pertinent challenge, extend, or develop them (Willig, 2008).
Typically (although not exclusively) a group interview has a single interviewer directing the questions.	Typically (although not exclusively) a focus group has more than one moderator to help facilitate group dynamics and take field notes or direct participatory activities, as appropriate.

Whilst there is some overlap between focus groups and group interviews (and focus groups are sometimes referred to as focus group interviews by researchers), there are differences. We outline some of those similarities and differences in Table 14.2. We also acknowledge that some of these differences are not absolute as some approaches have theoretical or practical aspects that transcend these descriptions.

Focus groups provide a space where members can develop a jointly elaborated account to offer insights into their lives or experiences (Wilkinson, 1998). This method allows you to ask questions in ways that explore how meaning is jointly constructed (Willig, 2008), which is valuable when the researcher also includes an analysis of the interaction between participants in the group (Willis et al., 2009). Focus groups are a useful way to encourage disclosures from participants by making use of group dynamics and encouraging group dialogue (Freeman et al., 2020). Thus, the synergistic effect can help elicit in-depth information and enable probing for additional information when unanticipated topics are explored by the group (Hoppe, Wells, Morrison et al., 1995).

Group dynamics comprise a central feature of focus groups, so consider how these might influence the kind of knowledge that might be generated through using this approach (Luke and Goodrich, 2019). Group dynamics may include factors that facilitate group cohesion. Because of this, focus group moderators need to respond to those group dynamics and consider how they manage them in practice (Luke and Goodrich, 2019). This is especially important when working to reduce the power and control of the researcher, which focus groups facilitate, as it is more difficult for moderators to impose their agenda onto the group and thus participants direct conversations, which can result in new information (Wilkinson, 1998).

One of the common questions asked about focus groups is about group composition and size. There are no simple answers as you need to adhere to the sampling adequacy indicators for your methodological approach (see Chapter 10 where we discuss this in more detail), but also you need to be able to address your research question with your method. There is some generic guidance available, but the coverage varies, and so it is vital to have a rationale grounded in your approach, aims, questions, and goals. The literature offers the following inconsistent advice:

- Focus groups should have no more than six participants so that all can remain active in the discussion (Willig, 2008).
- Typically focus groups recruit three to eight participants per group as an optimal number (Hoppe et al., 1995).
- Focus groups usually consist of six to twelve participants (Stewart and Shamdasani, 2015).

As we have noted, qualitative health researchers often engage vulnerable populations in their work and explore sensitive health topics. If this is the case, you will need to think about the appropriateness of focus groups for your project and whether that influences your group size. If your topic is especially sensitive, you may find that participants are more reluctant to disclose and talk in front of others, and interviews may be more suitable, although there may be advantages in individuals feeling less isolated by having the opportunity to speak with others with similar identities or experiences (Willig, 2008). Farquhar and Das (1998) noted some important things to remember when conducting focus groups, which we outline in Box 14.9.

Box 14.9

Important things to remember about focus groups (Farquhar and Das, 1998)

Here we invite you to consider practical ways to manage any sensitivity in focus groups:

- There will be a complex interplay of power between focus group moderators and participants, and the characteristics and demographics of all parties may need some consideration and matching as appropriate and where possible.

- Focus groups allow the co-creation of dialogue between participants and between participants and the moderators, so an environment of inclusivity and collaboration is necessary.
- Personal disclosures from the focus group moderators may help participants feel safe and mitigate stigma, but there is a risk of it sounding patronising, so care needs to be taken in what moderators reveal about themselves.
- Where topics are sensitive, the moderator should strive to be sensitive to the comfort and discomfort of group members; it can be helpful to acknowledge any embarrassment.
- Participation in the group might become distressing as participants share stories, and a specific topic may raise some painful experiences and memories. On this basis, sources of support should be identified for participants as part of the ethical considerations relating to the research project.

Designing a schedule of questions for an interview or focus group

Whether you are undertaking interviews, group interviews, or focus groups with your participants, you will need to do some planning and have a schedule of questions, topics, and thematic clusters that map against your research agenda. This will help guide your role as a researcher – whether that is in the interviewer or moderator role. Do not be too prescriptive in your schedule, regardless of the approach. The more open the approach is, the fewer questions you need.

Most qualitative interview designs and focus groups require the researcher to plan broad and open questions, although closed questions may help some participants become comfortable (Roulston, 2010). As Roulston pointed out, open questions allow participants to formulate extensive answers in their own words without being restricted. In planning, it can be helpful to check that your questions will provide the participants with space to elaborate on their responses. You may want to consult the literature to help guide the clusters of topics addressed in how your questions are ordered and framed.

In terms of practical considerations, keep your guide short, ideally no longer than a page, as this is not a list of specific questions, but rather specifies areas around which your questions are organised (Gaskell, 2000). This is because for many types of interviews/focus groups (but not all), you need to be responsive to your participant/s and allow the interview to be led by them, to a greater or lesser extent, using active listening to generate follow-up questions about what they have said. With your schedule of questions, it can help to have some ideas about how you will encourage your participants to continue talking or to elaborate on their responses, and different prompts can be helpful to have to hand. Consider these ways of encouraging participants to elaborate:

- Could you expand on that?
- Can you give me an example of a time when [participant's words]?
- You said [participant's words]. Is there anything more you want to say regarding this? [Or similar question]
- So, what I understand from that is [reformulation of participant's point].

- Hmmm (nodding); right; okay; um-hum.
- Could you explain more about what you mean by that?
- In what ways do [participant's words] help?
- Could you tell me more about [participant's words]?
- What else do you think may be important for me to know about your experience or views regarding this [refer to focus of the interview question]?

General guidance for your interview or focus group

As we move toward closing this chapter, we provide you with some general tips for doing qualitative health research using interview or focus group methods. In a recent contribution, McGrath, Palmgren, and Lijedahl (2019) offered a synthesis of pedagogical messages about conducting interviews and we note these in Box 14.10 as relevant to interviewing and focus groups. Thus, whilst these practical offerings by McGrath et al. were designed for researchers undertaking an interview study, we would argue that they can also be useful when conducting focus groups too.

Box 14.10

Important things to remember about interviewing (McGrath et al., 2019)

Here we reiterate the 12 tips for undertaking interviews provided by McGrath et al. (2019):

- Tip 1 – be certain that interviews or focus groups are the appropriate data collection method for your design.
- Tip 2 – do some planning with consideration of your research question and the wider literature, especially when developing your interview/focus group schedule.
- Tip 3 – spend some time developing a guide and test this out through a pilot stage.
- Tip 4 – ensure you consider power dynamics in your data collection and take steps to manage this.
- Tip 5 – build rapport with your participants, i.e. by spending time with them before the data collection begins.
- Tip 6 – recognise that you are a co-creator of the data as an instrument of data collection and so a reflexive position is necessary.
- Tip 7 – talk less and listen more by allowing your participants the space to think, talk, and elaborate.
- Tip 8 – reshape and alter the interview/focus group guide as you become experienced with the process of talking with participants.
- Tip 9 – you may need to manage participants' emotions or distress so be sensitive to participant reactions and body language.
- Tip 10 – transcribe an interview or focus group as soon as possible after it has taken place as a means of familiarising yourself with the recording.
- Tip 11 – check through your data as trustworthiness is part of ensuring quality in research.
- Tip 12 – initiate your analytic phase early so you can immerse yourself in the analysis at a relatively early stage in the project.

Author reflections and concluding remarks

From Philip

With a background in social work, for me, there was an intuitive appeal to interviewing as a research method. It afforded a way to use some of the skills I had developed as part of my professional experience and training. Mental health care is, by and large, talk-based work. I was pleased to conduct interviews as part of some of the initial research projects I did as a professional in training, and I have since had the opportunity to use a range of interview approaches and supervise professionals using them in their own research inquiries, much more than focus groups. This experience has reinforced to me the value of an interview-based approach in different types of health and social care research, as well as the need for flexibility and ways interviews can be (profitably) combined with other methods, such as participant observation.

I have also learnt the value of carefully considering interview schedules and questions. When completing a practice-based research project with limited time and resources, it can be easy to overlook the importance of this aspect of research planning. However, the ramifications can be significant. For example, one might end up with lots of rich, experience-based data, but this may not be useful in answering the research question one set out to investigate. Equally, with a poorly conceived interview schedule, participants may not be forthcoming if they think they have misunderstood an interview question or are concerned that the researcher does not properly understand their experience. Practising interviewing can be valuable. Role-playing interviews with colleagues and other researchers can be instructive, as can attending workshops or seminars that help you to get to grips, in a practical way, with a particular approach to interviewing.

References

Adams, C., and van Manen, M. (2008). Phenomenology. In L. Given (Ed.), *The Sage encyclopedia of qualitative research methods, volume 2* (pp: 164–169). Thousand Oaks, CA: Sage.

Anderson, C., and Kirkpatrick, S. (2015). Narrative interviewing. *International Journal of Clinical Pharmacy, 38*(3), 631–634.

Archard, P. J. (2020a). Psychoanalytically informed research interviewing: Notes on the free association narrative interview method. *Nurse Researcher, 28*(2), 42–49.

Archard, P. J. (2020b). Reflections on the completion of a psychoanalytically informed interview study involving children's services professionals. *Social Work & Social Sciences Review, 21*(3), 107–126.

Archard, P. J., and O'Reilly, M. (2022). Psychoanalytic therapy and narrative research interviewing: Some reflections. *Nurse Researcher.* https://doi.org/10.7748/nr.2022.e1844.

Bauer, M. (1996). *The narrative interview: Comments on a technique for qualitative data collection. Papers in social research methods (Qualitative Series No 1)*. London: London School of Economics and Political Science.

Bevan, M. (2014). A method of phenomenological interviewing. *Qualitative Health Research, 24*(1), 136–144.

Birch, M., and Miller, T. (2000). Inviting intimacy: The interview as therapeutic opportunity. *International Journal of Social Research Methodology, 3*(3), 189–202.

Boutain, D., Evans-Agnew, R., Liu, F., and Rosemberg, A.-M. (2018). Creating emancipatory dialogues about identity and health by modernizing interviews. *Advances in Nursing Science, 41*(4), 305–315.

Brinkmann, S. (2007). Could interviews be epistemic? An alternative to qualitative opinion polling. *Qualitative Inquiry, 13*(8), 1116–1138.

Cartwright, D. (2004). The psychoanalytic research interview: Preliminary suggestions. *Journal of the American Psychoanalytic Association, 52*(1), 209–242.

Corbin, J., and Morse, J. (2003). The unstructured interactive interview: Issues of reciprocity and risks when dealing with sensitive topics. *Qualitative Inquiry, 9*(3), 335–354.

Cunliffe, A., and Scaratti, G. (2017). Embedding impact in engaged research: Developing socially useful knowledge through dialogical sensemaking: Embedding impact in engaged research. *British Journal of Management, 28*(1), 29–44.

Del Busso, L. (2007). Embodying feminist politics in the research interview: Material bodies and reflexivity. *Feminism & Psychology, 17*(3), 309–315.

DeVault, M. L. and Gross, G. (2012). Feminist qualitative interviewing: experience, talk, and knowledge. In S.N. Hesse-Biber (Ed.), *Handbook of feminist research: theory and praxis.* (2 ed., pp. 206–236). Thousand Oaks: Sage.

Edwards, D., and Potter, J. (1992). *Discursive psychology.* London: Sage.

Farias, L., Rudman, D., Magalhães, L., and Gastaldo, D. (2017). Reclaiming the potential of transformative scholarship to enable social justice. *International Journal of Qualitative Methods, 16*(1), 1–10.

Farquhar, C., and Das, R. (1998). Are focus groups suitable for sensitive topics? In R. Barbour and J. Kitzinger (Eds.), *Developing focus group research: Politics, theory and practice.* Thousand Oaks, CA: Sage.

Flewitt, R. (2014). Interviews. In A. Clark, R. Flewitt, M. Hammersley, and M. Robb (Eds.), *Understanding research with children and young people* (pp. 136–153). London: Sage.

Finesurrey, S. (2019). Conducting interviews. In A. Tyler-Mullings, M. Gotta, and R. Coughlan (Eds.), *Ethnographies of work.* New York, NY: Manifold.

Freeman, S., Skinner, K., Middleton, L., Xiong, B., and Fang, M. (2020). Engaging hard-to-reach, hidden, and seldom-heard populations in research. In A. Sixsmith, J. Sixsmith, A. Mihailidis, and M. Fang (Eds.), *Knowledge, innovation and impact: A guide for the engaged health researcher* (pp. 81–91). Cham, Switzerland: Springer.

Gaskell, G. (2000). Individual and group interviewing. In M. Bauer and G. Gaskell (Eds.), *Qualitative researching with text, image and sound* (pp. 38–56). London: Sage.

Giorgi, A. (1997). The theory, practice, and evaluation of phenomenological method as a qualitative research practice procedure. *Journal of Phenomenological Psychology, 28*(2), 235–260.

Goffman, E. (1981). *Forms of talk.* Oxford: Basil Blackwell.

Hoggett, P., Beedell, P., Jimenez, L., Mayo, M., and Miller, C. (2010). Working psychosocially and dialogically in research. *Psychoanalysis, Culture & Society, 15*, 173–188.

Hollway, W., and Jefferson, T. (2013). *Doing qualitative research differently: A psychosocial approach* (2nd ed.). London: Sage.

Holmes, J. (2017). Reverie-informed research interviewing. *The International Journal of Psychoanalysis, 98*(3), 709–728.

Hoppe, M., Wells, E., Morrison, D., Gillmore, M., and Wilsdon, A. (1995). Using focus groups to discuss sensitive topics with children. *Evaluation Review, 19*(1), 102–114.

Husserl, E. (1970). *The crisis of European sciences and transcendental phenomenology: An introduction to phenomenological philosophy* (Carr D., Trans.). Evanston, IL: Northwestern University Press.

Johnston, M. (2016). Men can change: Transformation, agency, ethics and closure during critical dialogue in interviews. *Qualitative Research, 16*(2), 131–150.

Kayes, D. (2002). Experiential learning and its critics: Preserving the role of experience in management learning and education. *Academy of Management Learning & Education, 1*(2), 137–149.

Kiyimba, N., Lester, J., and O'Reilly, M. (2019). *Using naturally occurring data in health research: A practical guide.* Cham, Switzerland: Springer.

Kvale, S. (1996). *Interviews: An introduction to qualitative research interviewing.* Thousand Oaks, CA: Sage.

Kvale, S., and Brinkmann, S. (2009). *Interviews: Learning the craft of qualitative research interviewing* (2nd ed.). Thousand Oaks, CA: Sage.

Lakeman, R., McAndrew, S., MacGabhann, L., and Warne, T. (2013). 'That was helpful… no one has talked to me about that before': Research participation as a therapeutic activity. *International Journal of Mental Health Nursing, 22*(1), 76–84.

Lizardo, O. (2017). Improving cultural analysis: Considering personal culture in its declarative and nondeclarative modes. *American Sociological Review, 82,* 88–115.

Lochmiller, C. (2023). Using empathy interviews and qualitative evidence to improve human resource development practice and theory. *Human Resource Development, 22*(1), 84–103.

Luke, M., and Goodrich, K. (2019). Focus group research: An intentional strategy for applied group research? *The Journal for Specialists in Group Work, 44*(2), 77–81.

McGrath, C., Palmgren, P., and Lijedahl, M. (2019). Twelve tips for conducting qualitative research interviews. *Medical Teacher, 41*(9), 1002–1006.

McKenzie, G., and Payne-Gifford, S. (2023). But how do you do a narrative interview? Social Research Association. https://the-sra.org.uk/SRA/SRA/Blog/Buthowdoyoudoanarrativeinterview.aspx.

Merleau-Ponty, M. (1962). *Phenomenology of perception* (Smith C., Trans.). London: Routledge.

Mezirow J. (1990). How critical reflection triggers transformative learning. *Fostering Critical Reflection in Adulthood: A Guide to Transformative and Emancipatory Learning,* 1(20), 1–6.

Morgan, D. (2018). *Basic and advanced focus groups.* London: Sage.

Nardon, L., Hari, A., and Aarma, K. (2021). Reflective interviewing – increasing social impact through research. *International Journal of Qualitative Methods,* 20, 1–12.

Nelsestuen, K., and Smith, J. (2020). Empathy interviews. *The Learning Professional, 41*(5), 59–62.

Nelson, J., Onwuegbuzie, A., Wines, L., and Frels, R. (2013). The therapeutic interview process in qualitative research studies. *The Qualitative Report, 18*(40), 1–17.

Nichols, A., and Maner, J. (2008). The good-subject effect: Investigating participant demand characteristics. *The Journal of General Psychology, 135*(2), 151–166.

Oakley, A. (1981). Interviewing women: A contradiction in terms? In H. Roberts (Ed.), *Doing feminist research* (pp. 30–61). London: Routledge and Kegan Paul.

Oakley, A. (2016). Interviewing women again: Power, time and the gift. *Sociology, 50*(1), 195–213.

Oliver, M. (1992). Changing the social relations of research production. *Disability, Handicap, & Society,* 7(2), 101–115.

O'Reilly, M., and Dogra, N. (2016). *Interviewing children and young people for research.* London: Sage.

O'Reilly, M., and Kiyimba, N. (2015). *Advanced qualitative research: A guide to contemporary theoretical debates.* London: Sage.

Orne, M. (1962). On the social psychology of the psychological experiment: With particular reference to demand characteristics and their implications. *American Psychologist,* 17, 776–783.

Potter, J. (2002). Two kinds of natural. *Discourse Studies,* 4(4), 539–542.

Potter, J., and Hepburn, A. (2012). Eight challenges for interview researchers. In *The Sage handbook of interview research: The complexity of the craft* (2nd ed., pp. 555–570). London: Sage.

Rinaldo, R., and Guhin, J. (2022). How and why interviews work: Ethnographic interviews and meso-level public culture. *Sociological Methods & Research, 51*(1), 34–67.

Rossetto, K. (2014). Qualitative research interviews: Assessing the therapeutic value and challenges. *Journal of Social & Personal Relationships, 31*(4), 482–489.

Roulston, K. (2021). *Interviewing: A guide to theory and practice.* Thousand Oaks, CA: Sage.

Roulston, K. (2010). *Reflective interviewing: A guide to theory and practice*. Thousand Oaks, CA: Sage.

Stewart, D., and Shamdasani, P. (2015). *Focus groups: Theory and practice* (3rd ed.). Newbury Park, CA: Sage.

Tanggaard, L. (2009). The research interview as a dialogical context for the production of social life and personal narratives. *Qualitative Inquiry, 15*(9), 1498–1515.

Troman, G., Gordon, T., Jeffrey, B., and Walford, G. (2006). Editorial. *Ethnography & Education, 1*(1), 1–2.

Walford, G. (2018). Interviews and interviewing in the ethnography of education. In G. W. Noblit (Ed.), *Oxford encyclopedia of qualitative research methods in education* (pp. 672–685). New York, NY: Oxford University Press.

Way, A. K., Kanak Zwier, R., and Tracy, S. J. (2015). Dialogic interviewing and flickers of transformation: An examination and delineation of interactional strategies that promote participant self-reflexivity. *Qualitative Inquiry, 21*(8), 720–731.

Weeks, J. (2020). What good is the ethnographic interview? In R. Mir, A. Fayard (Eds.), *The Routledge companion to anthropology and business* (pp. 64–79). New York: Routledge.

Willig, C. (2008). *Introducing qualitative research in psychology* (2nd ed.). Milton Keynes: Open University Press.

Wilkinson, S. (1998). Focus groups in health research: Exploring the meanings of health and illness. *Journal of Health Psychology, 3*(3), 329–348.

Willis, K., Green, H., Daly, J., Williamson, L., and Bandyopadhyay, M. (2009). Perils and possibilities: Achieving best evidence from focus groups in public health research. *Australian and New Zealand Journal of Public Health, 33*(2), 131–136.

Wimpenny, P., and Gass, J. (2000). Interviewing in phenomenology and grounded theory: Is there a difference? *Methodological Issues in Nursing Research, 31*(6), 1485–1492.

Wolgemuth, J., and Donohue, R. (2006). Toward an inquiry of discomfort: Guiding transformation in "emancipatory" narrative research. *Qualitative Inquiry, 12*(5), 1012–1021.

Wooffitt, R., and Widdicombe, S. (2006). Interaction in interviews. In P. Drew, G. Raymond, and D. Weinberg (Eds.), *Talk and interaction in social research methods* (pp. 29–49). London: Sage.

CHAPTER 15

Qualitative health research and digital technologies

> **Learning objectives**
>
> This chapter enables the reader to:
>
> - Recognise the value of digital technologies in qualitative health research.
> - Identify core concepts in the digital context.
> - Assess the benefits and limitations of data collection using internet-mediated communication.
> - Reflect on the implementation of ethical principles in digital environments.

Introduction

Given the ubiquitous nature of digital technology in the modern world, the digital environment is now a topic of importance in contemporary texts on research methods. There is growing interest in using methods mediated by the internet and forms of digital technology. These methods require a different approach, extensions or modifications of ethical parameters, and considerations regarding the clinician-researcher role and positionality. The portability of handheld, mobile devices also create many possibilities for research innovation and given that much of modern life is mediated by the internet and other forms of technology, many research participants are at least familiar with digital devices and platforms.

In this chapter, we guide you through some of the benefits and challenges this kind of work entails. We also contextualise some of the ways in which you might use digital technology to support your research. However, we focus only on qualitative research and provide a basic overview of some of these issues, as this chapter is intended as a starting point to guide decisions rather than a comprehensive review. We would encourage you to engage in more in-depth reading of relevant literature should you elect to use digital methods. Also, while we acknowledge the great advances in digital wearables, Artificial Intelligence (AI), and machine learning, we focus our attention for this chapter on harnessing internet-mediated communication methods for data collection as these are currently most common in qualitative health research.

Understanding the digital environment
In approaching the digital environment as a research context, an understanding of key terminology is required.

- **Digital media** – this is a term used to describe a range of electronic data which includes audio and video, as well as text, images, and databases. Thus, digital media refers to the devices that store data as well as the communication methods transmitting data, and communications like email, text messages (SMS), instant messages (IM), and video-conference calls (O'Reilly, Dogra, Levine, and Donoso, 2021). Digital media is a broad term which encompasses technological devices, applications, social media and social networking platforms, internet-mediated gaming, and so on. Digital media can afford useful means to recruit participants and converse with them, as well as providing a way of collecting a range of different kinds of data for a research project.
- **The internet** – refers to the huge global network that links computers through telecommunication media (see Granic and Lamey, 2000). The internet connects millions of people through machines and is self-organised (Granic and Lamey, 2000). The internet constantly evolves as there is a continuous input of information (O'Reilly, Dogra et al., 2021).
- **Social media** – refers to websites and applications designed to promote sharing among its users. Many social media platforms are constituted through social networking sites (SNS), which are services mediated by the internet that enable users to create a public profile within the system, share connections with other users, and view their connections (boyd and Ellison, 2007). Broad definitions of social media recognise a wide range of types, including chatrooms, social networking, wikis, and microblogging, of which you are likely be familiar, for example, X (i.e. Twitter™), WhatsApp™, WeChat™, Snapchat™, Instagram™, YouTube™, Facebook™, and so on.
- **Information and Communication Technologies (ICT)** – refers to the technical means to manage information as well as facilitate communication, including software and hardware. ICT includes technologies like broadcast media and the processing and transmission of audio and video data, stressing the role of communication in information technology (UNESCO, 2013).

In thinking about digital media, social media, and communication technology, there are other related terms you will encounter in your reading that are relevant to the research context. Again, as above, we provide you with a simple overview of definitions.

- **Information literacy** – this is a concept that originated in the field of library and information studies, referencing the importance of access to information as well as how

- **Media literacy** – denotes the education individuals receive about their use of digital media and recognises the importance of people being able to understand, critically assess, and appropriately use media (UNESCO, 2013).
- **Digital literacy** – refers to the ability of an individual to engage with digital media and technology, networks and communication tools, and their ability to understand and use that information in multiple formats so they have competencies to perform tasks in the digital world (UNESCO, 2013).
- **Digital capital** – refers to the "accumulation of digital competencies" in terms of the user being able to communicate, stay safe, create content, and solve problems (Ragnedda, 2018, p. 2367). Put differently, individuals accumulate capital they utilise to negotiate their daily lives in terms of resources, knowledge, skills, and connections valued by society (Grant, 2007). In this way, digital capital references privileges associated with active technology use, in terms of observable social resources such as employment promotion, increased salary, and greater social supports (O'Reilly, Dogra et al., 2021).
- **Digital divide** – is an idea that transcends simple access to technology and refers to inequalities in skill levels, support, and ambitions to engage with the digital environment (van Deursen and van Dijk, 2019). The digital divide recognises challenges in access to the internet and devices, ownership of portable devices, access to education regarding digital competencies, inequalities, and privileges of immersion in the digital world, as well as connectivity to the internet and broader community knowledge and support (Law, Vostanis, and O'Reilly, 2022). It is a divide that can compound risks for those who are more vulnerable and exacerbate existing systemic and structural inequalities (Odgers and Jensen, 2020).

The rise of internet-mediated methods in research

As technology becomes increasingly embedded in people's daily lives, there is clearly value in harnessing this for the purposes of research. Notwithstanding critical arguments about the digital divide and digital inequality, there nonetheless remain valuable opportunities for health researchers. As we noted, we focus our attention mostly on using internet-mediated methods for data collection rather than technology more broadly.

We recognise that digital communication methods have utility in recruitment and participant retention and encourage you to critically reflect on how this may be beneficial but challenging for your research. Reflect, for example, on how much you rely on email as a form of communication, and how this is a common modality to send information to participants during the recruitment process, but how this might also serve to exclude certain participants from your study, potentially creating issues in relation to confidentiality. Similarly, in some studies, participant retention matters a great deal if there is ongoing engagement with participants or even if there is just a need to communicate findings to participants later. Digital methods tend to be utilised in contemporary research over traditional postal correspondence. Additionally, researchers might use WhatsApp™ or text messaging to stay in touch with participants at various points during a research project.

Most commonly, digital methods are harnessed for data collection. Broadly, "internet-mediated research" denotes the process of acquiring research data from participants using methods that require internet access (Pitman, Osborn, and King, 2015). Pitman et al. argued, however, that if researchers adopt methods using the internet to conduct their data collection without reflection and critical thinking, then the quality of their research can be compromised. Therefore, in the spirit of how this book has been developed and our foregrounding of reflective research practice, we encourage you to engage in the activity in Box 15.1.

Box 15.1

Reflecting on the benefits and challenges of internet-mediated research

In this chapter, we will be working through some of the different ways in which the internet might be harnessed to collect data for research. In so doing, we consider some of the benefits as well as some of the challenges. Before you read the rest of the chapter, we invite you to critically reflect on your own views of digital methods and to compile a list of the advantages and disadvantages for your project (and perhaps for qualitative research in general). Write these in your research diary and add to your notes as you read the chapter.

The influence of the COVID-19 pandemic

It was only recently that the world faced an unprecedented health crisis of COVID-19. This pandemic disrupted all systems of society, including economic, education, health, and political systems. It had a profound impact on the delivery of healthcare services, creating a need to rethink how care is accessed and provided by remote or digital means, with a range of practical and ethical implications (Damsgaard and Phoenix, 2022, Martinez-Martin, Dasgupta, Carter et al., 2020). The pandemic also had a considerable impact on the gathering of research data (Torrentira, 2020), and arguably led to a new digital revolution in research (Nind, Coverdale, and Meckin, 2021).

The pandemic created an environment whereby researchers needed to be more creative, innovative, and practical in the way they conducted research, especially data collection. The qualitative research community became inventive as people all over the world had to adjust, making more opportunities for digital data collection possible. Public health restrictions and the expectation of physical distancing to prevent transmission of the virus also meant that researchers were prompted to engage more with digital means such as video-conferencing and social media (Boland, Banks, Krabbe et al., 2022). However, facing this need to adapt, researchers needed to be more reflexively mindful of any unnecessary burden on participants, their digital literacy (as well as the researcher's), and any issues related to the absence of logistical support (Townsend, Nielsen, Allister, and Cassidy, 2020). Indeed, COVID-19 created many opportunities and challenges for qualitative health researchers. In Box 15.2, we provide an experiential example of how researchers adapted during the pandemic, as Professor Panos Vostanis reflects on his research during that time.

> **Box 15.2**
> **Practitioner reflection by Professor Panos Vostanis**
>
> Professor Vostanis has a professional background in child and adolescent psychiatry. Professor Vostanis's contribution is through the World Awareness for Children in Trauma (WACIT) research programme.
>
> The broad objective of the World Awareness for Children in Trauma (WACIT) is to design, implement, and evaluate capacity-building interventions and services for vulnerable children and young people in low-resource settings, predominantly in the Global South (Vostanis, 2019). Research is conducted in partnership with local non-governmental organisations (NGOs) and academic institutions. Qualitative studies include scoping, process, and impact evaluation.
>
> Three such studies were completed during the COVID-19 pandemic and involved multiple countries, which increased their complexity and emerging challenges. The first study explored available informal and structural mental health support through young people with lived experience in eight countries (Sheikh, Jacob, Vostanis et al., 2024; Vostanis, Ruby, and Jacob, 2022). This started around the time of the onset of COVID-19 and faced evolving health and safety measures around the world, without a precedent for the research team. The other two studies addressed COVID-19-related issues, i.e. how children and young people in five Global South countries coped with the pandemic (Haffejee, O'Reilly, Vostanis et al., 2022; Vostanis, Haffejee, Getanda et al., 2023), and how an emotional literacy intervention could be adapted and delivered digitally in Brazil (Freeland, O'Reilly, Fleury et al., 2022). Overarching lessons emerged from these three studies on factors that enabled the successful completion of the research.
>
> ### *Partnerships*
>
> The research network was established over many years and through different projects and their emerging challenges. This enabled trust-building and communication that was valuable for adapting to the unprecedented and unpredictable situation of the pandemic, without compromising the research.
>
> ### *Local knowledge and flexibility*
>
> Health and safety guidelines constantly changed during this period, with variations within and across countries. By working through a local host organisation, we were able to adapt data collection to face-to-face or remote approaches without compromising research or ethics standards. Children, parents, and professionals were given the option of attending local community venues (for example, in Kenya and Pakistan) if they felt safe and safety measures were being followed.
>
> ### *Peer researchers*
>
> The involvement of community members, especially those with lived experience, is viewed as increasingly important in influencing all aspects of the research process,

especially engagement with participants and data collection. In our first study, young peer researchers with lived experience of anxiety and depression were essential in approaching participants, who might have otherwise been more reluctant to participate because of COVID-19 restrictions. Peer researchers were active in proposing and designing creative and youth-centric approaches to data collection (Spuerck, Stankovic, Zeenat Fatima et al., 2023).

Fast-tracked research training, support, and supervision

The research team had to adapt to remote internal and external meetings and, crucially, researcher training in interviewing, transcribing, and data coding (O'Reilly, Haffejee, Eruyar et al., 2024). Although we lost some spontaneity of face-to-face interactions, we discovered the additional benefits of mixing researchers from different cultures, backgrounds, and countries who would otherwise have trained in silo. This necessity enriched our research experience and offered cross-country validation.

Technology

Despite the well-established digital divide between Global South and North (Law, Vostanis, and O'Reilly, 2023), we also challenged a few myths and enhanced participation by understanding and maximising digital platforms, mainly through mobile phones rather than computers, accessed by young people living in disadvantage. Again, peer researchers played a key role in guiding us to the most appropriate modes.

Online data collection

The methods you use for data collection that can be mediated by the internet are wide-ranging, including email, video-conferencing, text messaging or instant messaging, social networking and social media, chat rooms, discussion boards, blogs, and so forth. Some of these may be naturally occurring in the sense that they are posted without a predefined research focus and thus constitute naturally occurring data, and some may be researcher-generated (see Chapter 13). Additionally, some internet-mediated data collection will involve synchronous communication between the researcher and participant(s), and others will involve asynchronously collecting data.

Different modalities of data collection

A key decision to make when planning data collection is choosing an appropriate modality. You need to consider whether you conduct your data collection face-to-face with all parties present in the same physical space, use the telephone and capture audio, or use digital platforms for data collection (there are many, including Microsoft Teams™, Zoom™, Google Meet™, FaceTime™, and WhatsApp™ video on). You will also need to decide whether you use video functions or audio functions only. Alternatively, you may choose to undertake an asynchronous interview, where there is time for the participant to respond to questions, such as over email, text message, or a messaging platform. You may consider using a blend of modalities. In this chapter, we invite you to think about some of the benefits and challenges of how and where you might collect data.

- Face-to-face

In-person, face-to-face interviewing and focus groups are still arguably the most common approaches to data collection in qualitative research. The synchronous communication in time and space, the ethos created by multi-modal communication possibilities, and a shared social space potentially with shared refreshments and possibilities for small talk, create a pleasant environment. In choosing to meet with participants in person, you will need to consider the nature of the space you select to ensure it is private enough to respect confidentiality but at the same time manageable for your own safety (issues we have discussed already in the book). The practicalities of distance also need to be accounted for, as some participants may not reside in locations where it is easy to meet in person.

You may be more innovative in using face-to-face meetings, particularly if you are conducting interviews or other methods where it is just the researcher and a single participant. You might want to walk and converse in an outdoor environment, or engage with a participant while they engage in an activity such as gardening. You are not necessarily restricted to a small room with two chairs and a table. Indeed, it can be advantageous to consult with your participants to give them some control over the space where they meet you to talk. This advantage notwithstanding, you will need to pay attention to the challenge of background noise and ensure you are able to record the conversation (O'Reilly and Dogra, 2016).

- Telephone

With so many digital options available, researchers can sometimes overlook the simplicity of telephone-based data collection, which is arguably better suited to methods where a single participant is communicated with at a given time. Early research regarding qualitative interviewing indicated that there is little difference in the quality of a telephone-based interview and an in-person, face-to-face interview (Sturges and Hanrahan, 2004). In judging whether to use the telephone to collect your data, you will need to ensure that this modality is in keeping with the depth of responses you are seeking to generate and whether the removal of multi-modal communication (e.g. eye contact) will influence participant engagement.

Using the telephone for data collection is a useful way of reaching a wider geographic sample for those participants who are comfortable with this medium (Opdenakker, 2006). Some researchers argue the telephone can reduce emotional distress due to the comfort of being in a personal environment and the comfort of virtual communication (Mealer and Jones, 2014). Indeed, there are participants who may have difficulty accessing a location for an interview, thus telephone options can create opportunities for participation. Research has indicated that some participants experience being interviewed by telephone very positively, reporting that it helps them focus on the audio rather than the visual and they feel less judged in the experience (Ward, Gott, and Hoare, 2015). Of course, finding suitable hardware to record the conversation is necessary.

- Digital video-conference platforms

A modality growing in popularity is video-conferencing platforms, such as Microsoft Teams™, Zoom™, and Google Meet™. Using such platforms, researchers can eliminate the challenges of geographical distance while still maintaining synchronous interactions, and in many cases both the visual and audio elements of the interaction (Bertrand and Bourdeau, 2010). Digital video-conferencing is a cost-effective way to reach multiple participants in many locations. These modalities can be used effectively for both interviews and focus groups. However, while video-conference platforms are familiar to many, you should ensure participants feel comfortable using them and have some private space when communicating with you, as some participants may sit in public spaces, which may influence their interaction and give rise to concerns regarding confidentiality being maintained (Jenner and Myers, 2019).

> **Key point!**
>
> Research evidence indicates that using videoconferencing for focus groups creates challenges in participant engagement, as not all participants will have a webcam or feel comfortable having their faces on screen with others, and so may only join by audio connection.
>
> (Matthews, Baird, and Duchesne, 2018)

Evidently, to use video-conferencing for research, participants need access to a digital device and an internet connection. Addressing digital inequalities has a long way to go, and societies still face critical issues related to ethics, leadership, governance and social captial, despite calls for reducing such inequalities to be a priority (Imran, 2023) and so you need to be mindful of digital inequalities and what they might mean for your research (Law et al., 2023). Engaging with your Public Patient Involvement and Engagement (PPIE) group for advice can be helpful in this situation, to consider participant proficiency with technology and action that may be taken to support participation (Lobe, Morgan, and Hoffman, 2020). It is also worth reflecting on how you will build rapport with your participants and engage them in the interview, giving them some control over its direction. It is challenging to make eye contact with people over a webcam (Bertrand and Bourdeau, 2010) and this might influence how you communicate with your participants. You may need to think about some of the practical issues you may face. For example, managing distress and safeguarding can be more complex. There are some useful things to remember if you choose to use a video-conferencing platform for your data collection, and these were outlined by Irani (2019) and Gray, Wong-Wylie, Rempel, and Cook (2020), which we summarise in Box 15.3.

> **Box 15.3**
>
> **Things to remember when using video-conferencing for data collection**
>
> If you choose to use video-conferencing as the modality to collect data, the following advice may be useful (Irani, 2019; Gray et al., 2020):
>
> - Consider the benefits and disadvantages specific to your project of different video-conferencing platforms, and compare their features, like recording capability, screen sharing, whether a personal account is required, and so forth.
> - The organisation you work for will likely have regulations about which video-conferencing platforms are permissible in research, which you can check with appropriate representatives.
> - Ensure that you are familiar with the platform you are using. Practice with it and explore its features. You may need to help your participants troubleshoot issues with it. Make sure you test the platform before the interview and trial it with a colleague to test the audio quality and practice recording.
> - Organise preliminary consultations with participants to ascertain their levels of comfort with the platform and their levels of digital literacy. You can send them some technical information in advance of collecting data.
> - You will need to decide whether to use the recording function associated with the platform or to use a separate portable encrypted recording device to place near your device speaker.
> - Remember that this is a professional interaction, even if you are at home. What you wear and what is visible behind you is important to consider in managing your professional identity.
> - Keep records of contact details for the participants in case the technology or internet connection fails. Furthermore, this may be necessary for safeguarding if a participant abruptly leaves the conversation due to becoming distressed.
> - You will need a plan for safe data storage if you record a video file and ensure that the platform is secure for the purposes of research and data security, as some platforms are not when using a connection between a mobile phone and a laptop or personal computer.
> - Consider turning off any other devices that are using the same Wi-Fi to ensure a stronger internet connection.
> - Make sure you confirm the participant's consent for the benefit of the recording and to remind them of core information on the information sheet.

- Email, instant messaging, or other text-based methods

One, other option available to you is to text-based methods, which are typically asynchronous in that there are usually some gaps (hours or days, but maybe weeks) between a question being asked and a response. However, there can be a more synchronous dialogue where times are agreed for a text interaction, although there is still a small gap when each party formulates their response.

QUALITATIVE RESEARCH AND DIGITAL TECHNOLOGIES

> **Key point!**
>
> Text-based interviews, such as via emails, text messaging, or instant messaging, tend to be asynchronous as there is usually a delay before the participant responds. However, there can be some synchronicity with these methods if the participant is actively waiting for the question to arrive and a chain of communication arises in situ.

Email interviews are a common method for data collection and are typically used with single participants individually; however, where there is consent, a group interview can use this method. To manage email interviews, it is likely you will be corresponding with several participants in any given time frame, with individual emails to each of them. If you choose to use email to ask your questions, then outline the parameters of the discussion with your participants, setting up a timeframe for responses and possibly including some instructions too (Meho, 2006). Thus, you need to ensure your email interview strategy is flexible so that you can capture their accounts and give them some control over the process (Hamilton and Bowers, 2006). You may also need to include some mechanism for ascertaining that your questions have been adequately understood (Berger and Paul, 2011). One benefit of using email is that it enables participants to take time in providing their responses at their own pace (Ison, 2009), which can be particularly advantageous when the topic is sensitive in nature (Cook, 2011) or if communication difficulties are associated with the participant group (Bowden and Galindo-Gonzales, 2015). You need to ensure you have thought about the privacy of this form of communication and that others do not have access to either your computer and email, or the participants'.

Instant messaging is a method widely available on various mobile platforms, enabling both synchronous and asynchronous communication (Kaufmann and Peil, 2020). Instant messaging affords another text-based way of undertaking an interview, but there are likely expectations that responses will be quicker and in a conversational typed sequence (although not necessarily so). There are many platforms that support "chat" messaging exchanges between interviewer and interviewee. Because the instant messaging interview is usually set up to occur in real time, it will tend to resemble a conversation in text form more than an email would (Flynn, 2004). Additionally, many messenger platforms have an automatic saving function, which means that your conversation is retained if the computer crashes or if either party loses their internet connection (Fontes and O'Mahony, 2008).

One popular and well-known messaging service is WhatsApp™. Participants and researchers can record audio messages, type messages, share pictures or videos, or have a WhatsApp™ call or video call if preferred. WhatsApp™ may well be familiar to participants and is a communication app highly rated for accessibility and usability (Sutikno, Handayani, Stiawan et al., 2016). WhatsApp™ is encrypted end-to-end and thus offers some level of privacy (Gibson, 2022). An advantage of using WhatsApp™ is that it provides information about the connectivity of the communication partner (including date and time), as well as having a desktop version available, allowing users to type messages on a laptop or computer rather than a mobile device (Kaufmann and Peil, 2020).

Benefits and disadvantages of internet-mediated methods

For convenience, we present some of the common benefits and disadvantages of internet-mediated methods in Table 15.1.

Table 15.1 Benefits and disadvantages of internet-mediated data collection

Benefits	*Disadvantages*
Using digital methods might provide ways to redress some of the asymmetry between researcher and participant where steps are taken to achieve this.	Researchers require training in using digital methods so they can address issues with technology and digital literacy (Mirick and Wladkowski, 2019).
Most digital methods are low-cost or no-cost (other than Wi-Fi costs) (Boland, 2022).	Certain methods reduce or limit the availability of multi-modal communication, as eye contact, hand gestures, and so forth are lost.
Using internet-mediated methods supports a degree of flexibility, and depending on choices, can provide verbal and non-verbal data, as well as an accessible medium (Irani, 2019).	As these methods rely on an internet connection, there can be lags, glitches, delays, or dropped calls that must be managed and can be disruptive, especially at sensitive moments (Jenner and Myers, 2019).
Geographical location is not an issue with these methods, and it is possible to recruit participants from other countries. There is a greater level of possible inclusion for many participants, although some may still be excluded in some way, because of digital inequalities.	Closing the interview or focus group can be more challenging online, as it relies on the "leave meeting" button, which, when clicked abruptly terminates the interaction, which can leave a sense of separation or finality (Engward, Goldspink, Iancu et al., 2022).
Many (if not all) internet-mediated modalities can be used on a range of devices, such as laptops, mobile phones, and tablets, which gives participants choice and affords them a level of comfort owing to this familiarity (Gray et al., 2020).	Some modalities require a personal account and password, and some participants may not be comfortable with this (Gray et al., 2020).

Ethical considerations in internet-mediated research

We provided you with a chapter on ethics earlier (see Chapter 8), and the guidance we provided there is pertinent to any research you conduct using digital methods. Additionally, however, there are some specific matters raised by this modality of data collection or by broader internet-related concerns that mean that considerations relating to research ethics in these spaces may need to be navigated in different ways. In using these methods, you will need to be aware of some of these ethical considerations as you are still likely to be guided by the traditional deontological principles of ethics associated with research (Lunnay, Borlagdan, McNaughton, and Ward, 2014). In applying your ethics framework, you will need to critically reflect on your project in terms of any ways in which ethical issues might require further attention because of using digital mediums and researching online (Sy, O'Leary, Nagraj et al., 2020).

Many ethical concerns arise because the researcher is in a different physical environment from that of the participant. This means in practice that they are more limited in what they can do if the participant becomes distressed or uncomfortable, and there are greater challenges in building rapport and displaying empathy (Moran and Caetano, 2022). This has implications for vulnerable participants and engagement with sensitive topics. There are some tensions in the literature as to whether digital methods facilitate or compromise research of this kind. For example, it has been argued that using the internet to collect data can be more comfortable for participants if the topic they are discussing is in some ways sensitive or embarrassing (Deakin and Wakefield, 2013). Conversely, an alternative argument is that face-to-face interviewing is potentially ethically safer for sensitive topics as a researcher can be more responsive and supportive in the room (Thunberg and Arnell, 2022). Thunberg and Arnell did argue, however, that online methods give the participants more control, as it is easier for them to leave when they want to, and the physical distance makes it easier to disengage.

The challenge of determining public and private online spaces

One of the central concerns with using internet-mediated research is the challenges of assuring privacy, managing intellectual property rights, acquiring trust, and the authenticity of data (Convery and Cox, 2012). Convery and Cox noted that using the internet creates challenges in determining differentiation between public and private spaces. This is because, in digital spaces, the boundaries between public and private spheres tend to overlap and be quite opaque (Watson, Jones, and Burns, 2007). Importantly, the method of data collection and the modality of collection will have implications for privacy. For example, a privately conducted interview between a researcher and participant is arguably clearer as private than accessing Facebook™ pages or blogs or chatrooms which may or may not be intended to be publicly accessible.

Entering digital spaces where people can comment may have posts that are partial or incomplete as what is accessed by the researcher may be determined by the participant or might be related to how "public" the sites are to outsiders (Engward et al., 2022). Individuals may disclose information relating to their health on certain websites, chatrooms, or discussion boards with an account and username, and thus may not fully understand the limits to privacy on those sites. Problematically, using online information for research may mean that participants become identifiable, which can have ethical implications for the protection of their identity (Engward et al., 2022). For research, participants should be assured of their privacy and their right to withdraw from a research study (within the limits outlined from the outset), but this can become more complicated in digital spaces (Boland et al., 2022). Indeed, researchers should be cautious about using online methods for data collection and avoid making assumptions about the "public" nature of some sites. A good example of this is social media and social networking sites, where some information may be made publicly available, intentionally but also unintentionally. Sites like Facebook™ and Instagram™ can have public-facing pages, but this does not necessarily mean the data is publicly available for research purposes. Data acquired through these social media sites can contain substantial personal information about people, and care needs to be taken in using this data as research data without appropriate consent.

There are risks that using material from these kinds of sites may be used to intimidate, bully, or humiliate individuals by persons known or unknown to them (Lunnay et al., 2014). Note, also, that there can be data security concerns with using certain platforms because of the legal terms and conditions that users sign when downloading the applications to their devices. Many digital providers, such as WhatsApp™, X (formerly Twitter™), Instagram™, and Apple Cloud™, have their own provider conditions regarding data ownership, data usage, and data storage, and so researchers cannot override those in relation to attempting to use the data for research purposes. Users often sign over their data rights when setting up their accounts (Kaufmann and Peil, 2020).

Informed consent

Informed consent is one of the cornerstones of ethical research practice, as individuals voluntarily agree to participate in research based on full information provided by the researcher. Researchers actively seek consent from participants to collect data from or produce data with them and outline the conditions under which that data will be collected, stored, shared, and destroyed. This process can be more problematic with research in digital environments, not only because of challenges regarding the public-private dichotomy but also in practical ways.

Accessing personal pages on social media will require permission from the page owners, but the number of posts from other individuals on those pages makes it complicated as further consent is needed from these individuals too. Likewise, on more "public" forums, like chat rooms, discussion boards, and blogs, it can be difficult to acquire consent from all those persons who are posting. It may be possible to send information via email lists offering participants a chance to withdraw from the research before it starts, or to actively seek permission from users to include their contributions as data (Eysenbach and Till, 2001). Having said this, even data collection methods that involve data generated at the behest of the researcher, using email or video-conferencing to undertake interviews, can be challenging to secure consent and create a written record. While an email with a digital statement of agreement to participate may be deemed acceptable (Gibson, 2022), where possible, participants should sign a form and send it back by post or photograph it with their signature to send as an email attachment. Importantly (as noted earlier), this should also be verbally confirmed at the start of any recording or data gathering.

Safeguarding online

Considering issues relating to safeguarding is as significant for digitally mediated forms of research as they are when using other approaches to research. As with other methods of data collection undertaken in person, such as interviews and focus groups, you will need to be transparent with participants about how any information will be used and the process that will be followed if they report anything that suggests a safeguarding concern or if they are, themselves, at risk of harm.

As is the case with other research approaches, it is also beneficial to encourage participants to identify a trusted "supporter", i.e. a family member or professional, whom you might liaise with, as a researcher, regarding any emergent concerns. You should also provide participants and their supporters with an alternative and secure means of contacting you, for example, a telephone number or email address (McCarthy, Teague, Rowe et al., 2021). As we have found with our own research, these means of contact can be invaluable for following things up if a connection is lost or a participant ends a call abruptly.

Author reflections and concluding remarks
From Michelle

Working with digital methods can be rewarding but is not easy. In my own work, I have only recently begun to fully embrace the opportunities and creativity that using these ways of collecting data can offer. The use of video-conferencing for interviewing participants was driven by the COVID-19 pandemic when our planned face-to-face approach had to be abandoned because of public health measures. Nonetheless, we did have some interesting experiences in our research. For example, in our Digital Ethics of Care research (see O'Reilly, Levine, and Law, 2021) we were interested in primary school children's views around digital citizenship and mental health, including moral decision-making, responsibility, kindness, and care in terms of digital conduct and its emotional impact on others. Because of the pandemic, our data collection was delayed, and when we did have access to schools again, we could not enter the physical spaces because of restrictions. Instead, we created a process of having the interviewer on Microsoft Teams and the children in the classroom with a teaching assistant (TA) for safeguarding, safety, and support. While the presence of the TA did have some disadvantages, having some support in this research relationship between the stranger (the interviewer) and the children seemed to help them relax and engage in the process of answering questions on quite sensitive areas of their lives (see O'Reilly, Adams, Batchelor, and Levine, in press, for further information regarding the methodology).

On reflection, we would not have tried these more creative ways of engaging young children in research had it not been for the restrictions in place at the time. Yet, these methods offered a valuable way of exploring their stories, allowing the children control over the recording device, control over how much they engaged with the interviewer in the virtual space, and enabling them to lead the interview conversation. In many ways, it was an empowering method. Notably, we did manage the ethics of this activity in traditional ways. Parent/guardian consent and child assent were taken by the school, and signed paper copies were passed to the research team. Safeguarding was also in the physical space via the TA. Furthermore, we used a separate encrypted recording device in the room with the children to maintain confidentiality.

References

Berger, R., and Paul, M. (2011). Using e-mail for family research. *Journal of Technology in Human Sciences*, 29, 197–211.

Bertrand, C., and Bourdeau, L. (2010). Research interviews by Skype: A new data collection method. In J. Esteves (Ed.), *Proceedings from the 9th European Conference on research methods* (pp. 70–79). IE Business School.

Boland, J., Banks, S., Krabbe, R., Lawrence, S., Murray, T., Henning, T., and Vandenberg, M. (2022). A COVID-19-era rapid review: Using Zoom and Skype for qualitative group research. *Public Health Research & Practice*, 32(2), e31232112.

Bowden, C., and Galindo-Gonzales, S. (2015). Interviewing when you're not face-to-face: The use of email interviews in a phenomenological study. *International Journal of Doctoral Studies*, 10, 79–92.

boyd, D. M., and Ellison, N. B. (2007). Social network sites: Definition, history, and scholarship. *Journal of Computer-Mediated Communication*, 13(1), 210–230.

Convery, I., and Cox, D. (2012). A review of research ethics in internet-based research. *Practitioner Research in Higher Education*, 6(1), 50–57.

Cook, C. (2011). Email interviewing: Generating data with a vulnerable population. *Journal of Advanced Nursing*, 68(6), 1330–1339.

Damsgaard, J., and Phoenix, A. (2022). World of change: Reflections within an educational and health care perspective in a time with COVID-19. *International Journal of Social Psychiatry*, 68(1), 177–182.

Deakin, H., and Wakefield, K. (2013). Skype interviewing: Reflections of two PhD researchers. *Qualitative Research*, 14(5), 603–616.

Engward, H., Goldspink, S., Iancu, M., Kersey, T., and Wood, A. (2022). Togetherness in separation: practical considerations for doing remote qualitative interviews ethically. *International Journal of Qualitative Methods*, 21, 1–9.

Eysenbach, G., and Till, J. (2001). Ethical issues in qualitative research on internet communities. *British Medical Journal*, 323, 1103–1105.

Flynn, N. (2004). *Instant messaging rules: A business guide to managing policies, security, and legal issues for safe IM communication.* Saranac Lake, NY: AMACOM.

Fontes, T., and O'Mahony, M. (2008). In-depth interviewing by Instant Messenger. *Social Research update*, 53. www.soc.surrey.ac.uk/sru

Freeland, L., O'Reilly, M., Fleury, J., Adams, S., and Vostanis, P. (2022). Digital social and emotional literacy intervention in Brazil: Participants' experiences. *International Journal of Mental Health Promotion*, 24, 51–57.

Gibson, K. (2022). Bridging the digital divide: Reflections on using WhatsApp Messenger interviews in youth research. *Qualitative Research in Psychology*, 19(3), 611–631.

Granic, I., and Lamey, A. (2000). The self-organization of the Internet and changing modes of thought. *New Ideas in Psychology*, 18, 93–107.

Grant, L. (2007). Learning to be part of the knowledge economy: Digital divides and media literacy. https://www.nfer.ac.uk/publications/FUTL96/FUTL96.pdf

Gray, L., Wong-Wylie, G., Rempel, G., and Cook, K. (2020). Expanding qualitative research interviewing strategies: Zoom Video communications. *The Qualitative Report*, 25(5), 1292–1301.

Haffejee, S., O'Reilly, M., Vostanis, P., Law, E., Eruyar, S., Fleury, J., Hassan, S., and Getanda, E. (2022). Disruptions, adjustments, and hopes: The impact of the COVID-19 pandemic on child well-being in five Majority World Countries. *Children & Society*, 37(1), 8–28.

Hamilton, R., and Bowers, B. (2006). Internet recruitment and e-mail interviews in qualitative studies. *Qualitative Health Research*, 16(6), 821–835.

Imran, A. (2023). Why addressing digital inequality should be a priority. *The Electronic Journal of Information Systems in Developing Countries*, 89(3), e1225.

Irani, E. (2019). The use of videoconferencing for qualitative interviewing: Opportunities, challenges, and considerations. *Clinical Nursing Research*, 28(1), 3–8.

Ison, N. (2009). Having their say: Email interviews for research data collection with people who have verbal communication impairment. *International Journal of Social Research Methodology*, 12(2), 161–172.

Jenner, B., and Myers, K. (2019). Intimacy, rapport, and exceptional disclosure: A comparison of in-person and mediated interview contexts. *International Journal of Social Research Methodology, 22*(2), 165–177.

Kaufmann, K., and Peil, C. (2020). The mobile instant messaging interview (MIMI): Using WhatsApp to enhance self-reporting and explore media usage in situ. *Mobile Media & Communication, 8*(2), 229–246.

Law, E., Vostanis, P., and O'Reilly, M. (2023). Insights from impacts of the digital divide on children in five majority world countries during the COVID-19 Pandemic. *Behaviour & Information Technology, 42*(15), 2696–2715.

Lobe, B., Morgan, D., and Hoffman, K. (2020). Qualitative data collection in an era of social distancing. *International Journal of Qualitative Research, 19*, 1–8.

Lunnay, B., Borlagdan, J., McNaughton, D., and Ward, P. (2014). Ethical use of social media to facilitate qualitative research. *Qualitative Health Research, 25*(1), 99–109.

Martinez-Martin, N., Dasgupta, I., Carter, A., Chandler, J., Kellmeyer, P., Kreitmair, K., Weiss, A., and Cabrera, L. (2020). Ethics of digital mental health during COVID-19: Crisis and opportunities. *JMIR Mental Health, 7*(12), e23776.

Matthews, K., Baird, M., and Duchesne, G. (2018). Using online meeting software to facilitate geographically dispersed focus groups for health workforce research. *Qualitative Health Research, 28*(10), 1621–1628.

McCarthy, L., Teague, B., Rowe, K., Janes, K., Rhodes, T., Hackmann, C., Samad, L., and Wilson, J. (2021). Practice-informed guidance for undertaking remotely delivered mental health research. *Nurse Researcher, 29*(2), 8–16.

Mealer, M., and Jones, J. (2014). Methodological and ethical issues related to qualitative telephone interviews on sensitive topics. *Nurse Researcher, 21*(4), 32–37.

Meho, L. (2006). E-mail interviewing in qualitative research: A methodological discussion. *Journal of the American Society for Information Science & Technology, 5*(10), 1284–1295.

Mirick, R., and Wladkowski, S. (2019). Skype in qualitative interviews: Participant and researcher perspectives. *The Qualitative Report, 24*(12), 3061–3072.

Moran, L., and Caetano, A. (2022). Biographical research through the looking glass of social distancing: Reflections on biographical interviewing and online technologies in pandemic times. *Irish Journal of Sociology, 30*(2), 209–213.

Nind, M., Coverdale, A., and Meckin, R. (2021). Changing social research practices in the context of Covid-19: Rapid evidence review. National Centre for Research Methods.

Odgers, C., and Jensen, M. (2020). Annual research review: Adolescent mental health in the digital age: Facts, fears, and future directions. *Journal of Child Psychology & Psychiatry, 61*(3), 336–348.

Opdenakker, R. (2006). Advantages and disadvantages of four interview techniques in qualitative research. *Forum Qualitative Sozialforschung/Forum: Qualitative Social Research, 7*(4). www.qualitative-research.net/index.php/fqs/rt/printerfriendly/175/391.

O'Reilly, M., Adams, S., Batchelor, R., and Levine, D. (in press). Exploring the practice of 10–11-year-olds as co-researchers: Using a hybrid approach in educational research to promote children as interviewers. *International Journal of Social Research Methodology*.

O'Reilly, M., and Dogra, N. (2016). *Interviewing children and young people for research*. London: Sage.

O'Reilly, M., Dogra, N., Levine, D., and Donoso, V. (2021). *Digital media and child and adolescent mental health: A practical guide to understanding the evidence*. London: Sage.

O'Reilly, M., Haffejee, S., Eruyar, S., Sykes, G., and Vostanis, P. (2024). Benefits and challenges of engaging Majority World Children in interdisciplinary, multi-qualitative method, mental health research. *International Journal of Social Research Methodology, 27*(2), 219–233.

O'Reilly, M., Levine, D., and Law, E. (2021). Digital ethics of care philosophy to understand adolescents' sense of responsibility on social media. *Pastoral Care in Education, 39*(2), 91–107.

Pitman, A., Osborn, D., and King, M. (2015). The use of internet-mediated cross-sectional studies in mental health research. *BJPsych Advances*, 21, 175–184.

Ragnedda, M. (2018). Conceptualizing digital capital. *Telematics & Informatics*, 35(8), 2366–2375.

Sheikh, A., Jacob, J., Vostanis, P., Ruby, F., Spuerck, I., Stankovic, M., Morgan, N., Mota, C.P., Ferreira, R., Eruyar, S., Yilmaz, E. A., Fatima, S.Z., and Edbrooke-Childs, J. (2024). What should personalised mental health support involve? Views of young people with lived experience and professionals from eight countries. *Administration & Policy in Mental Health & Mental Health Services Research*, 51, 753–768.

Spuerck, I., Stankovic, M., Zeenat Fatima, S., Yilmas, E., Morgan, N., Jacob, J., Edbrooke-Childs, J., and Vostanis, P. (2023). International youth mental health case study of peer researchers' experiences. *Research Involvement & Engagement*, 9(33).

Sturges, J., and Hanrahan, K. (2004). Comparing telephone and face-to-face qualitative interviewing: A research note. *Qualitative Research*, 4(1), 107–118.

Sutikno, T., Handayani, l., Stiawan, D., Riyadi, M., and Subroto, I. (2016). WhatsApp, Viber and Telegram: Which is the best for instant messaging? *International Journal of Electrical & Computer Engineering*, 6(3), 909–914.

Sy, M., O'Leary, N., Nagraj, S., El-Awaisi, A., O'Carroll, V., and Xyrichis, A. (2020). Doing interprofessional research in the COVID-19 era: A discussion paper. *Journal of Interprofessional Care*, 34(5), 600–606.

Thunberg, S., and Arnell, L. (2022). Pioneering the use of technologies in qualitative research – a research review of the use of digital interviews. *International Journal of Social Research Methodology*, 25(6), 757–768.

Torrentira, M. Jr. (2020). Online data collection as adaptation in conducting quantitative and qualitative research during the COVID-19 pandemic. *European Journal of Education Studies*, 7(11), 78–87.

Townsend, E., Nielsen, E., Allister, R., and Cassidy, S. (2020). Key ethical questions for research during the COVID-19 pandemic. *The Lancet Psychiatry*, 7(5), 381–383.

UNESCO. (2013). *Global media and information literacy (MIL): Assessment framework: Country readiness and competencies*. Paris, France: United Nations Educational Scientific and Cultural Organization. http://unesdoc.unesco.org/images/0022/002246/224655e.pdf.

van Deursen, A.J., and van Dijk, J.A. (2019). The first-level digital divide shifts from inequalities in physical access to inequalities in material access. *New Media & Society*, 21(2), 354–375.

Vostanis, P. (2019). World awareness for children in trauma: capacity-building activities of a psychosocial program. *International Journal of Mental Health*, 48(4), 323–329.

Vostanis, P., Haffejee, S., Getanda, E., Eruyar, S., Hassan, S., and O'Reilly, M. (2023). Risk factors for mental health and wellness: Children's perspectives from five Majority World Countries. *Health, Risk & Society*, 25(7–8), 304–323.

Vostanis, P., Ruby, F., Jacob, J., Eruyar, S., Getanda, E., Haffejee, S., Krishna, M., and Edbrooke-Childs, J. (2022). Youth and professional perspectives of mental health resources across eight countries. *Children & Youth Services Review*, 136.

Ward, K., Gott, M., and Hoare, K. (2015). Participants' views of telephone interviews within a grounded theory study. *Journal of Advanced Nursing*, 71(12), 2275–2785.

Watson, M., Jones, D., and Burns, L. (2007). Internet research and informed consent: An ethical model using archived emails. *International Journal of Therapy and Rehabilitation*, 14(9), 396–403.

CHAPTER 16

Transcription and data management

Learning objectives

This chapter enables the reader to:

- Identify the benefits and challenges of using audio or video recording devices.
- Critically assess the ethical concerns that accompany recording data.
- Recognise different issues relating to data protection and data storage.
- Recognise that transcription is an active, not passive, process.
- Critically assess whether to commission a professional transcriptionist or undertake their own transcription.

Introduction

As we recognised in the previous chapter, we now live in a society where digital technology is integrated in our everyday lives and has created opportunities and challenges for collecting data in qualitative research. Increased quality in technology has afforded avenues for fieldwork capturing richness and depth through quality recording. Developments with digital technology do, however, raise ethical challenges (as we noted previously) and considerations for planning regarding data protection when collecting, storing, transferring, and sharing data on digital devices. Nonetheless, the higher quality of recording devices has had implications for transcription, at least making the technical aspect of the task more straightforward.

Transcription processes are not always something that researchers think too much about, and some people think of it as a mere administrative activity. There are, nonetheless, other areas related to transcription you can consider as a qualitative researcher, as transcription is an active process and not merely an administrative or mechanical one, and many methodological approaches see transcription as a step in the analytic process. Although researchers spend time familiarising themselves with the audio or audio-visual recordings, it is standard research practice to produce a textual version of those recordings to facilitate the analysis and to provide a mechanism for disseminating the research. In this chapter, we guide you through some of the considerations and decisions that you are likely to need to think about in relation to the process of transcription and data management for your research project.

Audio and video recording

Technological advances, along with greater cost-effectiveness of digital (visual and audio) recording devices, have created opportunities for qualitative researchers to capture their data with greater quality in sound and visual appearance (where appropriate). For most qualitative methods, it is appropriate to record the data on an audio or audio-visual device. Even for textual data or other forms of data, such as drawings, photographs, and handwritten documents, these are typically stored on digital devices like laptops, cloud-based systems, or hard drives. Having an accurate record of the data that can be frequently returned to for the purposes of analysis is considered essential in contemporary qualitative health research.

> **Key point!**
>
> Having good quality recordings enhances data management and analysis.
>
> (Halcomb and Davidson, 2006)

Many modern devices have large storage capacity, which means that high-quality files can be held for analysis (Paulus, Lester, and Dempster, 2013). Furthermore, the accessibility of the internet and internet-mediated communication has removed many of the barriers of geographic location and distance between researchers and participants (Hinchcliffe and Gavin, 2009), although this may erode the distinction between formal and informal environments, which can serve to blur professional boundaries (Heath, 2011).

When deciding to record your verbal discourse, whether that be in naturally occurring activities, interviews, focus groups, or captured by other methods, you will need to determine if you are going to capture data as an audio recording or video recording. Commonly, qualitative researchers have tended to favour audio recordings, as historically participants tended to be more comfortable not having their face and body on camera. Yet, over time with the growth of social media, the internet, modern surveillance, and people becoming more accustomed to being recorded during their normal daily activities, more research has used video recording. There are several things to consider when making your choice between audio and video capture, many of which we have previously noted (O'Reilly and Kiyimba, 2015):

TRANSCRIPTION AND DATA MANAGEMENT

- Bear in mind the reflexivity of the participants and of the researcher as they engage with the technology. Researchers should be thoughtful about the interaction between the researcher and the participant and recognise the interaction is mutually constituted and any response from participants is contextually situated. Using video can also be a mechanism to encourage later reflection (see also Iedema, Forsyth, Georgiou et al., 2007).
- There can be a blurring of the distinction between naturally occurring and researcher-generated data in some contexts.
- There are ethical sensitivities in recordings which may be intensified with the use of video. Having a digital record of what the participants said and did carries risks in relation to participant identification and confidentiality. There can also be matters to consider in relation to what is considered "on or off the record" (see O'Reilly, Parker, and Hutchby, 2011).
- There are also technical and practical considerations that need to be thought through. It may be helpful to think about the visibility or intrusiveness of the recording device (Bottorff, 1994). There are smaller and smaller devices available, but participants must be aware of the presence of a device, and consent should be recorded.
- There are various perspectives on whether the presence of a recording device alters the behaviour or discourse of participants. Most people are quite familiar with being recorded in various aspects of their lives and tend to be less concerned with the presence of a device. Also, research evidence indicates that people quickly become accustomed to the presence of a device when they are being recorded (see Speer and Hutchby, 2003).
- In contemporary society, there is often a preference for quick and immediate data collection with convenient tools for recording, such as mobile phones, but their use raises practical and ethical issues that should be reflected upon (Lau and Bratby, 2024).

There are many considerations that arise from this list, and we invite you to spend some time thinking about this further by trying the activity in Box 16.1.

Box 16.1

Activity on using audio or video recording devices

Based on your plans for your own research project, consider the following:

- What is more appropriate for your participants and topic: video or audio recordings?
- What are the potential advantages of your decision?
- What might the disadvantages be?
- What concerns might be raised for the safe storage and protection of the recordings?

Encryption

> **Key point!**
>
> If you are recording on an audio or video device, or if you are storing textual or visual data on a digital device, you will need to ensure the data are protected with encryption. You may also need to password protect stored data.

As part of ethical research practice, it is likely you will inform participants of the steps taken to protect the data to ensure their anonymity (or pseudo-anonymity) and confidentiality. There are various ways to protect data, and your organisation may provide safe storage space on a drive for you, and you may have access to experts in data security who can offer guidance. There are devices with built-in encryption that require a password to access, which may be helpful, and there are hard drives with strong levels of encryption for storage. You do need to be cautious when using some software or cloud-based systems about the levels of security these offer, and whose data is considered the property of should you store personal participant data there.

Practical issues with recording

You may believe that the process of recording your participants talking (in an interview, focus group, or natural activity) is straightforward: you buy a device, position it in an appropriate place, and press record to capture the data. This is far from the whole story, though, and there are multiple considerations that you may need to prepare for and think about in your planning. A good example of this is the kind of environment you are recording in. As we noted in Chapter 12, there are issues of your safety and the safety of the participants, which may have implications for finding entirely private, quiet spaces. Some researchers (out of necessity or planning) may collect their data in noisier or busier environments, and the recording may miss important facets of the data (Plowman and Stephen, 2008). For thinking about some of these considerations, we provide a list of things to consider in your planning in Box 16.2.

> **Box 16.2**
>
> **Things to remember when planning your recording**
>
> There are important things to plan for in your recording of data:
>
> - Think about where you place your recording device. You do not want it to be intrusive, but it does need to capture the sound (and image). This can seem, on first impression, quite simple. However, there is great scope for interference if, for example, you place it on a desk where papers are being moved or close to a window where there is noise outside.
> - Ensure the device is recording the data you want it to and not something else (by accident).

- Make sure you test your device and practice with it. Be familiar with its functions and what it is capable of.
- Check the battery life of your recording device and make sure it is sufficient. Plug into the mains if possible (and take a power source with you).
- Where possible, ensure your device has encryption software on it so that the data are protected while stored on the device. Transfer the data from the device to a more secure portal at the first opportunity.
- It is advisable to have a second recording device where costs allow so that you have two devices recording from different angles and in different parts of the environment to promote better data capture.
- Have your recording device in a fixed position where possible to aid quality. Of course, if you are trying to capture moving participants in natural environments, body cameras might be more suitable, but there may be limitations in what images are captured and quality of sound.
- If you are using internet-mediated devices to record (Teams™, Zoom™, smartphones, etc.), you need to be mindful of any policy, legal, or data issues that this might bring with the short- and long-term storage of the data.
- Keeping some short notes on what is said in an interview, as it is ongoing, or shortly after, can serve as something of a substitute if there are issues with the quality of the interview recording.
- Think about how you will keep the recording and recording device safe immediately after gathering data, for instance, after completing an interview.

Data management plans, data storage, and data privacy

We have already referred to some of the considerations necessary as they relate to storage and privacy in the previous sections, but because of the importance of these, and the legal issues associated with data protection, we are concluding this section by bringing your attention back to data storage and data privacy.

Key point!

When collecting data from participants, it is a good idea to create a data management plan for any data gathering and to iteratively update and develop this plan as you go. Your organisation may have a template, but you can also create your own.

There is a clear crossover between ethics, integrity, and legalities in the management of data, and it can be helpful to seek expert advice in addressing any questions you have about data recording, data storage, data management, data protection, data transfer, and data sharing. This is because data storage and retrieval are central in a world of digitisation (Brown, 2002). For example, we would encourage you to think about the following:

- Is the device encrypted? Your data should be stored on devices or systems that have high levels of encryption. Ask for advice from an IT specialist to ensure the right level of security for your project.
- Where are you storing your data? Is it secure to prevent it from being hacked into and the data stolen or easily accessed by others (who are unauthorised to do so)? In considering where data are kept for the duration of the project (after data collection on an encrypted device), your organisation may already have rules about where you can store research data. If not, this would be a good time to pull together a team to devise some appropriate policies and procedures that can serve to keep anyone conducting research in your organisation safe.
- Are the data protected? You should take steps to anonymise or disguise your raw data if possible. You will need to keep any demographic or personal data, including consent forms, separate from the raw data so that participant identities are not compromised (but these will, of course, need to be securely stored as well).
- How long will you be storing the data? You need to be clear with your participants about how long the original recordings will be retained and how long any related anonymous transcripts will be kept. Your funding body or organisation may specify this as part of their guidelines.
- Who is responsible for destroying the data at the end of the storage period? Just as important as storage is the destruction of data at the end of the allotted timeframe. Make sure you are clear on who is responsible for this, and how it will be destroyed.
- Who owns the data? By storing your data on some platforms, you no longer own the data, so be mindful of where you put it. Also, if you work for an organisation, check who owns which parts of the data and associated research outputs. This is important to establish, for example, in the case of someone leaving the organisation and questions such as whether they will still have access to the data and how.
- Are you sharing the data? Often, research is undertaken in teams, and different members may be in different organisations or even different countries. You may need a data-sharing agreement and a confidentiality agreement, or something similar. You may need legal advice to draw this up.

Transcription as an interpretive activity

In qualitative research, it is common practice to create a transcript of the recordings to represent the data, as taking extracts of these provides an accessible version of the data for wider audiences when disseminating the findings (Peräkylä, 1997). Notably, however, the process of transcription is not a neutral one, and neither is it that easy. In fact, early researchers did not widely consider the issue of transcription because of assumptions that the process was transparent (Lapadat, 2000). In the reporting of much qualitative research, transcription often seems to be a taken-for-granted aspect of the way a study was undertaken and is not often well-addressed (Point and Baruch, 2023) and yet transcription is arguably an interpretative process (Clark, Birkhead, Fernandez, and Egger, 2017). This is to say that transcription is not simply a technical tool, and researchers need an understanding of the role they occupy in transcribing data (Shelton and Flint, 2021).

The transcription process provides a way for researchers to immerse themselves in their data, which can help to develop insights (Vanover, 2021). Moreover, researchers need to be aware that transcription involves a level of judgement (Rossman and Rallis, 2011) and this judgement is interpretive in nature (Hammersley, 2010). The kinds of decisions that are typically made relate to the level of detail in the transcript. For example, if half words are transcribed accurately or are completed for ease of reading. Similarly, decisions about transcribing discourse makers (Schiffrin, 2012), such as ums, erms, and ahs, and paralinguistic features, like pitch and tone, as well as coughs, sneezes, and laughter may be made.

When thinking about the process of transcription, you need to be mindful that your transcription decisions are tied to the theoretical perspectives that are embedded in your research, and this, in turn, is tied to the methodology and methods of your work (Creswell and Poth, 2018). For example, some methodologies require a particular transcription convention. Thus, you will have to make some decisions about what your transcripts represent, which aspects of communication you are representing as text (Davidson, 2009) and how those decisions reflect the theoretical foundation of your research (Point and Baruch, 2023). By tying your decisions relating to transcription to theory, and considering transcription an active and interpretive process, the quality of your transcription becomes pertinent, and the quality of transcription becomes an aspect of rigour in qualitative research (di Gregorio, 2021).

One way in which the transcription process and decisions are tied to theory and rigour is in the level of detail you opt to embrace and report in transcripts (Point and Baruch, 2023). Some researchers view the practice of doing transcription as being on a continuum between naturalism and denaturalism (Oliver, Serovich, and Mason, 2005). Naturalism refers to where the transcript retains the features of natural talk including paralinguistic features, like gesture, sneezing, coughing, intonation, pauses and so (Oliver et al., 2005). That is, the researcher actively elects to attend to the rich, multimodal aspects of the talk and includes paralinguistic features as these are argued to convey interactive meaning (Hepburn and Bolden, 2013). By comparison, with denaturalism, there is minimal description where the talk is "tidied up" for readability. This is usually used where the detail is not essential for the analytic process.

> **Key point!**
>
> You need to convey an understanding of the practice of transcription by disclosing a rationale for all your transcription decisions.
>
> (Skukauskaite, 2012)

In practice, you need to make decisions such as your page layout, the width of your margins, the font, typeset, and so forth, as well as decisions about the inclusion of paralinguistic features, intonations, pauses, and so on (Lapadat, 2000). However, deciding to capture all this detail (should you require it) can be challenging if there is background noise in your recording or you use poor-quality equipment.

QUALITATIVE HEALTH RESEARCH

We now encourage you to reflect on your learning by addressing the reflective activity on decisions relating to transcription in Box 16.3.

Box 16.3

Reflecting on transcription decisions

Based on your learning in this chapter, reflect on decisions you make regarding transcription and write down in your research diary how you will approach transcription and what further reading you feel you need to do to ensure this approach is appropriate for your project and can be linked coherently to the methodological and theoretical framework on which the study is based.

Using technology as a transcription aid

In the contemporary context, one option open to you with transcription is to use dictation software or software built into recording platforms to transcribe for you. This is an appealing option, as transcription is a notoriously labour-intensive process. With a modest, exploratory qualitative research project, transcription costs to fund a professional transcriptionist can take up a significant chunk of a research budget, and so decisions need to be made on a pragmatic basis. In the modern world, there are a range of technologies that can turn speech into text. These "intelligent speech recognition systems" are developing and increasing in their sophistication and so open up possibility for research and transcription (Eftekhari, 2024). One advantage of using computer software to produce a textual representation of your recordings is that it circumvents some of the potential problems related to managing transcriptionist safety and emotional well-being (as we discussed in Chapter 12). There is now a range of automatic speech recognition software that you might choose to use to transcribe your digital recordings (Matheson, 2007), and some quite sophisticated software that converts audio files into text (di Gregorio, 2021). Thus, technology can now reduce the amount of time taken by researchers to produce an initial transcript (Bokhove and Downey, 2018). Notably, some video-conferencing platforms have a transcription option available where a transcript is simultaneously produced as people talk.

There are also negatives to using software to transcribe for you and a range of things that need to be considered if you choose this option. First, you need to check carefully what the security of the service you are using is if you are paying for an online service. These services could be based in any country in the world and may have different legal parameters for data security than you are required to abide by in the country where you have gained your institutional ethical review approval for the research you are doing. If you are using built-in software on your device, this may not apply. If you do use an intelligent speech recognition software, then you need to be aware that these often mean you need to use the technology company's third party platform (Eftekhari, 2024), and this may be problematic in terms of your data storage and data privacy obligations. After data security, the next consideration when using computer software to convert audio to text is accuracy. Even the best software available makes errors, which can significantly change the meaning of what the participant said (e.g. "ice-cream" versus "I scream"). There are no shortcuts to this process, which involves carefully listening to the original recording while reading the draft transcript, and this is especially important as many qualitative approaches consider transcription to be part of the analytic process. Do this when you do not have any distractions around you and you are not (too) tired, as it is easy to skip mistakes or read what you think you heard. Ideally, you will have someone else check the quality of the transcription as well. An inaccurate transcript can be highly problematic, as this is what your analysis, findings, discussions, and recommendations will be based on. In this way, the researcher only really uses automated transcription as a starting point and takes ample time to check through what is produced (Point and Baruch, 2023).

Translation in transcription
Much dissemination activity, that is, in terms of journal articles, books, and conference presentations about research, is in English. Yet much qualitative research and transcripts are produced in languages other than English and in countries where English is not the primary language. Historically, this was not especially well dealt with in the literature although there is growing attention being paid to this issue (Nikander, 2008). Nikander observed that this can raise problems for those researchers who collect data in their native language and transcribe that data in their native language as they face challenges in translating the work for dissemination purposes.

We previously identified two central matters to think about in relation to this concern (O'Reilly and Kiyimba, 2015):

1. The data may be collected via an interpreter. Hence, where the researcher speaks one language and the participants speak another, a professional interpreter may be needed. However, this creates challenges of precise interpretation and issues of accuracy in translation. There is a risk of misunderstanding, bias, or loss of fidelity.
2. The data may be collected in another country where the researcher and participants are native to that country and speak their natural dialect, which then needs translation for international audiences.

In regard to both these matters, the researcher must decide whether to represent the original language in the dissemination as well as the translation, and whether to translate the words literally. Many researchers choose this tri-part transcription representation way of working. This is where they first present the original language. On the next line, they provide a literal translation, word-for-word. The final line provides the translation with meaning so that the English version is comprehensible.

A foundational concern in translating data is that there may be implicit assumptions that the process of translation is objective and neutral (Wong and Poon, 2010). Transcription itself may be seen as mechanical, neutral, and passive, but as we have shown in this chapter, that is not the case. The researcher must think about the practical and theoretical issues that are pertinent to the way they present their translated transcripts (Nikander, 2008) as the omission of a phrase or even a single word can influence data interpretation, the construction of meaning, and how the experience or perspective of the participant is represented (Wong and Poon, 2010).

Considerations in commissioning transcription services
While we have guided you through some of the decisions you need to make in transcription, arguably one of the most important decisions you will make is whether you undertake the task yourself or commission a professional transcriptionist to create the initial version of a transcript for you. On one hand, there is value in doing your own transcript as you can build knowledge of your data and begin the analytical process (Braun and Clarke, 2013). On the other hand, this must be balanced against the time and resources available for your project (Richards, 2015).

As noted, transcription can be a laborious and time-consuming task, and this may influence a researcher's decision to outsource the task, at least for the initial verbatim version (Bokhove and Downey, 2018; Point and Baruch, 2023). Indeed, there is no doubt that transcribing takes a long time. Even someone with transcription skills can take 6–10 hours to transcribe a one-hour-long interview and even longer for multi-party conversations like focus groups (Saunders, Lewis, and Thornhill, 2019). For approaches with considerable detail, like conversation analysis (which uses the Jeffersonian method – Jefferson, 2004), the literature suggests it can take one hour to transcribe one minute of data even when the person has expertise and experience in the transcription approach (Wagner, 2018).

Evidently, there are advantages to doing your own transcription. It ensures that you fully engage with your recordings and provides a valuable opportunity for you to familiarise yourself with your data (Point and Baruch, 2023), which can be aligned with a view of transcription as a step in the analytic process (Braun and Clarke, 2022; Lapadat, 2000). Moreover, by undertaking transcription yourself, you are likely to bring more value to the process than by outsourcing it to an external party (Point and Baruch, 2023). As we have shown, transcription is an interpretive process and thus there is a good reason that you should undertake the transcription yourself (Lucas, 2010), as you have the knowledge and expertise yielded during the process of data collection (Halcomb and Davidson, 2006).

If you do elect to commission an independent transcriptionist, then you will have a responsibility to provide that person with clear written guidelines regarding what you expect, ask them to note their reflections as they transcribe, and you should have a confidentiality agreement with them (Bazeley, 2013). You will need to be active in supporting and communicating with your transcriptionist (Lucas, 2010). Indeed, Bazeley emphasised that the externally produced transcript is simply the first iteration and, as the researcher, you will need to add detail and go through each transcript checking for accuracy. Bazeley recommended that the researcher review and edit the transcripts while listening closely to the data. As noted, you may need to add in paralinguistic features, repetitious speech, intonation, laughter, coughing, sneezing, and pauses. You may also want to think about whether you include half words or words like "um", "erm", and so on.

> **Key point!**
>
> If you choose to commission a professional transcriptionist to produce the first representation of your data, then you need to be mindful of the sensitivity of the content. We included a section on transcriptionist safety in Chapter 12 and advise you to acquaint yourself with this again prior to commissioning them to complete this work.

Author reflections and concluding remarks
From Michelle

I have undertaken a lot of research that involves discursive psychology and conversation analysis, which meant that I have conducted a lot of Jeffersonian transcription, the ultra-detailed transcription system associated with conversation analysis. Over time, this has to some extent, become a little easier with the rise of technology but remains time-intensive. Nonetheless, I view the Jeffersonian approach to transcription as a valuable step in the analytic process, and so I do this part myself.

If I go back to my first truly memorable transcription task, it was during my PhD. As a student, I was guided to do my own transcription by my supervisor (a progenitor of discursive psychology, Derek Edwards). Furthermore, as a student, I simply could not afford to pay someone else to do that task for me, and neither were there many technological options to faciltiate. Back then, when I collected my data, my video recordings were on old-fashioned analogue VHS tapes, and so each time I pressed pause, the recording would jump a couple of seconds. I spent an inordinate amount of time going backward and forward through the tape. I spent hours and hours and hours of my life transcribing 22 hours of family therapy, each session with multiple speakers.

One thing I did learn during that time was that it was easier to capture the words spoken first, then go back and layer it with paralinguistic details, then go back again and add the Jeffersonian level of detail, and then go back again and check for accuracy. In my later research, with the benefit of research funding, I therefore tend to commission a professional transcriptionist to produce that first level, simply the words as spoken. This is still expensive and takes time, and, of course, once the transcript comes back, there are still three levels to go.

For me, the bottom line is that transcription is active, it is interpretive, it is tied to your methodology and theory, and there are no shortcuts. It will take you time, even if you pay for that initial version or if you use technology to produce it.

References

Bazeley P. (2013). *Qualitative data analysis: Practical strategies*. London: Sage.

Bokhove, C., and Downey, C. (2018). Automated generation of "good enough" transcripts as a first step to transcription of audio-recorded data. *Methodological Innovations*, 11(2).

Bottorff, J. (1994). Using videotaped data recordings in qualitative research. In J. Morse (Ed.), *Critical issues in qualitative research methods*. (pp. 244–261). London: Sage.

Braun, V., and Clarke, V. (2013). *Successful qualitative research: A practical guide for beginners*. London: Sage.

Braun, V., and Clarke, V. (2022). *Thematic analysis: A practical guide*. London: Sage.

Brown, D. (2002). Going digital and staying qualitative: Some alternative strategies for digitizing the qualitative research process. *Forum: Qualitative Social Research*, 3(2), Article 12.

Clark, L., Birkhead, A. S., Fernandez, C., and Egger, M. J. (2017). A transcription and translation protocol for sensitive cross-cultural team research. *Qualitative Health Research*, 27(12), 1751–1764.

Creswell, J., and Poth, C. (2018). *Qualitative inquiry and research design* (5th ed.). Thousand Oaks, CA: Sage.

Davidson, C. (2009). Transcription: Imperatives for qualitative research. *International Journal of Qualitative Methods*, 8, 35–52.

di Gregorio, S. (2021). Voice to text: Automating transcription. In C. Vanover, P. Mihas, and J. Saldaña (Eds.), *Analyzing and interpreting qualitative research: After the interview* (pp: 97–112). Thousand Oaks, CA: Sage.

Eftekhari, H. (2024). Transcribing in the digital age: qualitative research practice utilizing intelligent speech recognition technology. *European Journal of Cardiovascular Nursing*, 23(5), 553–560.

Halcomb, E., and Davidson, P. (2006). Is verbatim transcription of interview data always necessary? *Applied Nursing Research*, 19, 38–42.

Hammersley, M. (2010). Reproducing or constructing? Some questions about transcription in social research. *Qualitative Research*, 10, 553–569.

Heath, C. (2011) Embodied action: Video and the analysis of social interaction. In D. Silverman (Ed.), *Qualitative research* (3rd ed., pp. 250–270). London: Sage.

Hepburn, A., and Bolden, G. (2013). The conversation analytic approach to transcription. In J. Sidnell and T. Stivers (Eds.), *The handbook of conversation analysis* (pp. 57–76). West Sussex: Blackwell Publishing.

Hinchcliffe, V., and Gavin, H. (2009). Social and virtual networks: Evaluating synchronous online interviewing using instant messenger. *The Qualitative Report*, 14(2), 318–340.

Iedema, R., Forsyth, R., Georgiou, A., Braithwaite, J., and Westbrook, J. (2007). Video research in health: Visibilising the effects of computerising clinical care. *Qualitative Research Journal*, 6(2), 15–30.

Jefferson, G. (2004). Glossary of transcript symbols with an introduction. In G. H. Lerner (Ed.), *Conversation analysis: Studies from the first generation* (pp. 13–31). Amsterdam: John Benjamins.

Lapadat, J. (2000). Problematizing transcription: Purpose, paradigm and quality. *International Journal of Social Research Methodology*, 3(3), 203–219.

Lau, A., and Bratby, M. (2024). Collecting qualitative data via video statements in the digital era. *Labour and Industry*, 34(2), 101–113.

Littlejohn, S., Foss, K., and Oetzel, (2017). *Theories of human communication* (11th ed.). Long Grove, IL: Waveland Press.

Lucas, K. (2010). A waste of time? The value and promise of researcher completed qualitative data transcribing. Northeastern Educational Research Association conference Proceedings, Paper 24. http://digitalcommons.uconn.edu/nera_2010/24.

Matheson, J. (2007). The voice transcription technique: Use of voice recognition software to transcribe digital interview data in qualitative research. *Qualitative Report*, 12(4), 547–560.

Nikander, P. (2008). Working with transcripts and translated data. *Qualitative Research in Psychology*, 5, 225–231.

Oliver, D., Serovich, J., and Mason, T. (2005). Mason constraints and opportunities with interview transcription: Towards reflection in qualitative research. *Social Forces*, 84, 1273–1289.

O'Reilly, M., and Kiyimba, N. (2015). *Advanced qualitative research: A guide to contemporary theoretical debates*. London: Sage.

O'Reilly, M., Parker, N., and Hutchby, I. (2011). Ongoing processes of managing consent: The empirical ethics of using video-recording in clinical practice and research. *Clinical Ethics*, 6(4), 179–185.

Paulus, T., Lester, J. N., and Dempster, P. (2013). *Digital tools for qualitative research*. London: Sage.

Peräkylä, A. (1997). Reliability and validity in research based on tapes and transcripts. In D. Silverman (Ed.), *Qualitative research: Theory, method and practice* (pp. 201–220). London: Sage.

Plowman, L., and Stephen, C. (2008). The big picture? Video and the representation of interaction. *British Educational Research Journal, 34*(4), 541–565.

Point, S., and Baruch, Y. (2023). (Re)thinking transcription strategies: Current challenges and future research directions. *Scandinavian Journal of Management, 39*(2), 101272.

Richards, L. (2015). *Handling qualitative data: A practical guide* (3rd ed.). London: Sage.

Rossman, G., and Rallis, S. (2011). *Learning in the field: An introduction to qualitative research*. London: Sage.

Saunders, M., Lewis, P., and Thornhill, A. (2019). *Research methods for business students* (8th ed.). Harlow: Pearson.

Schiffrin, D. (2012). *Discourse markers*. Cambridge: Cambridge University Press.

Shelton, S., and Flint, M. (2021). Dichotomies of method and practice: A review of literature on transcription. *Qualitative Research Journal, 21*(2), 177–188.

Skukauskaite, A. (2012). Transparency in transcribing: Making visible theoretical bases impacting knowledge construction from open-ended interview records. *Forum: Qualitative Social Research, 13*(1), Article 14.

Speer, S., and Hutchby, I. (2003). From ethics to analytics: Aspects of participants' orientations to the presence and relevance of recording devices. *Sociology, 37*(2), 315–337.

Vanover, C. (2021). Transcription as a form of qualitative inquiry. In C. Vanover, P. Mihas, and J. Saldaña (Eds.), *Analyzing and interpreting qualitative data: After the interview*. London: Sage.

Wagner. J. (2018). Conversation analysis: Transcriptions and data. In C. Chapelle (Ed.), *The concise encyclopedia of applied linguistics*. Hoboken, NJ: Wiley-Blackwell.

Wong, P.-H. J., and Poon, K.-L. M. (2010). Bringing translation out of the shadows: Translation as an issue of methodological significance in cross-cultural qualitative research. *Journal of Transcultural Nursing, 21*(2), 151–158.

CHAPTER 17

Using clinical skills in research

> **Learning objectives**
>
> This chapter enables the reader to:
>
> - Identify the value that clinical skills have for research.
> - Consider the similarities and differences between psychological therapy and research.
> - Recognise the potentially beneficial impact of participating in qualitative research.
> - Critically assess the challenges of bringing clinical skills to data collection.
> - Ascertain the limits of using clinical skills in research contexts.
> - Identify the value of academic and clinical partnerships for research.

Introduction

Researchers who are practicing health professionals possess both research skills and clinical skills but may be more experienced in clinical practice than research activity. For the clinician-researcher, the boundaries and overlap between clinical work and research must be accounted for to ensure role clarity. This topic of role differentiation was acknowledged in Chapter 9 where we spoke about dual roles, and the matter of insider–outsider status in research. This current chapter extends that consideration, focusing on relationship boundaries and the role of a clinical sensibility and clinical skills in research, including benefits and challenges of this. The chapter also includes some discussion of positionality building on our earlier discussion, as well as more broadly considering the value of communication skills in research and the necessity of building rapport with participants.

We acknowledge there is a difference between naturally occurring and researcher-generated qualitative data. Whilst a researcher may have some contact with participants during the consent gathering stage when naturally occurring data are used, they do not engage directly with the participant much after that. The focus of this chapter, therefore, primarily relates to researcher-generated data collection, where the researcher is in direct contact with the participant. The exception to this would be a situation where a clinician-researcher is using recordings of their own clinical practice with clients (naturally occurring) for research purposes. In this instance, the clinician-researcher is completely in the role of clinician during the interaction with the client that is being recorded. We also note that in this chapter, we do not focus on participant observation. In instances where research involves observation, the goal is not to communicate with the participant so as not to disrupt what they would naturally be doing.

Communicating with participants
Communicating with patients/clients requires a great deal of skill to promote alignment and engagement in the clinical relationship (Lester and O'Reilly, 2021). At a basic level, communication involves the speaker, the recipient, and the message. However, beyond this, effective communication is highly complex, integrating verbal and nonverbal elements, human warmth, rapport, trust, and listening (Karim, McSweeney, and O'Reilly, 2021). Just as communication is a vital element in healthcare work, it is also fundamental in qualitative research. Qualitative research uses communication as its data.

There is no universal definition of communication, and it is a term difficult to capture in a precise way (Littlejohn, Foss, and Oetzel, 2017). What is more, not all people communicate in "typical" or normative ways. There are tensions in the research literature about how to refer to social interactions where one or more of the interlocutors has a health condition that is consequential to the way they communicate (Wilkinson, 2019). Adaptations in research practice and design, as well as researcher flexibility, are often necessary to promote participation and inclusion. There is a literature on "atypical communication" and this has implications for how clinical practitioners consult with those individuals (see George and O'Reilly, 2023). Atypical communication generally refers to individuals for whom communication has not developed in a normative way or whose development of speech, social communication skills, vocabulary, verbal and written fluency, literacy and/or language has been impacted (Fletcher and O'Toole, 2016).

In qualitative health research, you may interact with individuals with a range of communication styles and abilities. As a clinician-researcher, your dual role may also be instrumental as your clinical skills can be advantageous in engaging with participants. This being so, as touched on earlier in the book, there are considerations that accompany making use of these skills to ensure that the practices of research and clinical care do not become inappropriately blurred and the boundaries between the two are differentiated. For example, a "therapeutic" style of listening in research interviews may mean that participants disclose more about personal experiences than they would have otherwise wished to (Long and Eagle, 2009).

> **Key point!**
> There is a risk of emotional intimacy which might take the guise of mutuality (Sinding and Aronson, 2003). This has been referred to as the problem of "faking friendships" in research.
> (Duncombe and Jessop, 2012)

Owing to these risks, a critical reflexive position aids the researcher in managing all kinds of research communication in terms of their position, power, and influence as a researcher and clinician. For your research, it is beneficial to think about how you communicate during recruitment to prospective participants, to ensure the terms of reference are clear to them.

Building rapport in interviews and focus groups

In clinical practice, the dyadic relationship between two parties is the mechanism by which the task-related goals of the interaction are accomplished, as well as the relational goals. Thus, rapport between the clinical practitioner and client/patient is essential for progressing the task focus of the interaction as it relates to the institutional outcomes of the health encounter. Likewise, in research, the researcher–participant relationship is central to the quality of the data collection process.

Part of the challenge of considering rapport in both contexts is that there is no shared definition or conceptualisation of the meaning of the term (English, Gott, and Robinson, 2022). Despite the lack of definition of rapport, it is accepted that a key component is a degree of trust between the parties involved (Lonneman, 2016). Where the researcher is directly involved in the data collection process, for example, individual interviews or focus groups, building rapport with a participant includes giving attention to creating a safe, conversational space for participants to share their experiences (Owens, 1996). Trust is a necessary ingredient to "good" research and how rapport is managed locally (Zhang and Okazawa, 2023).

> **Key point!**
> There are additional challenges in creating rapport in virtual spaces, particularly those that rely on or involve a written or textual chat-based component. In this case, articulation of affect in the form of using emoticons may help to convey certain sentiments, which in turn may aid in supporting the relationship.
> (Park, 2023)

Recent perspectives regarding rapport in research foreground the value of an iterative approach that considers it to evolve over time, for instance, not just through a single interview, but developing from the outset of interacting with the participant (Prior,

2018). From this perspective, it is helpful to take an interdiscursive approach to rapport (Agha, 2005), especially in research projects that entail a longer or more involved engagement of participants through the process (Shahri, 2023). In Shahri's account, an interdiscursive orientation means attending to links between speech events, whereby positive rapport is something understood as a collaboratively accomplished experience dependent upon a dynamic flow of interaction. Given the dynamic and situated nature of rapport and the challenge of finding a definition that fully captures its meaning in the context of research, we encourage you to reflect further by engaging with the activity in Box 17.1.

> **Box 17.1**
> **Reflective activity on building rapport**
>
> Consider a recent experience building rapport in your clinical practice as a health or care professional. This might be a brief event, for instance, building rapport during a single assessment appointment or consultation. Equally, it could be a lengthier process, for example, getting to know a young person and planning work together for psychological therapy. After you have recalled this experience, try to think about it in terms of the specific steps involved, what you thought at the time, your actions, and how these actions were responded to by the individual/s you were working with. What did you find was beneficial in the specific context?
>
> After you have done this, consider a hypothetical example of building rapport for your own research (either research you are undertaking or planning to undertake) and consider these questions:
>
> - Are there any ways in which the skills you used as a practitioner may translate to the way you develop rapport in research relationships?
> - What aspects may be beneficial and which are potentially unhelpful?
> - Are there any issues this gives rise to in terms of the boundaries between your role and identity as a clinician and researcher?
> - How might these be navigated whilst undertaking the research?

The (quasi-)therapeutic qualities of research participation

One of the oft-cited benefits that research participants volunteer as a reason for agreeing to participate in a qualitative study is that it can be experienced as therapeutic to speak about their experiences, views, and feelings to an interested listener during an interview or focus group. The recognition of some of the overlaps between participating in qualitative research and accessing psychological therapy is not new, with various scholars addressing the issue (see, for example, Bourne and Robson, 2015; Rosetto, 2014). The degree of opportunity for the participant to describe their experiences freely will depend on how structured the interview schedule is, and consequently how much emphasis is on the researcher's agenda versus the participant's. Researcher-generated data collection methods require participants to self-disclose in a not dissimilar way to therapy (Birch and Miller, 2000). As has been acknowledged elsewhere in this book, some researchers also actively seek to make a difference with their research and have their findings applied to practice to bring about change.

If there is an overlap between qualitative research with participants and clinical health practice, areas of overlap need to be considered in practitioner-initiated research. In the research literature, there are instances where the qualitative researcher role is compared to that of a counsellor, particularly in the context of giving participants space to express their emotional experiences (McCosker, Barnard, Gerber, 2001). Indeed, expression of emotion and reflection on emotional experience tends to be central to both endeavours (LeChanaye and McCarthy, 2022). In this respect, qualitative researchers arguably stand to benefit from having counselling skills to help them manage the sensitivity of their research. At the same time, when collecting data in the role of a researcher, this is a different role than that of a therapist or counsellor, and thus the interview should be convened in a way that manages the participant's expectations. A researcher with psychotherapeutic training can engage in reflection on their practice to avoid drifting into providing therapy to participants (Owens, 1996).

The relationship between participant and researcher constitutes the vehicle through which a researcher can engage in empathic and active listening to ensure participants feel heard and understood (Myers, 2000). However, in creating an environment conducive to research-relevant disclosure, it is necessary to reflect on role boundaries and the function of the relationship (LaChenaye and McCarthy, 2022). A clinical practitioner who is skilful in conducting clinical interviews may not immediately think about the differences in the context of a research interview. This is where there is value in reflecting on the different purposes of research versus clinical interviews (Hunt et al., 2011). For example, clinical work may be more focused on eliciting facts, whereas research may be more interpretive (Borbasi, Chapman, and Read, 2002). This distinction has some validity, although we would contend that this depends on the type or epistemological underpinning of either. For example, in psychoanalytic forms of psychotherapy, the encounter is orientated to the client's subjective experience.

Thus, in terms of relationship building, the practice of counselling is based on a pre-existing understanding of relational engagement with clients, and whilst research has strengths in developing the co-construction of meaning and encouraging reflections, there are limitations to how far researchers can explore (LaChenaye and McCarthy, 2022). Kagle and Giebelhausen (1994) discerned ways in which the therapeutic relationship is different from other types of relationships, specifically in terms of the client's vulnerability and the therapist's influence. Our perspective is that the client's "vulnerability" relates to the degree to which the client allows themselves to be vulnerable with the therapist, which is related to the degree to which the client feels safe to talk about the things that are most painful for them. The influence of the therapist comes from their role in helping guide the client to make sense of their situation. This is typically considered a collaborative journey where considerations of "power" or "influence" are navigated in such a way as to allow the client to find their own sense of value and import in the process.

USING CLINICAL SKILLS IN RESEARCH

> **Key point!**
>
> Clinical practitioners involved in data collection should avoid being complacent and assuming their clinical interview experience will provide them with sufficient knowledge and competencies in research interviewing.
>
> (Hunt, Chan, and Mehta, 2011)

The value of clinical skills in undertaking qualitative research

As we have recognised in our writing, there are some issues you may wish to consider when reflecting on how your clinical skills might require adaptation with regards to managing the research relationship. There are, however, benefits to research when it is undertaken by a clinician and attendant challenges are appropriately addressed. Indeed, many of the communication and interviewing skills that clinical practitioners have are transferable to the research context, including the practised use of asking open-ended questions and attending to the subtle non-verbal cues provided (Britten, 1995). Aligned with this, clinicians and researchers must both manage power differentials involved in the process of communication. Although in the healthcare interaction the practitioner may be considered to be the expert on the way in which the medical profession understands an "illness" or medical condition the participant has been diagnosed with, the patient is the expert on their experience of it (Hunt et al., 2011). Hunt et al. proposed five strategies that can support clinician-researchers in conducting data collection. Notably, these steps relate to researcher-generated data collection involving direct communication with participants, such as interviews. These steps do not, therefore, relate to naturally occurring data collection, ethnographic studies, or participant observation. Acknowledging that caveat, we outline the steps proposed by Hunt et al. (2011) in Box 17.2.

> **Box 17.2**
>
> **Practical steps for data collection (Hunt et al., 2011)**
>
> There are several steps that clinician-researchers can take to facilitate the process of data collection:
>
> 1. **Acknowledge and critically reflect on any previous interviewing experience** – it can be challenging to transition from one style of interviewing to another, and not make assumptions that clinical skills directly translate into research activity.
> 2. **Preparation for the research data collection** – before consulting with the first participant, prepare for the encounter and be clear about the topics and the script of questions, including any probes.
> 3. **Manage power** – avoid giving the participants mixed messages, and carefully attend to the power dynamics within the interview.
> 4. **Attend to language and verbal cues** – during the process of data collection, pay attention to participants' use of language, terminology, and verbal cues.
> 5. **Evaluate in an iterative way** – it is necessary to reflect on progress in an ongoing manner and to pay continued attention to quality.

"Practice-near" research and professional transformation in doing research

"Practice-near" is a term associated with different forms of social work, health, and welfare research. This research is best defined as linked by the twin aims of:

1. "Getting closer to practice".
2. Building "research-mindedness" amongst practitioners.

(Froggett and Briggs, 2009, p. 370)

With the latter dimension, this is less in terms of supporting an ethos of evidence-based practice, but rather about supporting critical reflection on practice and care delivery, aided by a research sensibility.

The term "practice-near research" developed from a seminar series funded by the UK Economic and Social Research Council between 2007 and 2009. As Hingley-Jones (2009) has described it, a key idea underpinning practice-near inquiry is that situating research in close proximity to practice enables "a greater complexity of experience to be understood by practitioners" (pp. 413–414). This can encompass a range of concerns, from "structural disadvantage" through to emotional experiences and "inner worlds". Typically, central to practice-near research is a focus on emotional depth and situated knowledge, and with this, a preference for qualitative methods (Froggett and Briggs, 2012; Hingley-Jones, 2009). Practice-near research is often associated with psychosocial approaches involving principles drawn from psychoanalytic therapy, with a focus on exploring unconscious and intersubjective processes in social phenomena (Archard and O'Reilly, 2024; Cooper, 2009; Froggett and Briggs, 2012).

Cooper (2009) provided an account of practice-near research as developed through a psychoanalytic framework, drawing on his own experience supporting social care professionals pursuing doctoral research. In his estimation, practice-near research is recognisable by the degree of emotional and physical proximity to the object of a research study. He described it as involving discovering "complex particulars" (Cooper, 2009, p. 432) and an engagement with the "messiness" of real-world situations through in-depth case studies and reflective research practice. Cooper emphasised a close consideration of psychological and social processes with an appreciation of the uniqueness of individual situations. To this end, he positioned the intersubjective relationship between the researcher's self and the subject(s) of study (e.g. participants, an organisation) as an important site of concern in qualitative research. Moreover, according to Cooper, the level of emotional intensity in research and emphasis on the researcher–researched relationship means practice-near research usually involves personal change for the researcher. In other words, in endeavouring to undertake research, a practitioner-researcher will find that they themselves learn things about themselves through the inquiry, though this is not the focus of the endeavour.

This is an important dimension to consider if you view your inquiry as aligning with a practice-near tradition of work. At the same time, it is worth acknowledging that, based on Cooper's conceptualisation, a health or social care practitioner doing research relating to their work does not mean it will necessarily be classified as practice-near (Archard and O'Reilly, 2024). Rather, the term may be reserved for research which utilises a psychoanalytically-based approach with a focus on psychosocial understanding.

Partnerships with academic scholars

One way to manage the complexities of clinical practitioners undertaking research is the promotion of partnerships with academic scholars. Partnerships between academic and clinical colleagues are also a principal vehicle through which applied health research gets "done" in health and care settings. As we have noted elsewhere in this book, research is typically a team-based endeavour, unless it is for an educational qualification, such as a PhD, and even then, it will involve a supervisory team (and potentially others) supporting the research. On this basis, even where academics have clinical skills, and where clinical practitioners have academic skills, it is still helpful to collaborate, share ideas, and develop new ways of working. Furthermore, collaboration between clinical practitioners and academic researchers can increase the successful translation of research into clinical practice (Williams et al., 2020). Williams et al. noted that these kinds of joined-up approaches to the generation of new knowledge can help close the translational gap.

For the realisation of effective collaborations with academic researchers and practitioners, it is worth bearing in mind that they may be invested in undertaking a particular research study for different reasons. For example, whereas a clinician may be interested in how the study findings may be used to inform service development at a local level, an academic may be more concerned with the "impact" of furthering the development of knowledge. In a similar vein, a research project responding to local service needs may be considered important by professionals and other stakeholders in the service but be a challenging commitment for an academic researcher in safeguarding time for a more modest, exploratory project that has limited funding and "reach" in terms of implications for policy, practice, and other research. There is a range of literature that can be consulted in considering partnerships with academic researchers (Austin and Carnochan, 2020; Fouché, 2015). This work highlights the importance of establishing shared concerns and terms of reference for collaboration, as well as ways in which space can be created for applied research endeavours, for example, having an academic researcher co-located in a service setting.

Clinical academic careers and the value of clinician-researchers

Some clinician-researchers undertake research projects as part of their clinical role, but some clinicians go further and actively seek to make research a more fundamental aspect of their role by pursuing a clinical academic career, undertaking research qualifications to facilitate this, such as a master's degree or a PhD. Clinical academic careers are an occupational pathway in which the clinical practitioner combines their clinical practice with research activities, enabling them to address issues or problems pertinent to their patients/clients and/or their organisation, often involving a teaching and research component as well as a clinical component (National Institute for Health Research, 2016). The clinical academic therefore utilises their research activity to support the development of transformative health services and to be at the centre of change to meet the health needs of the communities they serve (NHS England, 2014).

Whether you are a research-active clinician or a clinical academic, both roles can have benefits for patients/service users, organisations, and healthcare professionals (including medicine and the allied health professions) (Harding, Lynch, Porter, and Taylor,

2017). For example, in occupational therapy, some research evidence indicates that clinical academic careers for practitioners lead to improved health outcomes for patients and efficiencies for organisations (Di Bona, Field, Read et al., 2019). Furthermore, clinician-researchers report valuing their personal development, job satisfaction, and contribution to evidence-based practice (Van Oostveen, Goedhart, Francke et al., 2017). To facilitate clinical academic career pathways and clinician-researcher development, clinician–academic partnerships between those working in higher education and those in healthcare organisations are beneficial as this offers a blend of expertise with mutual benefit (O'Reilly and Kiyimba, 2015; Strickland, 2017).

Despite the well-established benefits of clinician-researchers and clinical academic careers, clinical practitioners report challenges in accessing and pursuing this type of career (Di Bona et al., 2019). Challenges include financial sacrifices, barriers related to the highly competitive nature of fellowships, and job insecurity (Green et al., 2018; Van Oostveen et al., 2017). Some occupational groups report uncertainties regarding how to navigate clinical academic career pathways due to a lack of support and encouragement (Di Bona et al., 2019). Indeed, during a ten-year review, the UK National Institute for Health Research (NIHR, 2016) recognised problems with progression following the attainment of a master's degree for specific occupational groups, especially in nursing, midwifery, and allied health professions. This is despite high levels of motivation among these practitioners to engage in research and pursue clinical academic careers, and the recognition that leading research projects has considerable benefits to healthcare organisations and clients (Trusson, Rowley, and Bramley, 2019).

Solutions to the ongoing problems associated with supporting and developing clinical academic careers and supporting clinician-researchers in the workplace are essential for future directions in healthcare. This is especially true in nursing, midwifery, and allied health professionals, as these groups have tended to be under-represented in clinical academic career opportunities and funding (Strickland, 2017). Indeed, providing opportunities to engage in research has been shown to increase the recruitment of staff and may potentially support retention (Raine et al., 2022). The review conducted by Raine et al. also demonstrated the importance of ensuring clinical academics and clinician-researchers have protected time and support or mentoring from experienced staff. On this basis, healthcare organisations can support the ongoing development of clinical academic career opportunities and provide support for interested staff, which will help to foster a research culture and demonstrate what clinical academics are able to bring to patient care, service provision, and the wider organisation (Bernhardt, Baillon, Corr, and de Vries, 2023).

Author reflections and concluding remarks
Our partnership
As authors, we three have collaborated over a two-year period writing this book. This involved the initial idea, planning a proposal for the book, writing individual sections and chapters, taking responsibility for different parts, and then reading through, developing, and refining different draft versions together. This was a task we engaged in using time (typically extracurricular) we had away from different professional

responsibilities, in clinical practice, doing research, and teaching and supervising others (for clinical practice and research).

Two of us (Michelle and Philip) began working together more recently, about five years ago, after Philip took up a practice role in the NHS Trust Michelle is affiliated with (LPT). Philip had finished his PhD about a year before starting this post and was interested in opportunities to do more research, and Michelle's name was mentioned by colleagues in child and adolescent mental health. Together, we collaborated on a range of different writing projects based on a shared interest in qualitative methodologies. Michelle acted as Philip's mentor and helped support him in pursuing other endeavours, including local audit and evaluation projects and gaining experience in writing applications for research funding, as well as developing as a researcher, in writing for publication. This book was, though, the first time Philip was able to work with Nikki.

Nikki and Michelle's working relationship goes back further. Having studied for their respective PhDs in psychology at the same university, they had been peers as students before any research collaboration. After qualifying, Nikki and Michelle took different paths for several years, with Michelle continuing in academia and Nikki working in health and social care. At the point when Nikki decided to retrain as a Clinical Psychologist, she was completing a clinical placement in a child and adolescent mental health service when they met again during a chance encounter in a car park. Having a shared interest in child and adolescent mental health and with a close familiarity with discursive approaches to qualitative research, they decided to form a research collaboration, which has continued for the past 14 years.

From Michelle

I have been working in a blended role as a traditional university academic Associate Professor alongside being a mentor and adviser to clinical practitioners in the health service for over 20 years. I obtained Chartered Psychologist status but have not completed specialised clinical training. However, I have had the privilege of working within a healthcare organisation with many professionals in different clinical specialities for a long time and have worked in vocational mental health roles and have some counselling qualifications. During my career, I have supported and mentored many clinical practitioners from physical health and mental health backgrounds to complete a range of projects, from modest to substantive in nature, from small-scale quality improvement projects and service evaluations to pilot studies and exploratory investigations, and large-scale funded research projects. This book is itself a testament to the strong relationships I have built with clinical practitioners and the value of team writing that bridges academic scholarship with clinical expertise.

During my career, I have enjoyed the collaborative nature of dialogue and reflection as ideas are brainstormed and interrogated. I have learnt many things through working with newly qualified clinical practitioners who are entirely new to research, as well as with experienced clinical academics who work at the level of professor within the university and NHS Trust. Each and every clinician-researcher I have worked with, mentored, and supported has taught me something new about blending research and clinical practice. Possibly, my most challenging and newest project is my work with Consultant Gastroenterologist, Dr M. Farhad Peerally (see Chapter 7). I was entirely a novice in the work of endoscopy, and it was my skills and expertise in health communication that brought me to the funded project (*funded by the MPS Foundation). In the short period I have been working on this research, I have learnt a huge amount about endoscopy processes and types, as well as their risks and patient safety implications. In return, I hope my expertise in qualitative methods, healthcare communication, and research ethics has provided something valuable to the gastroenterology team.

As I move forward in my career, I genuinely want to continue to make a difference to clinician-researchers. I have supervised so many clinical practitioners through their PhDs and master's degrees and supported more small projects than I can keep count of. I have mentored many early career and senior practitioners and watched from the sidelines as they have flourished in developing their research skills and built a stronger and more meaningful career with research at the centre. It has been a pleasure to support their report writing, conference presentations, in-house business cases, educational theses, and published writing and to be part of something so important in healthcare. I continue to push hard for a research culture within the NHS Trust I am affiliated with, and I am pleased to see the benefits that this has across services.

From Philip

In some writing on practice-based research in social work, there is discussion of front-line professionals being "reluctant researchers" (Dodd and Epstein, 2012). I would actually say it is the other way around for me: I am something of a reluctant practitioner. Having gained experience with supporting healthcare research during my undergraduate degree and professional training, I very much wanted this to be part of my working life and saw research as key part of the social work profession helping the communities it serves. Also, in working in a clinical role in a CAMHS team for several years, I know I am stimulated by ideas regarding researchable topics and how material generated in practice, i.e. case records, might be used for the purposes of empirical research; indeed, I might even say I am overstimulated by this, in that I struggle to *not think* about research in these areas.

I would also say that my experience of clinical practice in CAMHS, after completing a PhD, enriched my understanding of research considerably. This was not just in terms of how research can be informed by – and inform – practice/direct care delivery, but also the practice of qualitative research. Experience supporting young people and their families has helped me refine my understanding of the interface between therapy and in-depth qualitative research interviewing, and possibilities around the transposition of ideas and practices between these contexts. I feel very fortunate to now be able to use this knowledge in supporting practitioner-researchers in my current teaching and supervisory roles, where I work with professionals undertaking research relating to their own practice-based interests.

From Nikki

I do not know what the statistics might show about whether more people start with a clinical career first and then move into research and academia, or whether more people do it the other way round. For me, I started as an academic. When my children were young, I completed my degree and doctorate in psychology and very much enjoyed the academic world of learning and expressing ideas about philosophy and how we understand what "truth" and knowledge are. I very easily related to what I learnt was a social constructionist epistemology, which views reality as a co-construction and agreement between multiple parties. I love this perspective both as an intellectual exploration and also as a lived experience in the way that I interact with people I meet.

Whilst part of me really loves the "ivory tower" academic world of ideas, I am also a pragmatist with a great love for people. After completing my PhD, I did not feel that academia alone was able to provide me with the grounded experience of real people's lives, so I spent a number of years working in a variety of "people helping" professions. Eventually, I felt the call to retrain as a Clinical Psychologist. This was not a small ask, as it meant doing *another* long doctoral-level training from scratch, as there was no "conversion" route available. Although it is not uncommon for me to meet other people who have done a similar thing, it really is not necessary or even desirable for most people to follow this kind of path! However, for me, it is the perfect balance. I get to be both an academic nerd and a real-life down-to-earth clinician. I know that my academic background helps me a great deal to understand the value (and limitations) of a culture of evidence-based practice in the world of clinical health provision. In addition, working with real people, with all their pain and struggles and fears and losses, makes me very motivated to get involved with research that will hopefully benefit more clients by educating clinicians.

The thing I have learnt about working with front-line health practitioners who are seeking to be more involved in research is to remember that it is just a bunch of skills that you can learn, the same way that you learnt your clinical skills. You might feel that you are more practical than academic, but with the right support and guidance, you can learn to write and speak in the language that the academic world communicates through.

References
Agha, A. (2005). Introduction: Semiosis across encounters. *Journal of Linguistic Anthropology*, *1*(1), 1–5.
Archard, P. J., and O'Reilly, M. (2024). Practice-near practitioner research. *British Journal of Mental Health Nursing*, *13*(1), 1–4.
Austin, M., and Carnochan, S. (2020). *Practice research in the human services: A university-agency partnership model*. New York, NY: Oxford University Press.
Bernhardt, L., Baillon, S., Corr, S. M., and de Vries, K. (2023). Developing a clinical academic career pathway in a Community and Mental Health NHS Trust. *Journal of Research in Nursing*, *28*(1), 72–84.
Birch, M., and Miller, T. (2000). Inviting intimacy: The interview as therapeutic opportunity. *International Journal of Social Research Methodology*, *3*(3), 189–202.
Borbasi, S., Chapman, Y., and Read, K. (2002). Perceptions of the researcher: In-depth interviewing in the home. *Contemporary Nurse*, *14*(1), 24–37.
Bourne, A., and Robson, M. (2015). Participants' reflections on being interviewed about risk and sexual behavior: Implications for collection of qualitative data on sensitive topics. *International Journal of Social Research Methodology*, *18*(1), 105–116.
Britten, N. (1995). Qualitative research: Qualitative interviews in medical research. *British Medical Journal*, *311*, 251–253.

Cooper, A. (2009). Hearing the grass grow: Emotional and epistemological challenges of practice-near research. *Journal of Social Work Practice, 23*, 429–442.

Di Bona, L., Field, B., Read, J., Jones, N., Fowler Davis, S., Cudd, P., and Evans, L. (2019). Weaving a clinical academic career: Illuminating the method and pattern to follow. *British Journal of Occupational Therapy, 82*(1), 60–64.

Dodd, S., and Epstein, I. (2012). *Practice-based research in social work: A guide for reluctant researchers.* London: Routledge.

Duncombe, J., & Jessop, J. (2012). "Doing rapport" and the ethics of "faking friendship". In T. Miller, M. Birch, M. Mauthner, and J. Jessop (Eds.), *Ethics in qualitative research* (2nd ed.). London: Sage.

English, W., Gott, N., and Robinson, J. (2022). The meaning of rapport for patients, families, and healthcare professionals: A scoping review. *Patient Education & Counseling, 105*(1), 2–14.

Fletcher, P., and O'Toole, C. (2016). *Language development and language impairment.* West Sussex: Wiley Blackwell.

Fouché, C. (2015). *Practice research partnerships in social work: Making a difference.* Bristol: Policy Press.

Froggett, L., and Briggs, S. (2009). Editorial. *Journal of Social Work Practice, 23*, 377–382.

Froggett, L., and Briggs, S. (2012). Practice-near and practice-distant methods in human services research. *Journal of Research Practice, 8*(2), 1–17.

George, R., and O'Reilly, M. (2023). Introduction: Atypical communication in healthcare. In R. George and M. O'Reilly (Eds.), *A healthcare professional's guide for managing atypical communication conditions: Meaningful conversations in challenging consultations* (pp. 1–14). London: Routledge.

Green, R. H., Evans, V., MacLeod, S., and Bharratt, J. (2018). A qualitative study of the perspectives of key stakeholders on the delivery of clinical academic training in the East Midlands. *Journal of the Royal Society of Medicine Open, 9*(2).

Harding, K., Lynch, L., Porter, J., and Taylor, N. F. (2017). Organisational benefits of a strong research culture in a health service: A systematic review. *Australian Health Review, 41*(1), 45–53.

Hingley-Jones, H. (2009). Developing practice-near social work research to explore the emotional words of severely learning-disabled adolescents in transition and their families. *Journal of Social Work Practice, 23*, 413–428.

Hunt, M., Chan, L., and Mehta, A. (2011). Transitioning from clinical to qualitative research interviewing. *International Journal of Qualitative Methods, 10*(3), 191–201.

Kagle, J., and Giebelhausen, P. (1994). Dual relationships and professional boundaries. *Social Work, 39*(2), 213–220.

Karim, K., McSweeney, E., and O'Reilly, M. (2021). Communication in child mental health: Improving engagement with families. In M. O'Reilly and J. Lester (Eds.), *Improving communication in mental health settings: Evidence-based recommendations from practitioner-led research* (pp: 17–35). London: Routledge.

Lester, J., and O'Reilly, M. (2021). Communication, mental health, and how language-based research can help in practice. In M. O'Reilly and J. Lester (Eds.), *Improving communication in mental health settings: Evidence-based recommendations from practitioner-led research* (pp. 1–14). London: Routledge.

Littlejohn, S., Foss, K., and Oetzel, J. (2017). *Theories of human communication* (11th ed.). Long Grove, IL: Waveland Press.

LaChenaye, J., and McCarthy, S. (2022). The intersection of counselling micro-skills and qualitative interviewing and reporting in the study of sensitive topics. *American Journal of Evaluation, 43*(2), 255–268.

Leslie, J., and Lonneman, W. (2016). Promoting trust in the registered nurse-patient relationship. *Home Healthcare, 34*(1), 38–42.

Long, C., and Eagle, G. (2009). Ethics in tension: Dilemmas for clinicians conducting sensitive research. *Psycho-Analytic Psychotherapy in South Africa*, 17(2), 27–52.

McCosker, H., Barnard, A., and Gerber, R. (2001). Undertaking sensitive research: Issues and strategies for meeting the safety needs of all participants. *Forum: Qualitative Social Research*, 2(1), Article 22.

Myers, S. (2000). Empathic listening: Reports on the experience of being heard. *Journal of Humanistic Psychology*, 40(2), 148–173.

National Institute for Health Research (NIHR). (2016) *Building a research career handbook*. http://www.nihr.ac.uk/documents/faculty/Building-a-research-careerhandbook.pdf.

NHS England. (2014). Five year forward view. https://www.england.nhs.uk/ourwork/futurenhs/.

O'Reilly, M. and Kiyimba, N. (2015). *Advanced Qualitative Research: A Guide to Contemporary Theoretical Debates*. London: Sage.

Owens, D. (1996). Men, emotions and the research process: The role of interviews in sensitive areas. In K. Carter and S. Delamount (Eds.), *Qualitative research: The emotional dimension* (pp. 56–65). Aldershot, UK: Avebury.

Park, J. (2023). How to build rapport in online space: Using online chat emoticons for qualitative interviewing in feminist research. *Qualitative Research Journal*, 24(3), 205–220.

Prior, M. T. (2018). Accomplishing "rapport" in qualitative research interviews: Empathic moments in interaction. *Applied Linguistics Review*, 9(4), 487–511.

Raine, G., Evans, C., Uphoff, E. P., Brown, J. V. E., Crampton, P. E., Kehoe, A., Stewart, L. A., Finn, G. M., and Morgan, J. E. (2022). Strengthening the clinical academic pathway: A systematic review of interventions to support clinical academic careers for doctors and dentists. *BMJ Open*, 12(9), e060281.

Rosetto K. (2014). Qualitative research interviews: Assessing therapeutic value and challenges. *Journal of Social & Personal Relationships*, 31(4), 482–489.

Shahri, N. (2023). Rapport in research interviews: An interdiscursive perspective. *System*, 119, 103165.

Sinding, C., and Aronson, J. (2003). Exposing failures, unsettling accommodations: Tensions in interview practice. *Qualitative Research*, 3(1), 95–117.

Strickland, K. (2017). Developing an infrastructure to support clinical academic careers. *British Journal of Nursing*, 26(22), 1249–1252.

Trusson, D., Rowley, E., and Bramley, L. (2019). A mixed-methods study of challenges and benefits of clinical academic careers for nurses, midwives and allied health professionals. *BMJ Open*, 9(10), e030595.

Van Oostveen, C. J., Goedhart, N. S., Francke, A. L., et al. (2017). Combining clinical practice and academic work in nursing: A qualitative study about perceived importance, facilitators and barriers regarding clinical academic careers for nurses in university hospitals. *Journal of Clinical Nursing*, 26(23–24), 4973–4984.

Wilkinson, R. (2019). Atypical interaction: Conversation analysis and communicative impairments. *Research on Language & Social Interaction*, 52(3), 281–299.

Williams, J., Craig, T. J., and Robson, D. (2020). Barriers and facilitators of clinician and researcher collaborations: a qualitative study. *BMC Health Services Research*, 20, 1–11.

Zhang, T., and Okazawa, R. (2023). Managing neutrality, rapport, and antiracism in qualitative interviews. *Qualitative Research*, 23(6), 1689–1713.

CHAPTER 18

Thematic approaches and coding data

Learning objectives

This chapter enables the reader to:

- Critically assess the benefits and limitations of a thematic approach to analysis.
- Differentiate between different types of thematic analysis.
- Create a coding frame from data.
- Identify themes from data.

Introduction

The most common approach to qualitative data analysis is thematic analysis. The coding style associated with thematic analysis is also foundational for a number of other qualitative methods. Hence, it is typically the case that educational programmes in qualitative research train practitioners in thematic analysis first. There are different ways of doing thematic analysis, and whilst they share similar conceptions and goals, there are some theoretical and practical differences that you need to be mindful of in deciding which approach you might use. Thematic analysis has been subject to much discussion over the years, particularly as we already noted, since the seminal paper by Braun and Clarke (2006) which provided a more systematic view of this popular approach to analysis. Braun and Clarke followed this paper with two textbooks (Clarke and Braun, 2013; Braun and Clarke, 2022). During this time, Braun and Clarke expressed concerns about the quality of the way the approach is used, especially the ways in which researchers apply theory in relation to thematic analysis, and misinterpretations of the process of coding and organising data thematically.

THEMATIC APPROACHES AND CODING DATA

Much work on thematic analysis has been undertaken recently, and in this chapter, we distil this into practical and relevant information for any health practitioner wishing to use this approach. In so doing, we draw heavily on the work of Braun and Clarke and recommend that you also read some of the original writings from these authors alongside this chapter. We devote this entire chapter to thematic analysis, in terms of coding and organising data thematically, for the following reasons:

1. There are different types of thematic analysis, each with their differences in the practices of performing this method.
2. Thematic analysis is often considered the most straightforward type of qualitative analysis to undertake, especially for neophyte qualitative researchers, and it is one that sets foundational knowledge for other approaches.
3. This approach to data analysis is more theoretically flexible than other approaches.

Types of thematic analysis
Thematic analysis enables the researcher to synthesise large amounts of qualitative data and offers a robust way of doing analysis. Put simply, thematic analysis is an analytic method to develop, analyse, and interpret patterns across a data corpus through a systematic process of coding data and developing themes (Braun and Clarke, 2022). Braun and Clarke emphasised that thematic analysis is conceptualised in two central ways: first, as a process whereby the researcher-as-analyst seeks to identify meanings that exist in the dataset, and second, as a process whereby the analyst brings their own subjectivity, situated understanding, and technical skill to the analysis, and is not neutral; that is, the analysis is shaped by them as a person and their existing knowledge.

> **Key point!**
>
> Thematic analysis is conceptualised as a method of data analysis rather than a methodology.
> (Braun and Clarke, 2022)

There are several different ways of doing thematic analysis, and a researcher should be clear about which form of this method they are using and why. Broadly speaking, the different kinds of thematic analysis are synthesised into three clusters, that is of coding reliability, codebook, and reflexive (Braun and Clarke, 2019, 2022) which we review in Table 18.1 based on Braun and Clarke's published writings.

Coding reliability thematic analysis
Coding reliability types of thematic analysis are based on a commitment to seeking an assumed, unbiased truth from the data set (Braun and Clarke, 2022). Braun and Clarke argued that researchers engaging in a coding reliability type of thematic analysis seek to establish accuracy in their coding.

Table 18.1 Different kinds of thematic analysis (See Braun and Clarke, 2022)

Thematic approach	Description
Coding reliability	These types of thematic analysis tend to lean on post-positivism as an epistemological foundation and seek to uncover the "truth" in people's accounts. These tend to take a structured coding style.
Codebook	These types of thematic analysis tend to involve a blend of deductive and inductive coding, accounting for what is known from available empirical and theoretical literature and the presuppositions of the researcher.
Reflexive	These types of thematic analysis centre the role of the researcher and their reflexive engagement with the data. With this, the researcher's subjectivity and the situated nature of the understanding are closely attended to. This is the type of thematic analysis detailed in Braun and Clarke's (2006) influential article.

> **Key point!**
>
> Coding reliability approaches involve producing a list of codes and themes that are tightly defined; thus, each code has a label, a definition, and instructions on how to identify them.
>
> (Braun and Clarke, 2022)

In coding reliability types of thematic analysis, there is a team of researchers who ideally code individually before sharing based on a "naïve" position in relation to the topic and research question. The goal is consensus, and some types utilise some form of statistical test to measure reliability (O'Connor and Joffe, 2020).

> **Key point!**
>
> The coding reliability approaches rely heavily on a measure of agreement between the coders, as this is seen as key to quality with this type of approach.
>
> (Braun and Clarke, 2022)

If you plan on using a coding reliability type of thematic analysis, you will need to work with a team where each person has sufficient time to code the data in a rigorous way, and to ensure that the coding across the team is reliable. The concept of reliability is aligned with quantitative research and is one of the principal quality markers for that kind of work. In this sense, some advocates of coding reliability types of thematic analysis argue that this form of coding and theming of data serves as a bridge between quantitative and qualitative approaches (see, for example, Boyatzis, 1998). Also in that sense, coding reliability forms of thematic analysis may be conceptualised as "small q" approaches in qualitative research (Kidder and Fine, 1987).

> **Key point!**
>
> Qualitative research is on a spectrum in terms of theoretical positioning, from small q approaches that lean more toward post-positivism to Big Q, which are more aligned with values associated with qualitative research and interpretive social science and depart from principles associated with positivism, with an emphasis on developing understanding that is inherently subjective and reflexive.
>
> (Kidder and Fine, 1987)

Braun and Clarke (2022) have, however, argued that coding reliability approaches to thematic analysis are compromised when quantitatively orientated scholars encourage positivist-empiricist ideas within methods training and reviewing qualitative work. As they succinctly acknowledged:

> It is problematic in promoting inter-coder reliability as an implicitly or explicitly "universal" – rather than paradigm-embedded – marker of quality, researcher subjectivity becomes problematically conflated with poor quality analysis, and the inference that subjective knowledge is necessary flawed. Reader, it is not! We suspect this embracing of such "good practice" guidelines reflects their easy-alignment with the positivist-empiricism that dominates much methodological training, and the wider under-valuing and lack of training of qualitative research across many disciplines.
>
> *(Braun and Clarke, 2022, p. 241)*

Braun and Clarke (2021) argued that it is too frequently the case for more reflexive, Big Q researchers to be asked by reviewers or editors to illustrate the reliability of their coding processes and demonstrate agreement in coding and theming of data. These requests are problematic because they rest on an assumption which renders the subjectivity of the analyst invisible and are based on an idea that there is a "truth" that can be discovered, which is contrary to many theoretical positions (Braun and Clarke, 2022).

Codebook types of thematic analysis
Codebook approaches to thematic analysis are placed somewhere between the Big Q of reflexive approaches and the small q of coding reliability ones. Codebook types of thematic analysis combine the values of the qualitative paradigm with a more structured approach to coding and theme development, and thus can be considered a Medium Q approach (Braun and Clarke, 2022). Braun and Clarke suggested that whilst the coding process is more structured than in reflexive approaches, researcher subjectivity is not problematised like it is in coding reliability types.

QUALITATIVE HEALTH RESEARCH

> **Key point!**
>
> The codebook approaches to thematic analysis aim to generate a codebook of codes and themes, which blends deductive and inductive codes, with some mapping of the coded data.
> (Braun and Clarke, 2022)

There are several codebook approaches to thematic analysis, including matrix analysis, framework analysis, network analysis, and template analysis. These approaches share similar processes and theoretical underpinnings but also have some differences in style and reporting (Braun and Clarke, 2022). Here, we provide you with some practical discussion on two of the most common codebook approaches, template analysis and framework analysis.

Template analysis
Template analysis provides a process for coding and theming data with a view to develop a template that visually represents the data and the relationship between themes. Template analysis was developed by King (2004) and colleagues (Brooks et al., 2014) to combine some of the flexibility associated with thematic analysis with a structured approach to coding. In this way, codes can be both descriptive and interpretive (King, 2004).

> **Key point!**
>
> Template analysis (and more broadly, codebook approaches) can be a suitable approach for professionals who are novice qualitative researchers, as it is a relatively straightforward approach and learning the tools is a foundation of skills for more complex methodologies.
> (Braun and Clarke, 2022)

As template analysis is a form of codebook thematic analysis, the coding process can be entirely inductive, but typically tends to blend inductive (data-driven) with deductive (researcher or theory-driven) coding processes (Braun and Clarke, 2022). This means that, when first developing the template from the data, some *a priori* codes may be identified in advance of engaging with the data by exploring related research literature and utilising knowledge in the development of the interview or focus group guide (King, 2004). However, not all or only the themes previously identified from the literature will be found in the data, and therefore it is necessary to also incorporate inductive coding (King, 2012).

The goal of template analysis is to visually represent the themes and the connections or relationships between and across them. The template reflects the coding framework, which is gradually built through engagement with the data. Typically, the template is constructed by generating a hierarchical coding framework to present a thematic structure, then applying the template to the entire data corpus and refining to it throughout the process (Braun and Clarke, 2022). The template offers a way for the analyst to hierarchically map patterned meanings from the data, allowing them to move from broader to more specific meanings and offer multiple levels of evidence for the analytic claims made. In this way, template analysis does diverge from the more reflexive forms of thematic analysis, as emphasised by Braun and Clarke (2022, p. 243):

> Unlike reflexive TA, template analysis does not involve two levels of analytic work – coding and theme development – and two distinct analytic entity outputs – codes and themes. Rather the terms code and theme are often used interchangeably, echoing the conflation of these terms in small q TA.

There are some limitations with template analysis (which are also applicable to other forms of codebook approaches), and it is worth bearing these in mind if you choose this kind of thematic analysis for your work. Braun and Clarke (2022) argued that there is a risk in emphasising the development of *a priori* codes and themes, as this may reduce open interpretation and the development of themes that are products of the analysis process. They further suggested that there is potentially excessive emphasis on structure and hierarchy, which may undermine the development of a more nuanced understanding of the data and ultimately reduce the depth of meaning.

This consideration notwithstanding, we would argue that codebook approaches still have a lot of value for clinician-researchers, and these forms of thematic analysis are a valuable way of organising large volumes of qualitative health data. Doing template analysis requires time and close engagement with data. In Box 18.1, we offer some practical steps on which to base template analysis of your own data.

Box 18.1

Doing template analysis (Brooks, McClusky, Turley, and King, 2014; King and Brooks, 2017)

There are several steps to undertake a template analysis, and these were presented by Brooks et al. (2014) and King and Brooks (2017) as entailing:

1. **Familiarisation** – become familiar with the accounts being examined. Read through the transcripts at least once and listen to the recordings several times.
2. **Preliminary coding** – develop a preliminary coding of the data. This is the same process as for other thematic approaches, and the researcher should go through all the data collected and highlight areas that contribute to understanding. For template analysis, coding is both deductive and inductive, and thus some *a priori* codes are generated from engagement with the literature and research agenda, and these can shape the coding framework produced. These *a priori* themes should be tentative and may be refined during the inductive coding process.
3. **Organisation** – organise the developing themes into meaningful clusters and start to work in defining how these relate to each other. This will include hierarchical relationships

where narrow themes are clustered within broad ones. There will be a development of integrative themes in template analysis where several clusters are grouped together.
4. **Defining** – define an initial coding template. In template analysis, the researcher will develop an initial version of the coding template based on early inclusion of transcripts to define the thematic structure.
5. **Modification and building** – apply that initial template to more of the data and begin modification. The relevance of new data to the template is identified, and the template is changed accordingly where new data do not fit the existing themes. Thus, new themes are inserted, and existing themes may be redefined or changed in some way.
6. **Completing** – finalise the template. Theoretically, there is no such thing as a final template as there could potentially be further refining and defining, but the template can be a final version for dissemination on a pragmatic basis. Integrative themes are created to illustrate the relationship between different aspects of the analysis.

For an overview of the experience of using this approach, see the account in Box 18.2 of Dr Sarah Hunt, a recently graduated PhD student who utilised this method of analysis in her research with refugee populations.

Box 18.2

Practitioner perspective of Dr Sarah Hunt

Dr Sarah Hunt (PhD) is a recently graduated PhD candidate at the University of Leicester who studies mental health, well-being, service needs, and health equity among refugees and asylum-seekers in host country post-migratory settings. Sarah's research focuses on systems response to the needs of refugees and asylum-seekers, identifying gaps in policy and practice from a health equity perspective.

Background: Health inequity is a complex problem that requires a systems approach (Baker, 2024). This case example represents a two-phase study design ($n = 100$) that involved a systems approach to explore the complex problem of unmet mental health needs among refugees and asylum-seekers living in England with the aim to enact change. To enact system change, the system must be understood by both its boundaries and the actors operating within it (Midgely and Midgely, 2000; Mingers, 2014). Focusing on the interplay between structure and agency, the influence of structures [rules and resources] on service provider and service user decision making and event outcomes (Giddens' 1984), produces valuable systemic insight (Arnold and Wade, 2017). In this study, a collaborative model of co-production was used to identify causes and enact change. Focus group discussions with stakeholders and refugees and asylum-seekers generated knowledge for action that informed a multi-sectoral co-production of a Theory of Change (ToC).

The application of template analysis: In this study, template analysis (TA) as a form of thematic analysis provided an analytical framework to examine interactional behaviours and event outcomes through a systems lens, establishing the "bigger picture". The methodological decision behind the application of TA (King and Brooks, 2017), lay in multiple analytical strengths suited to qualitative psychological research. TA takes a structured yet flexible approach; a template can be adapted as new themes are identified, and from a systems perspective, TA highlights systemic issues. For example, often using *a priori* themes, the researcher codes data according to a predefined template (the "*initial template*") systematically identifying recurring themes [in this study, barriers to access] across multiple perspectives and further and iteratively developing the template. Furthermore, from an epistemological position, TA is a good fit for research that seeks to identify underlying causality; thus, TA can be used from a realist position (Brooks et al., 2014). I present here the application of TA in the present study, whereby the overarching methodological approach was systems thinking, and the epistemological stance was critical realism. The analytical steps undertaken to produce a causal explanation for the problem of unmet needs were guided by six stages of TA, as described by King and Brooks (2017).

During the development of the initial template [Stages 1–4], the use of a researcher diary and data audit table is helpful to refer to throughout what is an iterative process, providing an auditable trail of researcher decision making. Preliminary coding can be done by hand or using software such as NVivo. Like other thematic approaches, the researcher codes to themes, clustering themes and exploring ways to organise themes. Key features of TA come into play during the development of the initial template. TA involves *hierarchical coding*, whereby top-level themes are selected by the researcher to focus on specific areas of interest. For example, in the present study, the referral system was a central focus [examining service interactions], which was considered significant to the research aims. Thus, sub-themes represent specific aspects of the referral system and process, such as assessment and therapeutic decision making. Another key tenet of TA is *parallel coding*, whereby the researcher applies the same perspective [data] to two different themes. In the present study, this was of much value. For example, themes had a cause-and-effect relationship; a lack of refugee trauma-informed practice prevented adequate assessment of needs, and inadequate assessment of needs prevented early intervention, an outcome that often results in crisis.

Finally, "integrative themes" the lateral relationship between and across themes whereby themes permeate a cluster, producing an integrative theme. To bring this to life in the present study, the problem of silo working was raised by all. It was identified as an undercurrent that exacerbated access barriers due to low knowledge of service partners, absence of referral pathways, and absence of knowledge exchange across services regarding the target population group. Having described the process of developing the initial template and the key tenets of TA, I present in the image below the iterative process of applying the initial template as a "coding frame" [Stages 5–6] whereby the researcher systematically applies the template to subsequent datasets, modifying the template each time to produce the next version that addresses the research question until saturation is reached.

QUALITATIVE HEALTH RESEARCH

Figure 18.1 Template analysis cycle

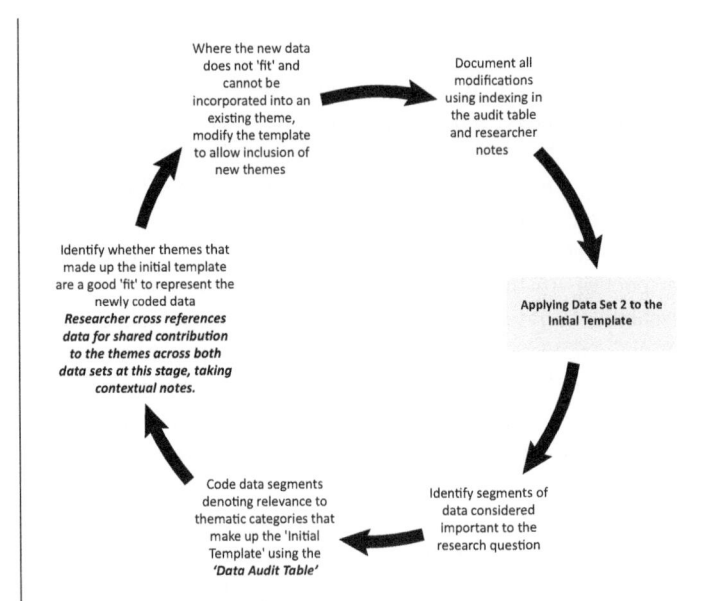

Summary: The image demonstrates the process of TA from the development on initial template and applying data to template, thereafter, modifying the template to produce the next version and documenting the process. There is no limitation on the number of template versions, a record of the development process however is critical to interpretation of the key outcomes important to the research aims.

* Image originally produced in Hunt, S. (2025). *A systems approach to addressing the complex problem of unmet mental health needs among refugees and asylum-seekers living in England.* PhD thesis. University of Leicester.

Once a "final template" is created, the researcher then applies the template to the whole dataset. This provides opportunity to ensure that the themes prioritised best answer the research question and the interpretation of the data provides a "holistic" perspective; that is, insight into "system behaviour" and co-determinants of system response to the mental health needs of refugees and asylum-seekers living in England.

Framework analysis

Another common form of codebook thematic analysis is framework analysis. Although this approach to thematic analysis has tended to be utilised in larger-scale social policy research, it has also become increasingly popular in health and medical research (Gale et al., 2013). Framework analysis was developed as an analytic method by Ritchie and Spencer in the late 1980s for analysing audit trails, with a key goal of articulating a framework (Ritchie and Spencer, 1994). The framework is used as a tool to assist with the analysis, similar to template analysis, where the template is the endpoint (Braun and Clarke, 2022).

> **Key point!**
>
> Developing themes is the basis for framework development, and like other types of codebook approaches, themes are developed at an early stage in the analytic process.
>
> (Braun and Clarke, 2022)

The framework method of thematic analysis is a systematic approach to coding data and organising it thematically. With the framework method, coding can be conducted deductively, inductively, or as a blend of both (Gale, Heath, & Cameron, 2013). Gale et al. (2013) detailed some concepts associated with the approach that researchers using it should be aware of. We outline these in Table 18.2.

Using the framework method requires many of the standard procedures associated with codebook analysis, notably, the creation of a codebook and a translation of this into a framework for organising the broader categories and generation of the core themes to address a research question. Therefore, there are several phases to undertaking framework analysis, and we provide some practical guidance in Box 18.3 based on the perspective of Gale et al. (2013).

Table 18.2 Core concepts of framework analysis (outlined by Gale et al., 2013)

Concept	Description
Analytic framework	Codes that are organised into categories jointly generated by a team of analysts. The framework develops a structure for the data in a way that refines and reduces the data corpus to answer a (research) question.
Analytic memo	Memos reflecting the investigation of a concept, code, or theme as part of the process of data analysis.
Categories	Codes are clustered into categories to reflect interrelated concepts. The identification of categories begins the abstraction of the data toward more general interpretations.
Charting	Charting the data by representing it within a framework or matrix. This may be in spreadsheet format to organise the data into columns and rows reflecting the categories and themes.
Indexing	The systematic application of codes from the framework to the data corpus.

Box 18.3
Doing framework analysis (Gale et al., 2013)

There are several steps you will need to take if you decide to use framework analysis as proposed by Gale et al. (2013):

1. **Transcribe the data**. Ensure your recording is high quality so that you can produce a verbatim transcript to represent the data. It is not typically required to have a high level of detail (such as intonation or timed pauses) as it is the content of the talk, i.e. the words used, that is most important.
2. **Familiarisation with the data**. Listen to the original recordings numerous times. Do not just rely on re-reading the transcript. This process of familiarisation helps strengthen the analysis. In larger multi-disciplinary research, the analysts may not be the people who undertake the data collection or transcription, and thus repeated listening becomes

essential. Keeping analytic memos at this point, and in subsequent stages of the analysis, is helpful as well.

3. **Coding the data**. Once the analyst feels confident in working with the data, a detailed coding process is required. Taking each transcript, line by line, the analyst needs to move each segment of talk into the codebook and apply codes to the content. Each code needs a code label, and more data can be moved under this code as the process unfolds. This coding can be inductive, where open coding is undertaken with anything of interest or relevance moved into the codebook and given a label. Alternately, it can be deductive, whereby the analyst approaches the coding with pre-determined concepts and ideas taken from the literature, theory, and/or prior knowledge, categorising the data using those labels.

4. **Developing an analytical framework**. Once the first few transcripts are coded in detail, the research team should meet and compare their labelling of the codes (if working as a team). At this point, some agreement on the set of codes to use needs to be reached, so that subsequent transcripts can be coded within that coding frame. At this point, also, codes may be grouped together into categories and a visual tree diagram can be created. This helps to create a working analytic framework, although it may take several iterations before the final framework is formulated.

5. **Application of the analytical framework**. This working framework is now ready to be applied, and this is accomplished by indexing subsequent transcripts using the existing categories and codes. Specialist computer software like NVivo or Atlas.ti may be used at this point to help organise the data.

6. **Charting the data into the framework**. Distilling large volumes of data in a serviceable way is helpful in this form of thematic analysis, as evidenced in charting the data in the framework, where spreadsheets are often used as a tool for this purpose. Effective charting means that you will maintain the integrity and meaning of the data, whilst reducing the volume into manageable messages.

7. **Interpreting the data**. Keep a notebook to help with early interpretations of the data and have regular team discussions (or with your supervisor(s) or peers). Whilst developing the framework, characteristics of the data and differences between the data can be noted, as well as the relationships between codes, categories, and themes. At this stage, it is useful to map connections between categories and themes to explore those relationships.

Reflexive thematic analysis

Reflexive thematic analysis is the approach to thematic analysis associated with the work of Braun and Clarke (2006, 2018, 2019, 2022). While there are different ways to undertake reflexive thematic analysis, there are many commonalities across the reflexive approaches (Braun and Clarke, 2022). Braun and Clarke (2019) reported that they termed their version of thematic analysis as reflexive because of a commitment to recognising the situated nature of the researcher's knowledge and the role of their subjectivity.

THEMATIC APPROACHES AND CODING DATA

> Reflexive research treats knowledge as situated, and as inevitably and inescapably shaped by the processes and practices of knowledge production, including the practices of the researcher. We therefore view researcher subjectivity, and the aligned practice of reflexivity, as the key to successful reflexive TA.
>
> *(Braun and Clarke, 2022, p. 12)*

For researchers using reflexive thematic analysis, it is essential to ensure that the research question is at the centre of the analytic inquiry so that the developed analytic narrative fully addresses that question (Braun and Clarke, 2022). Although this does not need to be fully defined at the outset of planning the research and is iteratively developed, it should form part of a conceptually coherent design, and this needs to be anchored to the theory and epistemology driving the work. Braun and Clarke (2022) observed that, like other forms of thematic analysis, reflexive thematic analysis is theoretically flexible but not theory-free, hence, researchers need to be transparent about the influence of theory on their interpretive process. As they have developed this analytic method further in recent years, Braun and Clarke (2021) are clear that reflexive thematic analysis should have rigour, transparency, and follow the robust process they have detailed. They argued that teams of researchers can engage with reflexive thematic analysis together, but if multiple coders are involved, this is not about reliability; rather, the purpose is to collaboratively realise more nuanced insights and richness in analysis, not to reach agreement about every code. Braun and Clarke (2022) have outlined ten core assumptions of reflexive thematic analysis, and we summarise these in Box 18.4. Of note in this process is that it starts with data and analysis, and full engagement with relevant literature occurs later in the process than some other forms of qualitative research.

Box 18.4

Ten core assumptions of reflexive thematic analysis (Braun and Clarke, 2022)

There are ten assumptions underpinning reflexive thematic analysis which you should remember and return to if this is the approach to thematic analysis you decide to use in your own work.

1. Researcher subjectivity is a principal tool guiding analysis, and knowledge generation is considered to be situated and subjective in nature. The researcher is the instrument in qualitative research.
2. Analysing the data is not an objective process, and analysis should be rich, insightful, complex, nuanced, and have depth.
3. Reflexive thematic analysis is possible as a single independent researcher. However, collaborative coding will enhance interpretation and reflexivity, not to ensure consensus but to support a richer, dialogic analysis.

4. Well-defined codes and themes are produced through a process of immersion in the data and depth of engagement with the data.
5. Patterns generated are anchored by a shared concept, meaning, or ideas. Themes are not summaries of a topic. A theme should be united by a central organising concept and this should be clarified by the analyst.
6. Themes are the analytic output. Themes are generated from the coding process but are not developed before engagement with the data in a deductive, *a priori* way. Engagement with the literature comes later in this type of analysis.
7. Themes do not *emerge* from the data as if they pre-exist; rather, the researcher actively identifies and produces them by systematically engaging with the data.
8. Analysis is always underpinned by theoretical assumptions, which need to be acknowledged.
9. Central to analysis is (researcher) reflexivity.
10. Data analysis requires creativity.

Here, we draw your attention to the seventh point in the assumptions list. Over the years, among researchers using different forms of thematic analysis, there has been some confusion as the method has gradually become more robust in terms of its contribution and available writings that researchers can refer to. The language used in relation to themes and codes and the process of doing analysis has not always been as clear as it might be, and pioneers like Braun and Clarke have worked hard to create resources for qualitative researchers to enhance the quality of research produced. One key area relates to the theoretical underpinning of codebook approaches and reflexive approaches as Medium Q and Big Q forms of qualitative work. Historically, it was frequently the case that analysts talked about themes "emerging" from the data without necessarily giving too much attention to how that might reflect a positivist position on truth. This is to say themes were written about if they could be simply pulled out (or found in) the data, as if they resided within those data, in manifest or latent form (Ely et al., 1997). The language of emergence is a misconception as themes do not possess agency, and the analytic process relies on researchers' interaction with the data (Varpio et al., 2017). Indeed, Varpio et al. have emphasised that using the term emerging themes reflects a positivist understanding that the truth can emerge objectively, and such passivity and "objectivity" are not congruent with theories around qualitative research where the researcher is deemed to play an active and interpretative role in the analysis.

Following the original procedures set out by Braun and Clarke (2006), as refined in later work (Braun and Clarke, 2019, 2022), there are six main stages involved in undertaking a reflexive thematic analysis. These stages are termed "phases" rather than steps to recognise that the boundaries between them are, in different ways, porous. We outline these in Box 18.5.

> **Box 18.5**
>
> **Phases in reflexive thematic analysis (Braun and Clarke, 2006, 2022)**
>
> There are several phases involved in doing a reflexive thematic analysis. These involve:
>
> 1. **Familiarisation with the data.** During this phase, you need to immerse yourself in your data by repeatedly listening to recordings and/or reading the text [if you have documents as data]. You will need to watch the video, listen to the audio recording, or work with the text, along with the transcripts, and make memos and notes regarding any analytic insights or identified patterns.
> 2. **Coding the data.** This should be done in a rigorous, systematic way by working through your data line-by-line, statement by statement. You can identify interesting, relevant, or meaningful data in relation to your research question and assign a code label to the chunk of data. This can be at an explicit surface meaning (semantic codes) or a more conceptual level of coding labels (i.e. latent codes). Coding should not just summarise the content but should reflect the researcher's analytic consideration of the data.
> 3. **Generate initial themes.** In this phase, an effort is made to identify shared patterns of meaning across the data, and codes can be clustered where a central idea provides a meaningful answer to the research question. The meaning is not hidden to be uncovered, but theme development is an active process constructed by the analyst. Themes are created and generated by the researcher and do not emerge; i.e. they are not "discovered" as if they pre-exist the process of analysis.
> 4. **Develop and review the initial themes.** The task for the analyst during this phase is to assess the fit of the initial candidate themes generated in the third phase to check the robustness of the analysis. The analyst reflects on whether the candidate themes make sense in relation to coded extracts of data and the entire data corpus. The themes should collectively capture the most important patterns of shared meanings. Whilst reviewing themes, the analyst needs to consider the character of each theme, the focus of the theme, and generate a central organising concept. Here the analyst can start to map the relationships between themes and existing knowledge in the field by engaging with wider, relevant literature.
> 5. **Refining, defining, and naming themes.** At this point in the process, the analysis is refined, and each theme should be demarcated and built around a strong core concept. During this phase, the analyst writes a brief synopsis of each theme, and each theme needs a final label that reflects the content.
> 6. **Writing up.** Writing up is an integral phase and requires the analysis and interpretation of the data. In reflexive thematic analysis, the analyst starts writing early on, during the third phase, weaving together the analytic narrative as they move through to this final phase. It is here in the final phase that the analyst writes a persuasive story about the analysis of the data and links this narrative to the aim(s) and question(s) of the research project.

Now that we have introduced you to the common types of thematic analysis, we invite you to consider which of these is more suitable to your own way of working and your own project. We recommend you engage with the reflective activity in Box 18.6 to begin to consider your decision.

> **Box 18.6**
>
> **Reflective activity on approaches to thematic analysis**
>
> We have introduced you to some differences between thematic approaches to data analysis, including views of inductive and deductive coding processes, interpretation, theory, and mapping of data. We invite you now to reflect on some of the differences between approaches and decide which is most appropriate for your own work. We recommend you create a table of benefits and disadvantages associated with each type and then map these against your own project. If you wish to do this in depth, it will be helpful to do some further reading on the topic.

A note about theory

Whatever form of thematic analysis is used, theory remains central to this analytic approach. Indeed, to describe thematic analysis as a theoretically flexible approach does not mean that it is (or can be) theory-free. There are various ways in which theory will shape your approach to thematic analysis. One way might be to conceptualise your project as shaped by certain theoretical assumptions; alternatively, you may construct it according to your aims and research questions, or you might orient it more to pragmatic decisions and what is realistically possible in the time available for the research (Braun and Clarke, 2022). Whatever you do and however you design your thematic analysis, you need to be mindful of your epistemological assumptions and any explanatory theory informing the way in which you work and collect your data.

> **Key point!**
>
> Qualitative research is not homogeneous, and therefore no single theory underpins it, although the different ways of doing research may share foundational assumptions.
>
> (Braun and Clarke, 2022)

In attending to this dimension of qualitative enquiry, we can broadly distinguish between approaches that are experiential and those that are critical, with the distinction relating to how language is conceptualised (Reicher, 2000). Experiential qualitative approaches are those that are focused on meaning-making and experience in the sense that they explore what people feel, think, do, and how they make sense of their experience (Braun and Clarke, 2022). Braun and Clarke have highlighted that an experiential qualitative approach is underpinned by a view of language as "a tool for communicating meaning", affording insight into the psychological state of the individual or their social world (p. 160). As Braun and Clarke argued, an experiential qualitative approach focuses on participants' worldviews and frames of reference, known as a hermeneutics of empathy.

Critical qualitative approaches take a different view. These approaches are more focused on meaning-making, negotiation, and social construction. The critical qualitative approaches are concerned with interrogating patterns of meaning and examining the effects and functions of patterns of language use and meaning (Braun and Clarke, 2022). Thus, language is understood in a very different way from the experiential approaches where communication is not seen as a way to convey a reality or truth, but instead as an integral part of the way in which reality and truth are constructed.

> **Key point!**
>
> Reflexive thematic analysis is the most theoretically flexible of all the approaches, as this kind can be used with both experiential and critical qualitative approaches. Thus, critical reflexive thematic analysis is different from experiential reflexive analysis based on theory. Theory, then, is not an analytical tool but is instead a conceptual basis for analysis.
>
> (Braun and Clarke, 2022)

The process of coding

Fundamental to any type of thematic analysis is the process of coding. There are differences in coding types depending on theoretical positions and the extent to which *a priori* knowledge informs the initial coding framework (deductive or inductive coding). From reading the earlier parts of this chapter, you will have found that the different approaches to thematic analysis lean more heavily toward deductive or inductive coding, with some approaches blending the two. Consequently, in coding, a dimension of the coding process and ultimately of theme development is where and how meaning is noticed, ranging from inductive (data-driven coding) to deductive (researcher or theory-driven coding) (Braun and Clarke, 2022). Braun and Clarke advocated, however, that deductive–inductive coding should be considered more as a spectrum than a dichotomous distinction, and that a blended approach using aspects of each can be productive. As they pointed out, when a researcher adopts a more inductive orientation to coding, the starting point is to engage with meaning and give voice to the participants to tell their stories but recognise that pure induction is never fully possible as a researcher inevitably brings theoretically based assumptions, perspectives, and meaning to the analysis. Furthermore, codes can be concrete or descriptive, or they can be more conceptual and capture more abstract constructs (see, for example, Hennink et al., 2017).

Coding is part of all types of thematic analysis and can also be foundational to other forms of qualitative analysis. It is through coding that the analyst gets close to the data, immerses themself in the worlds of the participants, and begins to organise the data in a meaningful way. In some thematic approaches, the purpose of coding is to locate evidence for the themes (Braun and Clarke, 2022). Braun and Clarke argued that the difference with reflexive thematic analysis is that this type of coding is not simply a process for theme development; rather, coding is the process for the generation of codes and code labels and is a process of tagging data with an appropriate label. Codes are an analytic output and entity generated from this.

Coding is, nonetheless, central to all types of thematic analysis, and creating codes is a focused and important part of the process. Some have argued that it is helpful to generate key words prior to coding, taking words from participants (Naeem, Ozuem, Howell, and Ranfagni, 2023). Naeem et al. argued that these key words should have realness (reflect participant experiences), richness (be rich in meaning) repetition (be significant), have rationale (linked to theory), repartee (insightful or evocative words), and regal (crucial to understanding). Naeem et al. proposed, then, that key words can help with code development, facilitate categorisation of data, support pattern identification and data comparison, and improve understanding during coding and theme development. Themes are then created from codes, which represent a second level in the data analysis process.

> **Key point!**
>
> Generating codes is considered the "building blocks of analysis", especially in reflexive thematic analysis where the code is the smallest unit of analysis.
>
> (Braun and Clarke, 2022)

Pertinent across the approaches in the coding process is the need to capture meanings in the data that relate to the research question, with codes focusing on certain sites of analytic interest (Braun and Clarke, 2022). There are three terms with this:

1. **Coding** – refers to the process of exploring how meanings are patterned in the data corpus and developing codes, and applying labels to them to assign specific segments of data.
2. **Code** – refers to an output of the coding process; a code comprises "an analytically interesting idea, concept, or meaning associated with particular segments of data; often refined during the coding process" (Braun and Clarke, 2022, p. 53).
3. **Code label** – refers to a clear and defined phrase attached to a segment of the data and, as such, is a shorthand tag for a code.

Practically speaking, there are different ways to code qualitative data. You might decide to do your coding manually using printed pages and highlighter pens or using a word processing software like Microsoft Word™, or you might use computer software like NVivo or Atlas.ti to assist in the process of organising the data. We offer some caution in relation to this software here and suggest that doing some manual coding as an initial step can be quite rewarding and a beneficial activity for the cogency of your analysis, whether using computer software or pen and paper methods. This practice enables you to engage fully with the data and move ideas about, change code labels, and transfer segments of data easily. Alternatively, computer software allows you to produce word clouds, diagrams, and frequency word counts, which may be helpful, and after creating a simple coding framework manually, you might choose to shift to using these tools.

> **Key point!**
>
> Arguably, coding is never fully complete as meanings are never final. That is, it would always be possible to spot new things in the data. However, there will be a point where, for different practical reasons and on account of the resources available, coding must conclude.
>
> (Braun and Clarke, 2022)

Creating themes and doing analysis

Once the dataset has been completely coded, you can create the themes and cluster your codes within those themes to finalise the organisation of the data corpus. Whilst the way in which you do this is similar across the thematic approaches, there are some differences to consider in relation to the process of constructing themes. For example, how a theme is defined differs according to the approach used. For instance, in coding reliability approaches, a theme is something that describes or interprets aspects of the phenomenon and refers to a pattern in the data (Boyatzis, 1998). In reflexive thematic analysis, a theme is considered more than just a "pattern" across the data; rather, it captures a range of data that is clustered and represents a shared idea, and in this way, denotes shared meanings, and conceptual patterns (Braun and Clarke, 2022). Notably, a theme is a result of an anaytical in depth process to represent the data in a meaningful way (Varpio, Young, Uijtdehaage, and Paradis, 2019).

Braun and Clarke (2022) emphasised that, in reflexive thematic analysis, themes are patterns of shared meaning, and these should be underpinned by a central organising concept. They argued that the central idea, meaning, or concept holding the theme together should be explicitly expressed – as a semantic theme, or alternatively, conceptually or implicitly evidenced – as a latent theme. As they noted:

> A topic summary is a summary of everything the participants said about a particular topic, presented as a theme. One of the main problems with topic summaries for us, and for reflexive TA, is that they unite around a topic, rather than a shared meaning or idea.
>
> *(Braun and Clarke, 2022, p. 77)*

In considering the act of creating themes, it is first necessary to generate your initial themes. This is because this initial creation of themes is a "generative" process and is an early step in the analysis as the analyst shifts their attention from the smaller units (the codes) to larger and more meaningful patterns (the themes) (Braun and Clarke, 2022).

> **Key point!**
>
> Initial creation of themes at the generative stage is referred to as creating candidate themes. Each cluster of codes forming a candidate theme needs to be closely examined on its own terms in relation to the aims and questions guiding the project.
>
> (Braun and Clarke, 2022)

At this practical stage of creating several candidate themes (which are provisional in nature), the analyst needs to begin to consider the story that might be told about the data corpus (Braun and Clarke, 2022). Braun and Clarke recommended that a useful way to achieve this is through a visual mapping technique, by drawing a thematic map where candidate themes can be considered in their own right, as well as how they may relate to one another as part of a story about the data.

> **Key point!**
>
> For reflexive thematic analysis, there are three levels of themes to report: 1) overarching themes, 2) themes, and 3) subthemes. The overarching theme draws together the themes and subthemes and demonstrates the broader conceptual idea being represented by the analyst and provides contextual information. The subthemes sit under the theme and represent a core idea of the theme.
>
> (Braun and Clarke, 2022)

Braun and Clarke (2022) emphasised that at the initial stage of theme development, there are some things that the analyst should be aware of, and we summarise these in Box 18.7.

> **Box 18.7**
>
> **Initial theme development (Braun and Clarke, 2022)**
>
> These are some things you will need to consider during your initial theme development:
>
> 1. Initial themes will not capture everything, and this is not altogether problematic. The initial themes will not reflect all the codes, and it is not the case that they ought to represent everything participants said, as this is an early phase in analytic development.
> 2. Each of the themes requires a central organising concept, as this clarifies the purpose of the analysis and determines the "essence" of what that theme is about and gives an indication to the audience of the material that "fits" within that theme. Thus, it relates to the sense made of the codes and affords clarity in understanding.
> 3. As an analysis iteratively evolves, the themes may change and be developed further.
> 4. At the initial stage of theme development, you may have a large number of themes. They may narrow down later as themes are merged or deleted, but there is no "correct" number of themes for a project.
> 5. Ensure you check if your candidate themes meet the basic criteria of your central organising concept and review each theme. You will need to be clear on the boundaries of each theme and check if there is sufficient data to evidence the theme created.
> 6. After initial theme creation, you will need to further develop your themes and ensure coherence across them.

Once you have developed your themes, are clear about what they capture and represent, and ensure they fit the central organising concept, you should be satisfied with your overall thematic framework and coding structure. You should have a clear idea of which codes fit within which themes and have your overarching themes, themes, and sub-themes based on that work (remember some thematic approaches use a slightly different language such as template analysis, where there is reference to codes, themes and integrative themes (Brooks et al., 2017) so use the concepts appropriate for your method). Once you have achieved this, the organisation of the data is complete enough to begin developing the analysis. The analytic task then is not to reveal or distill the data, but instead, through analysis, to tell your (anticipated) audience a story to make sense of what is going on in your data and provide clear take-away messages. The way in which you carry out your analysis and present it will be tied to the type of thematic analysis you are reporting. Some types of thematic analysis primarily offer descriptions of patterns within the data to make sense of the overall issues at stake for the data. For others, there is a greater level of interrogation and theorising.

For those approaches that are more interpretive, like reflexive thematic analysis, interpretation is based around participant meaning and the interpretation of data should be located within the wider context, treating the data and participants as embedded in the contexts that are "inflected in the data" (Braun and Clarke, 2022). Indeed, as Braun and Clarke (2022, p. 214) have observed:

> there is no simple or pure description; we always interpret from a position – or, perhaps more accurately, an aggregate of positions. This means interpretation is inevitably a political act.

In presenting your analysis, you are building the analytic story using the themes as a way of signposting the reader through the main messages. You will need to use direct quotations from your data. Remember, these should not be left to tell the story for you, but instead are evidence for the point you are building.

Author reflections and concluding remarks
From Nikki
Although, initially, the distinction between being theory-flexible and theory-free may take a little while to grasp, it makes thematic analysis particularly interesting for both new and experienced researchers alike. Typically, one's training as a healthcare practitioner is steeped in a positivist medical paradigm. In other words, there is a "right" answer to a problem. If a patient is displaying a range of symptoms, there is a "correct" diagnosis and treatment plan. Often people who have a medical background prefer to approach research in a similar way, seeking to find the answers to what interview participants actually believe, for example. Similarly, in approaching data analysis and clustering codes into themes, preference for this approach takes the position that the researcher themselves is a tool to perform the function, but not an active agent in making thematic choices. In other words, themes appear to be latent and discoverable by the researcher. From this position, objectivity is prized, and analysis focuses on agreement between coders or "inter-coder reliability", with any kind of researcher "bias"

being sought out and, wherever possible, eliminated. If this is the approach to data collection and analysis that you prefer, and that fits with your training and your perspective on the objectivity of information, then make sure that you acknowledge that this is the theoretical foundation from which you are approaching your coding and analysis.

However, even within healthcare, there are some practitioners who have a different view. With a social constructionist paradigm, the clinician-researcher may consider that there are many ways of understanding something, many ways of understanding reality or truth. From a realist/positivist perspective, this way of looking at things can appear flawed because of its subjectivity. However, from within this paradigm, there is a perspective that each person is experiencing the world slightly differently and creating an agreed-upon accepted reality from those different vantage points. The humanness of the researcher, as much as the participants, is embraced as something valuable in the research process, not as something to try to eliminate. All the more so for the clinician-researcher. If we accept that decisions about codes and themes cannot be anything but influenced by who the researcher is, we settle into reporting this in the research as a part of the process. As a clinician-researcher, you may have particular insider knowledge which shapes the way you formulate codes and themes and cluster them together into overarching themes. It is always important to consider the possibility of circularity in research (finding what you set out to find because that is what you were looking for), which is why, even if using a deductive approach for part of the process, allowing space for inductive inquiry mitigates against this risk. Nevertheless, even during an inductive stage, the clinician-researcher is likely to be more aware of certain topics or ideas due to their insider status, and therefore more easily notice those things in the participants' words.

Putting aside the consideration of circularity for a moment, an awareness of this can be treated as a beneficial aspect of the reflexive type of thematic analysis. One of the reasons is that the final written article produced from the analysis may highlight themes that are translatable back into the clinical world. The language chosen to describe themes may be more relatable to the practitioners reading the research, and the way that codes have been grouped into themes may make more intuitive sense to the practitioners reading the findings. Whichever approach to thematic analysis you use, know that one is not necessarily better than another, but they are different and have different strengths and limitations. The main take-home message is to know which position you are starting from, acknowledge that to yourself and your audience, and make it clear to your readers when you present your findings.

References

Arnold, R. D., and Wade, J. P. (2017). A complete set of systems thinking skills. *Insight*, 20(3), 9–17.

Baker, D. W. (2024). Achieving health care equity requires a systems approach. *Joint Commission Journal on Quality & Patient Safety*, 50(1), 1–5.

Boyatzis, R. (1998). *Transforming qualitative information: Thematic analysis and code development*. London: Sage.

Braun, V., and Clarke, V. (2006). Using thematic analysis in psychology. *Qualitative Research in Psychology*, 3, 77–101.

Braun, V., and Clarke, V. (2013). *Successful qualitative research: A practical guide for beginners*. London: Sage

Braun, V., and Clarke, V., (2019). Reflecting on reflexive thematic analysis. *Qualitative Research in Sport, Exercise & Health*, 11(4), 589–597.

Braun, V., and Clarke, V. (2021). One size fits all? What counts as quality practice in (reflexive) thematic analysis? *Qualitative Research in Psychology*, 18(3), 328–352.

Braun, V., and Clarke, V. (2022). *Thematic analysis: A practical guide*. London: Sage.

Brooks, J., McClusky, S., Turley, E., and King, N. (2014). The utility of template analysis in qualitative psychology research. *Qualitative Research in Psychology*, 12(2), 202–222.

Clarke, V., and Braun, V. (2018). Using thematic analysis in counselling and psychotherapy research: A critical reflection. *Counselling & Psychotherapy Research*, 18(2), 107–110.

Ely, M., Vinz, R., Downing, M., and Anzul, M. (1997). *On writing qualitative research: Living by words*. London: Routledge.

Gale, N., Heath, G., Cameron, E., Rashid, S., and Redwood, S. (2013). Using the framework method for the analysis of qualitative data in multi-disciplinary health research. *BMC Medical Research Methodology*, 13(117).

Hennink, M., Kaiser, B., and Weber, M. (2017). Code saturation versus meaning saturation: How many interviews are enough? *Qualitative Health Research*, 27(4), 591–608.

Kidder, L., and Fine, M. (1987). Qualitative and quantitative methods: When stories converge. In M. Mark and L. Shotland (Eds.), *New directions for program evaluation* (pp. 57–75). San Francisco, CA: Jossey-Bass.

King, N. (2004). Using templates in the thematic analysis of text. In C. Cassell and G. Symon (Eds.), *Essential guide to qualitative methods in organisational research* (pp. 256–270). London: Sage.

King, N. (2012). Doing template analysis. In G. Symon and C. Cassell (Eds.), *Qualitative organizational research* (pp. 426–450). London: Sage.

King, N., and Brooks, J. (2017). *Template analysis for business and management students*. London: Sage.

Midgley, G., and Midgley, G. (2000). Systems thinking for the 21st century. In G Midgley (Ed.), *Systemic intervention: Contemporary systems thinking* (pp. 1–17). Boston, MA: Springer.

Mingers, J. (2014). *Systems thinking, critical realism and philosophy: A confluence of ideas*. London: Routledge.

Naeem, M., Ozuem, W., Howell, K., and Ranfagni, S. (2023). A step-by-step process of thematic analysis to develop a conceptual model in qualitative research. *International Journal of Qualitative Methods*, 22.

O'Connor, C., and Joffe, H. (2020). Intercoder reliability in qualitative research: Debates and practical guidelines. *International Journal of Qualitative Methods*, 19.

Reicher, S. (2000). Against methodolatry: Some comments on Elliott, Fischer, and Rennie. *British Journal of Clinical Psychology*, 39(1), 1–6.

Ritchie, J., and Spencer, L. (1994). Qualitative data analysis for applied policy research. In A. Bryman and R. Burgess (Eds.), *Analysing qualitative data* (pp. 173–194). London: Routledge.

Varpio, L., Ajjawi, R., Monrouxe, L., O'Brien, B., and Rees, C (2017). Shedding the cobra effect: Problematising thematic emergence, triangulation, saturation, and member checking. *Medical Education*, 51(1), 40–50.

Varpio, L., Paradis, E., Uijtdehaage, S., and Young, M. (2020). The distinctions between theory, theoretical framework, and conceptual framework. *Academic Medicine*, 95(7), 989–994.

CHAPTER 19

Common analytic approaches

Learning objectives

This chapter enables the reader to:

- Identify different analytic approaches in qualitative research.
- Differentiate between interpretative phenomenological analysis, grounded theory, narrative analysis, psychoanalytically informed analysis, discourse analysis, and conversation analysis.
- Critically assess the value of the different analytic approaches.
- Recognise practical steps involved in analysing qualitative data.

Introduction

There are various methodological approaches for doing qualitative research which we introduced you to in Chapters 12 and 13. Notably, different methodologies specify different processes for data collection and analysis. Thus, the data analysed may be a video/audio of an interaction, or original medical notes or it could be a representation of the original data in the form of a transcript or field notes. The different approaches to research design and data gathering are associated with certain types of analysis. These analytic approaches are complex, and it is not possible for you to learn how to do these types of analysis from a single book chapter. Instead, you will need to engage in further reading, and likely also undertake specialist training courses to learn how to do these methods of analysis in a rigorous way.

COMMON ANALYTIC APPROACHES

> **Key point!**
> It is helpful to engage with others using the same form of analysis as you by hosting or attending data analysis sessions where you can share ideas and learn together.

In taking steps to specialise in a specific form of analysis, you first need to decide which analytic approach to use and have a basic understanding of the alternatives. Remember, as we have noted in this book, the method of data analysis you select should be congruent with your theoretical framework, epistemology, methodological approach, and data collection method. Building on the previous chapter, which specifically addressed thematic analysis, this chapter provides you with a practical overview of the most common types of qualitative data analysis. In reading this chapter we strongly recommend you revisit Chapter 6 where we introduced you to the methodologies to which these approaches to analysis are anchored.

Interpretative phenomenological analysis

Interpretative phenomenological analysis (IPA), as one would expect from its label, is a form of analysis informed by phenomenology. Phenomenology is "a philosophical approach to the study of experience" (Smith, Flowers, and Larkin, 2009, p. 11). Smith et al. (2009) noted that there were two key philosophers who were originally associated with phenomenology, Husserl and Heidegger, and, as an approach, IPA is influenced by both. As a qualitative methodology and analytic approach, IPA aims to explore the personal lived experiences of participants, understanding those experiences and participants' active sensemaking of their personal and social worlds (Smith, 2004).

> **Key point!**
> IPA analysis employs the "double hermeneutic", which refers to the researcher's attempts to make sense of participants making sense of their own experiences.
> (Smith, 2004)

Those practising IPA advocate an interpretive position and work to detail a "thick description" of the lived experiences of participants, focusing on the participant's interpretation rather than the researcher's (Sandberg, 2005). Accordingly, a key assumption of IPA is that researchers interpret data through the lens of their own experiences, which are ultimately influenced by their own biography (Smith, 2004). They do so in relation to the participant's lived experience and thus share "a space of inquiry" (Engward and Goldspink, 2020). Researchers see, hear, and feel aspects of their experiences; they are not merely observers or processor of data, but active contributor to the interpretation of the data.

> **Key point!**
>
> For IPA, one core concept is personal experience – that is, the phenomenon being explored. Another is interpretation, that is, the ways in which people make sense of or interpret that experience.
>
> (Tomkins, 2017)

In practice, researchers making use of IPA are interested in the phenomena of the participants' "life-worlds", expressly, what life is like for them, as well as an interpretation of those phenomena in terms of what they mean (Tomkins, 2017). IPA requires the analyst to undertake a series of analytic steps and utilise a "multi-step investigative process that steers the analyst and analysis through the transition from the collected raw data to the identification of interpretative themes" (Engward and Goldspink, 2020, p. 3). Smith et al. (2009) identified six steps to doing IPA, which were intended as general guidelines, and we outline these in Box 19.1.

Box 19.1

Practical steps to doing IPA (Smith et al., 2009)

Smith et al. (2009) outlined the following six steps involved in IPA:

1. Read through the transcripts multiple times to familiarise yourself with the data. Listen to the audio or watch the audio-visual whilst reading the transcripts to check for accuracy of transcription.
2. Develop the prototype themes for each case and make initial notes in an exploratory way. These themes should stay close, that is, link directly, to the data.
a. Goldspink and Engward (2018) added another aspect to this, which was to attend to reflexive echoes, emphasising the importance of reflexivity during analysis.
3. Develop themes and create summaries.
4. Search for connections across these initial themes within each case, considering connections that may not be immediately obvious.
5. Move to the next case.
6. Begin to look for patterns within the case and across cases.

At this point in the analytic process, you can begin your interpretation of the data, which is not a simple task, can have variable levels of depth, and some interpretations can be speculative (Tomkins, 2017). Commitment to a structured approach enables the researcher to have a deeper understanding, to comprehend the participant's perspective more fully, and achieve a detailed representation of the phenomenon being researched, moving from the specific to the shared, from the descriptive to the interpretative (Engward and Goldspink, 2020).

If you are interested in using this approach, we would recommend you read the book by Smith et al. (2009) to help you understand IPA practice.

- Smith, J. A., Flowers, P., and Larkin, M. (2021). *Interpretative phenomenological analysis: Theory, method, and research* (2nd ed.). London: Sage.

Grounded theory analysis

Grounded theory (GT) refers both to the method of inquiry as well as outcomes from this form of inquiry (Charmaz, 2005). As an analytic approach, it developed from the seminal work of Glaser and Strauss (1967), who recognised the value of blending data gathering and analysis (Willig, 2008) with the goal of developing explanatory theories of social processes grounded in data (Glaser and Struass, 1967). Contemporary grounded theorists adhere to these founding principles whilst also seeking to further explore social processes and understand the multiplicity of interactions that lead to variations in those processes (Heath and Cowley, 2004). Glaser is recognised as having created the original version of grounded theory (Heath and Cowley, 2004), with Strauss and Corbin later reformulating this (Annells, 1996). Since then, there has been further diversity within grounded theory analytic approaches in qualitative research (Heath and Cowley, 2004). As such, you will need to be clear which variant of grounded theory you are following.

> **Key point!**
>
> Some grounded theorists have based their analysis in symbolic interactionism (Starks and Trinidad, 2007) and others in social constructionist (Burck, 2005) or constructivist (Charmaz, 2005) thinking.

When performing a grounded theory analysis, the researcher works to realise the goal of developing an overarching theory (Biggerstaff, 2012), which requires identification and integration of categories within the data (Willig, 2008) using constant comparative analysis (Charmaz, 2006). There are some useful guides to undertaking grounded theory analysis, and Charmaz and Thornberg (2021), in their discussion of ensuring good quality when following this approach, offer some useful pointers. We outline these steps in Box 19.2. We note, in this form of analysis, engagement with relevant research literature tends to occur later in the process of analysis.

> **Box 19.2**
>
> **Quality assurance in performing a grounded theory analysis (Charmaz and Thornberg, 2021)**
>
> Performing a grounded theory analysis requires time and effort. We outline some steps here:

- Typically, researchers using grounded theory analysis begin by familiarising themselves with the transcripts, field notes, and recordings (of interviews or focus groups usually) so they are close to the data. Remember that data collection and data analysis occur synchronously in grounded theory, so, as part of a research project, alongside analysing transcripts, you will continue to collect data, transcribe, and code new data.
- The first transcript and recording (and any other data format) from the first participant is initially coded – which can be word-by-word, line-by-line, or incident-by-incident. Charmaz and Thornberg recommended using line-by-line coding as this prompts the analyst to look (very) closely at the data. This rigour also helps in understanding the participant's perspective on their experiences. Whilst undertaking this coding, you will need to write memos about the codes and any questions you have. This is an intermediate step between coding and writing the first draft of the analysis. In writing these memos, the codes can be defined by their properties or characteristics.
- Look for any unstated assumptions or presuppositions of the participant, as well as checking your own assumptions. [Note: Multiple coders can assist in pointing out any blind spots].
- Consider how the codes are connected to other codes. Some codes are concrete and descriptive, whereas others may be more analytic. At this point, it can be useful to look for similarities and differences within and across the data, especially as more transcripts are added and coded.
- After this, define your codes as focused codes, which expedite the analytic process whilst staying close to the data and help you generate tentative analytic categories. The names of the categories and codes should reflect the data. In this way, the coding process moves from open coding (sometimes called initial coding) to selective or focused coding to theoretical coding.
- Grounded theory is a comparative method, and there needs to be sufficient data to make comparisons between fragments of data and the codes labelled. Comparisons between the codes then lead to comparisons between the categories, and eventually to the final core category or categories against the existing literature.
- At this point, a systematic search of the literature is useful to facilitate comparative analysis.
- The conceptualisation of the data is translated into a final theory.

If you are interested in using grounded theory approaches, we would recommend a practical article that differentiates some of the differences between various grounded theory approaches by Chun Tie, Birks and Francis:

- Chun Tie, Y., Birks, M., and Francis, K. (2019). Grounded theory research: A design framework for novice researchers. *Sage Open Medicine*, 2(7)

Narrative analysis
Narrative analysis is a preferred form of analysis for researchers who are interested in making sense of people's lived experiences via the stories they tell. To explore how

those people make sense of those stories (Thorne, 2000), narrative analysis involves the systematic exploration of narrative data (Riessman, 2008). Narrative analysis is a form of analysis underpinned by narrative theory grounded in an assumption that people, as social beings, are born into and live in a "storied world" (Murray, 2003). There are different types of narrative analysis; indeed, it can be said that narrative analysis is an umbrella term with different variants, both in terms in the process and goals of the different types. Riessman (2008) and other scholars have outlined the main types of narrative analysis, and a brief description of these is provided in Table 19.1.

Researchers engaged in narrative analysis will have different epistemological positions, such as symbolic interactionism or social constructivism (Riessman, 2008), and the theoretical foundations shape the way in which the analysis is conducted. There is diversity in narrative inquiry, but a fundamental principle is to support research participants in telling their stories in their own way (Crossley, 2000). The focus of narrative analysis is language, and meaning is created using linguistic devices to explore the

Table 19.1 Variants of narrative analysis (Gubrium and Holstein, 2009; McAdams, 2013; Riessman, 2008).

Variant of narrative analysis	General description
Thematic narrative analysis	The focus of this variant of narrative analysis resides with what is said by the participant, that is, the content of the narrative. In this form of narrative analysis, common thematic elements of talk are identified, but the analysis itself remains participant centred.
Structural narrative analysis	The focus of this variant of narrative analysis is on how a narrative is spoken. Thus, the narrative form is considered, including the function of clauses, organisation in units of discourse, and other structural features.
Dialogic narrative analysis	This is a more interpretative approach to narrative analysis which focuses on the contexts that shape the person's narrative. In this way, the narrative is viewed as multi-voiced, shaped by past language use, but also co-constructed in the present conversation. Attention is paid to how talk performs social action.
Visual narrative analysis	The focus of this form of narrative analysis is on images, and how images can be made and interpreted with participants.
Rhetorical narrative analysis	The focus of this form of narrative analysis is the identification of oppositions (good versus bad) and incomplete arguments that occur in people's stories; that is, how they rhetorically position themselves and the things they tell stories about.
Interactional narrative analysis	The focus of this form of analysis is on the interactions between persons, which serves to create stories. Stories are analysed in terms of how they are constructed during interactions that occur naturally or in interactions with the researcher (e.g. in the interview).
Personal narrative analysis	The focus of this form of narrative analysis is primarily on the internalised and iteratively developing stories of individuals.

structural aspects of language, including "stanzas" that are the basic building blocks, which form "strophes", which in turn make up the whole story (Gee, 1991).

When undertaking narrative analysis, and in selecting the type of narrative analysis that suits your project, be mindful of these considerations so that your work is rigorous and will stand up to scrutiny. Furthermore, in decisions regarding the approach, the researcher needs to choose whether to take the position of story analyst, where the researcher communicates analytic findings in a realist way, or the position of storyteller, where the story is communicated in the form of a creative analytical practice which presents the narrative *as* story (Smith, 2016).

Like most forms of qualitative analysis, any guidance on how to go about doing the analysis is simply a guide, rather than a prescriptive set of procedures to apply. Indeed, narrative analysis does not have a linear step-by-step procedure. Nonetheless, efforts have been made to provide support to those new to narrative analysis (Smith, 2016). Smith has provided some guidance for narrative researchers, which we outline in Box 19.3.

Box 19.3

Practical steps when doing narrative analysis (Smith, 2016)

Be mindful that there are different types of narrative analysis when using the guidance provided by Smith (2016):

- **Getting the story** – you need to analyse stories, and so apprehending this is an important first step in the process.
    - ☐ Decide what you are defining as a "story" and what the narrative is. You will need to clearly define the core concepts of your analysis.
    - ☐ Decide whether to collect big and/or small stories. Interviews are the most common way researchers collect stories, but you may use autobiographies, vignettes, diaries, letters, media, visual material, the internet, or other sources of material.
    - ☐ If not available in written form already, you need to transcribe your stories as a verbatim transcript, as part of the analytic process. This is not just a technical exercise, but a constructive process where you have an opportunity to immerse yourself in and think about the narrative.
    - ☐ Writing is part of this process where you should be capturing your thoughts through notes and memos, refining your ideas throughout the analytic process.
- **Getting to grips with stories** – requires a full engagement with the participant narratives.
    - ☐ Indwelling. This is sometimes referred to as familiarisation in other analytic approaches, and you should read/listen to the data many times and make initial brief notes during that time.
    - ☐ Identify stories in the data by working with the transcripts. It can be helpful to look for key junctures or new beginnings in the talk where there are shifts in the content or where a new part of the story becomes apparent.
    - ☐ Identify the narrative themes and the thematic relationships, considering what is said and the content of the person's story. A narrative theme is a pattern that is

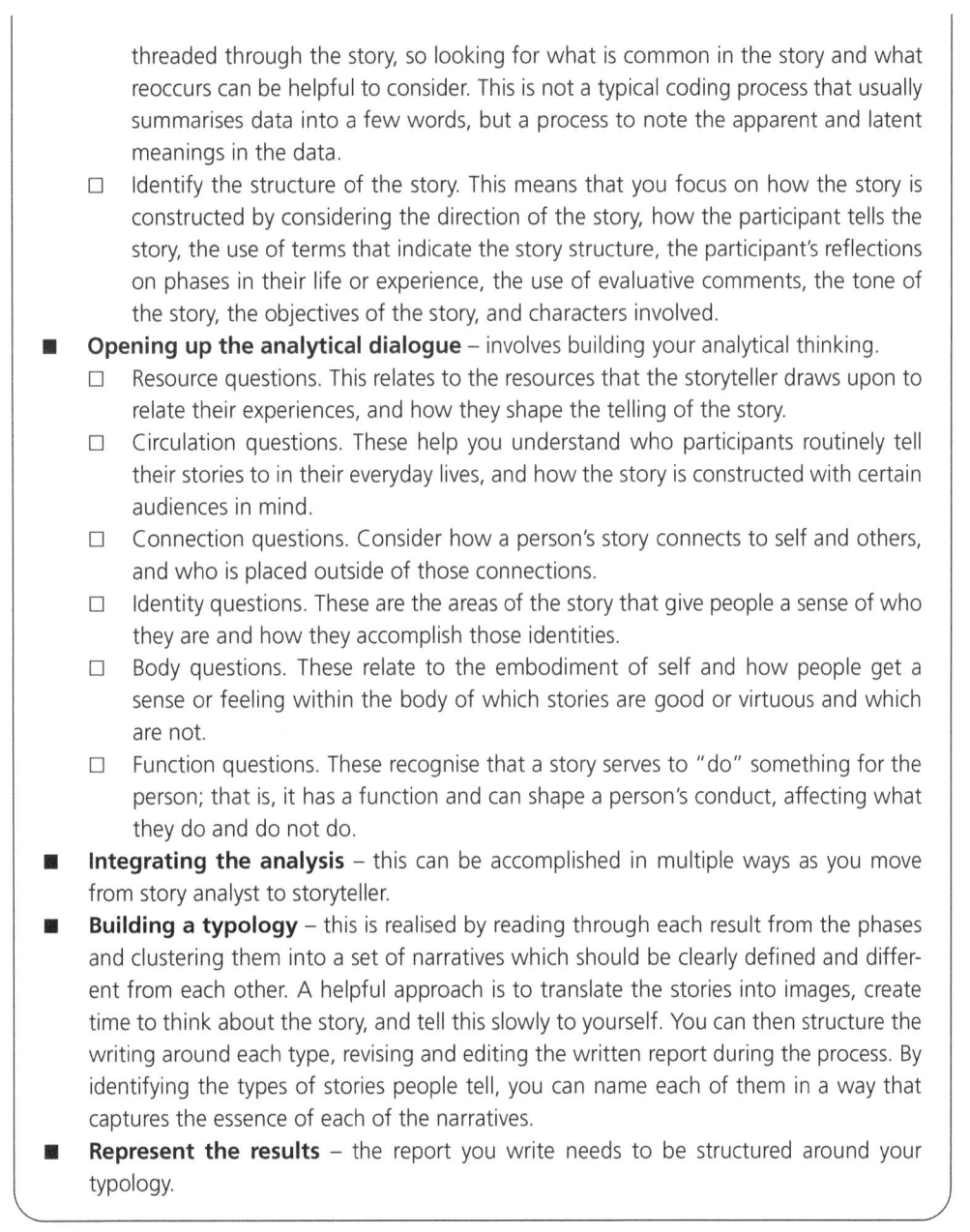

threaded through the story, so looking for what is common in the story and what reoccurs can be helpful to consider. This is not a typical coding process that usually summarises data into a few words, but a process to note the apparent and latent meanings in the data.
- ☐ Identify the structure of the story. This means that you focus on how the story is constructed by considering the direction of the story, how the participant tells the story, the use of terms that indicate the story structure, the participant's reflections on phases in their life or experience, the use of evaluative comments, the tone of the story, the objectives of the story, and characters involved.
- **Opening up the analytical dialogue** – involves building your analytical thinking.
  - ☐ Resource questions. This relates to the resources that the storyteller draws upon to relate their experiences, and how they shape the telling of the story.
  - ☐ Circulation questions. These help you understand who participants routinely tell their stories to in their everyday lives, and how the story is constructed with certain audiences in mind.
  - ☐ Connection questions. Consider how a person's story connects to self and others, and who is placed outside of those connections.
  - ☐ Identity questions. These are the areas of the story that give people a sense of who they are and how they accomplish those identities.
  - ☐ Body questions. These relate to the embodiment of self and how people get a sense or feeling within the body of which stories are good or virtuous and which are not.
  - ☐ Function questions. These recognise that a story serves to "do" something for the person; that is, it has a function and can shape a person's conduct, affecting what they do and do not do.
- **Integrating the analysis** – this can be accomplished in multiple ways as you move from story analyst to storyteller.
- **Building a typology** – this is realised by reading through each result from the phases and clustering them into a set of narratives which should be clearly defined and different from each other. A helpful approach is to translate the stories into images, create time to think about the story, and tell this slowly to yourself. You can then structure the writing around each type, revising and editing the written report during the process. By identifying the types of stories people tell, you can name each of them in a way that captures the essence of each of the narratives.
- **Represent the results** – the report you write needs to be structured around your typology.

If you are interested in using narrative analysis, we would recommend a practical chapter that describes narrative analysis in detail, with specific practical guidance about how it is used:

- Smith, B. (2016). Narrative analysis. In E. Lyons and A. Coyle (Eds.), *Analysing qualitative data in psychology* (2nd ed., pp. 202–221). London: Sage.

Psychoanalytically informed analysis

A psychodynamic or psychoanalytically informed analysis is concerned with generating insights into unconscious experience, or, specifically, with exploring unconscious processes involved in social experience (see, for example, Holmes, 2013). There are areas of contact, even overlap, between psychoanalytically informed analysis and discourse and narrative analysis, notably in terms of a concern for the "storied" nature of human experience and the way language serves to construct spoken accounts of experience (Hollway and Jefferson, 2013). These approaches are also associated with research that is described as psychosocial and grounded in a transdisciplinary concern for avoiding psychological or sociological reductionism in social science enquiry.

There are ongoing debates as to the possibility and necessity of clinical psychoanalytic training and skill for realising a psychoanalytically based analysis in a defensible way (Archard, 2020a, 2020b). These issues notwithstanding, a psychoanalytically informed analysis is typically based on data rich in detail, enabling claims to be made regarding unconscious processes, including defence mechanisms, with the researcher and participant being considered "defended subjects" in research (Hollway and Jefferson, 2013). To accomplish this type of analysis, different arrangements may be necessary depending on the method used, for example, interviews or participant observations. To focus on interviewing here, it would be expected that the researcher engaged in a psychoanalytically informed analysis would make use of data capturing the interview dialogue, that is, in the form of interview transcripts, and records of their own experience undertaking interviews (Hollway and Jefferson, 2013). Combining these data sources is considered key in engaging with intersubjective processes in interviews, in accord with a psychoanalytic view of affective states and felt emotion as mobile and transferrable, passing between the parties involved.

> **Key point!**
>
> For psychoanalytically informed analyses, a key consideration is the portability of ideas derived from clinical psychotherapeutic practice and the use of a sensibility that parallels aspects of psychotherapy.

Debates about how such unconscious and intersubjective processes can be investigated for the purposes of research are wide-ranging, with some researchers suggesting that too much is assumed by other researchers about the parallels between psychotherapeutic practice and research (see, for example, Frosh and Baraitser, 2008; Hoggett et al., 2010). Moreover, the approach to analysis will vary, arguably considerably, according to the tradition of psychoanalytic theory and practice drawn upon (see Frosh and Emerson, 2005; Lapping, 2011). However, as a starting point, Hollway and Jefferson (2013) have provided some valuable ideas and practical recommendations about how a psychoanalytically informed analysis might be realised, and we detail these in Box 19.4.

COMMON ANALYTIC APPROACHES

Box 19.4

Practical steps for psychoanalytically informed analysis (Hollway and Jefferson (2013)

Based on Hollway and Jefferson's (2013) approach, there are several steps involved in a psychoanalytically informed qualitative analysis where interview material is used (Archard, 2020b). Following them, you would:

1. Use data that is derived from interviews that are interviewee-centred and open-ended, i.e. where open questions or requests are used with participants (for example, "tell me about your experience of ..."). As noted in Chapter 14, for Hollway and Jefferson, this means the material generated can be considered in terms of its "associative" qualities, i.e. the process of association in the participant's mind in response to a particular question or prompt.
2. Alongside this, you use data from your fieldnotes or "process" notes. These notes capture aspects of the interview that would not be apprehended by audio recording alone, that is, the emotional "atmosphere", body-language, your subjective experience of the encounter as researcher, and so on.
3. Spend time immersed in the data, listening to the interview recordings multiple times, and reading and re-reading the interview transcripts and notes. Hollway (2011) advised that there are advantages to transcribing interviews yourself, as this helps increase familiarity with the dataset and provides an opportunity to contemplate aspects of communication that you perhaps did not consciously pick up when carrying out interviews.
4. Engage in both a line-by-line coding of the material and consider the "gestalt" of all that is communicated in a particular interview or series of interviews (with their approach, Hollway and Jefferson recommended that two interviews be completed per participant). Engaging with this "gestalt" entails considering processes of "association" in what is said, that is, the sequencing of an account and the "emotional logic" of what is said. There is a consideration of seemingly inconsequential communication, which may indicate something of unconscious significance, that is, in terms of the repetition of particular words, mis-phrasings, slips of the tongue, and so on.
5. Develop "pen portraits" to provide summary accounts of individual participants. These make use of material from both the interview transcripts and process notes to develop coherent theoretically based formulations and incorporate speculative consideration of psychodynamic processes.
6. Use these pen portraits in the construction of a report for the findings of the analysis. In constructing this write-up, return to the original data to ensure avoidance of drifting into an excessively speculative, "wild" analysis.

The act of interpretation, that is, of attributing meaning to data or material, is an ongoing, iterative process in psychoanalytically informed research. Drawing on a framework enables you to carefully consider the robustness of the analysis being carried forward, and how it may be appropriate to be more tentative in any claims made. Actively make use of the support available to you to process your own experience in undertaking the analysis, that is, through supervision or other supportive, reflective spaces where you can consider the meaning of the research material.

QUALITATIVE HEALTH RESEARCH

Whilst psychoanalytically informed analytic approaches in qualitative research are arguably best used, i.e. ethically and effectively, by researchers with clinical experience in psychoanalytic therapy, even with this experience, care needs to be taken to ensure this approach is deployed in a considered way. For example, there needs to be sufficient data available to ground claims regarding unconscious processes as part of an analysis (Archard, 2020a, 2020b).

In Box 19.5, we offer the perspective of Massimiliano Sommantico, a psychoanalyst and psychologist, on using this approach in research.

Box 19.5

View of Dr Massimiliano Sommantico on the free association narrative interview method

Dr Massimiliano Sommantico is a psychologist, psychoanalyst registered with the Italian Psychoanalytic Society and International Psychoanalytical Association, and Associate Professor of Dynamic Psychology at the University of Naples Federico II.

From my point of view as a psychoanalyst and researcher, I have found the free association narrative interview method (FANIM), ever since reading the authors' [Hollway and Jefferson] first works, very stimulating and enriching. This is particularly related to the fact that FANIM stimulates the clinician's reflection on the questions of reflexivity and countertransference, which are central in the analytical exchange between patient and analyst, and also in conducting psychoanalytically informed qualitative research. Furthermore, within the theoretical landscape of psychosocial studies, FANIM stimulates the reflection of a psychoanalyst by conceptualising subjective experience as a dynamic and constant interaction between inner psychic and outer social and cultural dimensions, which manifests through both unconscious or emotional states, and conscious communication. In this vein, in using FANIM, data collection and analysis consider felt emotions and spoken words, as well as the intersubjective dynamics between interviewer and interviewee, proposing a similarity to a psychoanalyst's work on the session's materials.

Moreover, FANIM is founded on three fundamental assumptions, which further bring it closer to clinical practice and psychoanalytic theory, specifically Kleinian: 1) unconscious intersubjectivity, understood in terms of a psychosocial analysis that makes dialogue a co-product of the unconscious, and which pays particular attention to the relational dynamics between interviewee and interviewer; 2) "defended subject" rather than unitary rationality, thus implying a specific emphasis on the defensive mechanisms enacted by the research subject, as well as by the researcher; and 3) free associations method, which opens up the possible emergence of latent content in the narrative, and which puts attention on the processes of signification inherent in the connections between the topics discussed during the interview. Finally, in conducting psychoanalytically informed qualitative research based on FANIM, the psychoanalyst and researcher keep in mind that that psychosocial subjects develop identity investments in their subject position over time and that they defend these positions in their narrative. Thus, the role of anxiety in driving investment in and defence of subject positionings becomes a strong theme in the data, once again stimulating the clinician's attention to the use of a method based on psychoanalysis but used in extra-clinical contexts.

If you are interested in using this approach, we would recommend you read Hollway and Jefferson's (2013) influential account:

- Hollway, W., and Jefferson, T. (2013). *Doing qualitative research differently: A psychosocial approach* (2nd ed.). London: Sage.

Discourse analysis

Discourse analysis is a broad term capturing a range of language-based approaches, including discourse analysis (sometimes called traditional discourse analysis), critical discourse analysis, Foucauldian discourse analysis, Bakhtinian discourse analysis, discursive psychology, and critical discursive psychology. Whilst there are theoretical and practical differences in these different discourse approaches to analysis, they are all bound by an interest in how social processes inform the ways knowledge claims are considered as factual representations of the world (Wooffitt, 2005). They also share a commitment to the assertion that language is performative and not simply reflective of mental processes (Lester, O'Reilly, and Steele, 2023).

What is more, whilst there are differences between discourse analytic approaches, one central theoretically founded consideration is the extent to which the discourse analyst is epistemologically concerned with "truth" and "power". Some approaches, like discursive psychology, align with a more micro-social constructionist approach that views power as being co-created via language and interaction (see Edwards and Potter, 1992; Lester et al., 2023; Wiggins, 2017). Other, more critical approaches are more macro-social-constructionist or Foucauldian in theoretical orientation, such as critical discourse analysis or critical discursive psychology (Wetherell, 2007; van Dijk, 2008). For more critically orientated discourse approaches, the goal tends to be to examine the role of discourse in the production of power within social structures to sustain and legitimise social inequality (Wooffitt, 2005), usually with an explicit socio-political position being adopted in the analysis (van Dijk, 2008).

Discursive psychology (not critical discursive psychology) has a different theoretical foundation and goal of analysis. This form of discourse analysis tends to favour naturally occurring data because of the belief that any speech act can only be meaningfully analysed in terms of the situated nature of the talk and the characteristics of the interlocutors (Edwards and Potter, 1992). Discursive psychology examines how talk is organised interactionally (leaning on the principles of conversation analysis) to capture the authenticity of the details of the interaction (Potter and Hepburn, 2012). Discursive psychology primarily seeks to study psychological topics, with a focus on discourse, and does not presuppose that mental states are fixed cognitive or emotional states, but rather conceives of them as constructed through social interaction (Wetherell, 2007). As such, as Wetherell has pointed out, researchers using discursive psychology seek to find new ways of theorising and studying forms of psychological knowledge as made evident in text and talk.

How discourse analysis is conducted varies depending on which approach you choose. To help you understand the process, we specifically provide some practical steps for doing a discursive psychology analysis, but note that the steps for other DA approaches do differ. Like other approaches summarised in this chapter, there is not a rigid stepwise procedure for this, and any recommendations must be taken simply as a guide. Lester, O'Reilly, Kiyimba, and Wong (2018) have provided some useful practical guidance on approaching this kind of work, drawing on the original work of Potter (2012) and we outline this in Box 19.6.

> **Box 19.6**
> **Practical steps for doing discursive psychology (Lester et al., 2018; Potter, 2012)**
>
> In doing discursive psychology, there are no prescriptive steps. However, there are some general guidelines:
>
> - Be thoughtful in the collection of data and management of ethics. This can be challenging when collecting naturally occurring data, especially when using video to capture the multi-modal aspects of interaction.
> - There are no hard rules about sample sizes for analysis in discursive psychology. Rather, it is necessary to build an interactional dataset related to a phenomenon of interest. The volume of data is considered in hours of talk or volume of text.
> - Data management is an integral part of the analytic process, especially as the project evolves, including collating digital files, transcripts, analytic notes, and providing a clear audit trail.
> - Data are usually transcribed following the conversation analytic transcription conventions of the Jeffersonian approach (Jefferson, 2004). This is an essential aspect of analysis as it aids familiarisation with the audio or audio-visual material and helps the analyst to hear not only what was said but also how it was said.
> - It is necessary for you reconsider and redevelop the open research questions guiding the analysis. In discursive psychology, research questions evolve iteratively, and it is through analysis that these become more defined.
> - The data are analysed in micro-details through a systematic examination of the entire data set.
> - The discourse action model can facilitate your close interrogation of the data (please note, this model was developed by Edwards and Potter, 1992). Edwards and Potter noted that this is not a traditional type of model and has three elements: action, fact and interest, and accountability. Action refers to the action-orientated nature of talk, in that talk is performative, such as inviting, complaining, persuading, and inviting. Fact and interest refer to the ways in which speakers manage their interest in what is said. Accountability refers to the process of managing the ways in which people claim, refute, or direct responsibility and blame to others in situ.
> - It is advised that you organise and participate in "data sessions" where groups of researchers with various levels of expertise and experience in using discursive psychology come together and explore a specific aspect of the data.

If you are interested in DP, we would recommend this book, which provides an overview (as well as the original Edwards and Potter, 1992 book):

Tileaga, C., and Stokoe, E. (2016). *Discursive psychology*. London: Routledge.

Conversation analysis

Conversation analysis (CA) is an approach to studying social interaction by attending to the details of talk-in-interaction, the sequential order of talk, and the ways in which people perform social actions with language (Sacks, 1992; Schegloff, 1987). The central tenet of CA is to examine the social organisation of activities that are produced through talk by a detailed analysis of sequential patterns of interaction (Hutchby and Wooffitt, 2008). Conversation analysts utilise data that is "naturally occurring" so they can explore the performative nature of language in situ (Kiyimba et al., 2019).

In the early days of CA at its inception, Sacks and his colleagues pioneered the approach, and most of the work studied seemingly mundane or ordinary conversations. Whilst Sacks sought to study institutional settings to start with rather than ordinary conversations, examining telephone calls to a suicide centre, he was primarily interested in the structures of conversation rather than the institutional nature of the talk (Sacks, 1992). Sacks seemingly did not intend for conversation analysis to become a formal analytic method (Silverman, 1998), and his original writings are transcripts of university lectures he gave about his observations of talk in everyday encounters. However, as the approach developed, more researchers became interested in using the principles he set out to explore formal conversations occurring between people within organisations, commonly referred to as institutional talk (Antaki, 2011; Lester and O'Reilly, 2018). Thus, from these beginnings, over time a distinction was made between "pure CA" and "applied CA".

Applied CA has been conceptualised in two distinct ways by ten Have (2001). It was argued by ten Have that, first, applied CA can be the application of findings from a pure conversation analytic study to the study of institutional interactions; and that, second, it can involve efforts to apply CA findings in the service of practical recommendations to organisations that have a bearing on practice. Indeed, as a clinician-researcher, you are likely to be interested in how the CA-based lessons about social interactions in healthcare settings might be applied to inform or change practices (see Lester and O'Reilly, 2019).

If you choose to use CA for your research project, this is a method that will require training, support from experienced researchers who use the approach, and a good deal of reading. Here we provide you with some core information about the building blocks of doing CA, its principles, and tools. The basic principles of CA provide you with the main tools you need to carry out an analysis, as these are related to the fundamental structures of conversation (Lester and O'Reilly, 2019). In the practical *Handbook of conversation analysis* there is a whole segment devoted to the fundamental structures of conversation (Sidnell and Stivers, 2013). It is these structures we introduce you to here as support for the practical steps.

In working toward providing a practical guide to CA, we introduce the basic tools or principles:

1. **Sequence organisation**. This rests on the core assumption of CA that in human interaction, talk is responsive to the conversational turn immediately prior to it (Heritage, 2011). It is through sequence organisation that the actions fundamental to talk-in-interaction are managed by the speakers (Heritage, 2005).

2. **Practices**. This refers to the feature of a turn which has a distinctive character, has a specific location within the turn or sequence, and has unique consequences for the meaning of the action implemented by the turn (Sidnell, 2013).
3. **Turn design**. This principle of CA relates to how a speaker constructs their turn in the unfolding social interaction, and how this is done so it can be understood as performing a social action (Drew, 2013). Drew noted that there are three principles that shape turn design: the location within the sequence where the turn is taken, the social action being performed, and the recipient of the turn who is being addressed.
    a. **Turn-taking, turn-sharing, and turn-allocation** – may occur differently in institutional settings compared to mundane ones. There are some systematic transformations in turn-taking procedures that have the potential to alter the speaker's opportunity for action (Heritage, 2005).
    b. **Adjacency pairs** – an aspect of turn design and turn organisation is that talk is mainly organised into adjacency pairs where there is a first-pair-part, and the next action is the delivery of the second-pair-part (Sacks, 1992).
    c. **Next-turn-proof-procedure** – as part of the turn-taking organisation, the next-turn-proof-procedure is used to evidence analytic claims (Sidnell, 2013). Sidnell demonstrated that the recipient's orientation to the original speaker's turn shows their understanding of the prior turn, which is displayed in the way their turn is constructed.
    d. **Turn construction unit** – refers to the production of turns in real time and the organisation of determining when a speaker completes their turn (Sacks et al., 1974). Thus, the turn construction unit (TCU) refers to the segments of interaction that make up a complete turn in the talk.
    e. **Transition relevance place** – is also relevant to the organisation of turns. A recipient apparently anticipates when a speaker is going to finish their turn. The completion of a prior TCU provides a transition relevance place (TRP), which is a socially understood point at which a change of speaker becomes possible (Clayman, 2013).
4. **Repair**. This is a set of practices used by speakers to manage apparent interruptions, mis-understandings, mis-meanings, or slips of the tongue. Repairs can change the shape and composition of spoken sentences (Schegloff, 1997). Schegloff (1987) noted that a repair may be used if a speaker misarticulates a word, if there is trouble hearing, or if there is a failure of a recipient to understand what has been said. There are different types of repair action, which Schegloff et al. (1977) described as self-initiated repair (repair initiated by the same speaker as the source of trouble), other-initiated repair (when the need for repair is indicated by the recipient but re-constructed by the speaker), self-initiated other-repair (when the speaker who was the source of trouble encourages the recipient to repair), and other-initiated other-repair (when the recipient of the trouble source initiates the repair and offers a trouble solution).
5. **Preference organisation**. The use of preference was introduced by Sacks (1992) in the context of invitations. That is, when invitations are issued, they are designed to elicit acceptance rather than declining them. Preference organisation is not about wanting to do something but refers to affiliation, accountability, and sanctions in talk (Seedhouse, 2004). Thus, the use of preference for conversation analysts differs from the traditional semantic interpretation.

Using CA has been a popular approach in health, and we provide the perspective of Dr Leanne Chrisostomou in Box 19.7 on the usefulness of this analytic approach for research in health.

> **Box 19.7**
>
> **View of Dr Leanne Chrisostomou**
>
> > Dr Leanne Chrisostomou works as both a clinician and an academic. She works for the NHS as a Researcher and an Assistant Psychologist. Leanne is also a Teaching Fellow at the University of Portsmouth. Her research interests include the interactional practices and instruments utilised to diagnose neurodevelopmental conditions.
>
> Applying my knowledge of everyday interactions through the framework of conversation analysis [CA], I have been able to question how everyday nuances within interaction are taken for granted in certain clinical health practices. For example, in my clinical role as a diagnostician, whilst partaking in autism assessments, I knew how certain interactional questions and comments made by an examiner were motivated to elicit certain behaviours associated with autism. Over time, I began to observe how patterns of interactional difficulties emerged within specific semi-structured interactional tasks. As a researcher of conversation analysis, I noticed how many of these interactional difficulties were situated in turns at talk that would not typically occur in everyday conversation. This knowledge of everyday talk allowed me to consider how these difficulties in specific clinical interactions might be avoidable if more was understood about how the participants were making sense of one another's turns at talk.
>
> Taking an applied CA perspective of my clinical work allowed me to focus my area of research on a specific part of practice. Applied CA (Antaki, 2011) enables the analyst to illuminate how certain question constructions, comments, and entitlements to talk all shape the instructional delivery of "institutional" practice. Applied CA also removes the status (such as clinician/patient, no condition/condition) of the co-interactants by describing only how the speakers co-construct meaning in interaction. This analysis of talk enables clinicians to consider how some communicative behaviours in conditions of "disordered talk" may, in fact, be strengths, or adaptations to compensate for areas of difficulty (Lam, Holden, Fitzpatrick et al., 2020; Russell, Kapp, Elliott et al., 2019).
>
> Therefore, as a clinician, I have found that orienting to the times when clinical interactions feel frequently discordant and incorporating a fine-grained analysis framework such as CA is likely to be invaluable and illuminating. Moreover, as my clinical training, academic training, personal values, and background will influence what I perceive and choose to research, CA provides clinicians with an analytic tool that aims to eliminate biases by pursuing the closest version of objectivity by only describing what happens within any interaction.

If you are interested in using CA, we would recommend a book that provides an overview of conversation analysis:

- Lester, J., and O'Reilly, M. (2019). *Applied conversation analysis: Social interaction in institutional settings*. Thousand Oaks, CA: Sage.

A summary of approaches to data analysis

As we have acknowledged already, opting to use one of the qualitative approaches to analysis that we have detailed will require you to do more reading, training, and engagement with other researchers with relevant expertise. Our intention in this chapter has been to introduce you to common ways of doing analysis and to give you a sense of the practical steps involved. We now guide you to the reflective activity in Box 19.8.

Box 19.8

Reflective activity in choosing an analytic approach

Deciding on which analytic approach to use for your project is not a decision that should be left, that is, put off, until after you have collected your data. Your data collection approach needs to be informed by your epistemology, any explanatory theoretical positions taken, and should be congruent with your methodology. In deciding on an analytic approach, it needs to be congruent with those other aspects of the project.

In this reflective activity we encourage you to consider the following questions:

- Based on your methodological framework, which of the analytic approaches might be suitable for your project?
- Based on your epistemology and theoretical position, which of the analytic approaches might be congruent with your perspective on the way in which knowledge can be produced?
- Based on the summaries in this chapter, which readings might you like to explore further?
- What are the key concepts you would like to search for in the methodological literature?
- What training is available where you are based, and how might you engage with that to enhance your knowledge and skills?
- What expert researchers might be available to give you further support – e.g. supervisors, people in your networks?

Author reflections and concluding remarks

From Nikki

When considering qualitative analysis, I am drawn to reflect on the position of privilege held by the researcher who handles the information provided by the research participants, whether that be via researcher-generated or naturally occurring means. The academic side of me has enjoyed the immense privilege of a university education and mentorship by some of the most brilliant minds in qualitative methodology. In many ways, I am grateful that I was an academic first, learning to understand and respect methodological rigour, and to align my beliefs and values with a compatible epistemological position. As a social constructionist, it makes sense to me that by agreeing together about something, we make it so, rather than the view that we stumble across realities that existed before we did. As such, I have a strong preference for naturally occurring data, whereby the situated nature of the discourse can be transparently included in analysis. However, I also see value in interview data and have been involved in numerous projects using this data collection method to access the narratives of those who volunteer to use that medium to say something that is important to them. The deliberate choice to report something in a research interview, especially one that allows a lot of latitude to the participant to talk about the topic in the way they choose, can be considered an intentional act of communication. The participant is hoping that something about what they have reported about their experiences will make its way to the big wide world.

When I first left academia to engage in clinical training, it was with a sense of disillusionment that in some academic circles data were being used to bolster individual careers. The idea of accessing "juicy" data was sometimes spoken about like a newspaper headline that would entice would-be readers. For this and other reasons, there are some populations of participants that become over-researched, in part because the unusual tends to provoke researcher curiosity. From my perspective, these projects are often initiated by the research community rather than the people who become participants. However, there is an opportunity to reverse this trend. In clinical settings, there are often groups of people who want to learn more about something related to their own community. One of the reasons for this book is to support people in those groups to team up with others who understand how the research process works, so they can learn more. Redressing this balance of power, so that those who may benefit from the research outcomes have more say in the design and focus from the beginning, I would argue, is an important step. The other matter is that of analytic interpretations.

It is well known that it is difficult for us to see or understand experiences that are outside our own worldview, and that we tend to fill in the gaps and recreate other people's experiences in ways that make sense to us according to our own worldview. The danger of this is that we can inadvertently colonise others in our attempts to explain them. This is the main reason that I really appreciate the double hermeneutic principle gifted to us in IPA. This approach explicitly illuminates the humanness of the researcher when it states that we are trying to make sense of the way our participants make sense of their worlds. In other words, we are applying an additional filter based on our own interpretative repertoires birthed from our own worldviews. Inevitably then, we report the intentions, feelings, values, opinions, or experiences of our participants through this filter of what makes sense to us. My worry is that we do not do our participants justice, because we do not, and perhaps cannot, understand or see things from their perspective. So, what is the answer? My view is that at least we acknowledge this. Let us be honest with ourselves and our readers that we have done our best from our own particular perspective to make sense of what our participants have shared.

References

Annells, M. (1996). Grounded theory method: Philosophical perspectives, paradigm of research, and postmodernism. *Qualitative Health Research*, 6(3), 379–393.

Antaki, C. (2011). Six kinds of applied conversation analysis. In C. Antaki (Ed.), *Applied conversation analysis: Intervention and change in institutional talk* (pp. 1–4). Basingstoke, Hampshire: Palgrave MacMillan.

Archard, P. J. (2020a). Psychoanalytically informed research interviewing: Notes on the free association narrative interview method. *Nurse Researcher*, 28(2), 42–49.

Archard, P. J. (2020b). Reflections on the completion of a psychoanalytically informed interview study involving children's services professionals. *Social Work & Social Sciences Review*, 21(3), 107–126.

Biggerstaff, D. (2012). Qualitative research methods in psychology. In G. Rossi (Ed.), *Psychology-selected papers* (pp. 175–206). London: InTech Open Science.

Burck, C. (2005). Comparing qualitative research methodologies for systemic research: The use of grounded theory, discourse analysis and narrative analysis. *Journal of Family Therapy*, 27(3), 237–262.

Charmaz, K., and Thornberg, R. (2021). The pursuit of quality in grounded theory. *Qualitative Research in Psychology*, 18(3), 305–327.

Charmaz, K. (2006). *Constructing grounded theory: Practical guide through qualitative analysis*. London: Sage.

Charmaz, K. (2005) Grounded theory in the 21st Century: applications for advancing social justice studies. In N. Denzin and Y. Lincoln (Eds.), *The Sage handbook of qualitative research* (Third edition). London: Sage. pp: 507–535.

Chun Tie Y, Birks M, and Francis K. (2019). Grounded theory research: A design framework for novice researchers. *Sage Open Medicine*, 2(7), 2050312118822927

Clayman, S. (2013). Turn-construction units and the transition-relevance place. In J. Sidnell and T. Stivers (Eds.), *The handbook of conversation analysis* (pp. (150–166). Chichester, West Sussex: Blackwell Publishing.

Crossley, M. (2000). *Introducing narrative psychology: Self, trauma and the construction of meaning*. Buckingham: Open University Press.

Drew, P. (2013) Turn design. In J. Sidnell, and T. Stivers (Eds.), *The handbook of conversation analysis* (pp. 131–149). Chichester, West Sussex: Blackwell Publishing.

Edwards, D., and Potter, J. (1992). *Discursive psychology*. London, UK: Sage.

Engward, H., and Goldspink, S. (2020). Lodgers in the house: Living with the data in interpretive phenomenological analysis research. *Reflective Practice*, 21(1), 41–53.

Frosh, S., and Baraitser, L. (2008). Psychoanalysis and psychosocial studies. *Psychoanalysis, Culture & Society*, 13, 346–365.

Frosh, S., and Emerson, P. (2005). Interpretation and over-interpretation: Disputing the meaning of texts. *Qualitative Research*, 5, 307–324.

Gee, J. (1991). A linguistic approach to narrative. *Journal of Narrative & Life History*, 1(1), 15–39.

Glaser, B., and Strauss, A. (1967). *The discovery of grounded theory: Strategies for qualitative research*. New York, NY: Aldine.

Goldspink, S., and Engward, H. (2018). Shedding light on transformational online learning using five practice-based tenets: Illuminating the significance of the self. *The Asia Pacific Journal of Contemporary Education & Communication Technology*, 5(2), 10–16.

Gubrium, J., and Holstein, J. (2009). *Analyzing narrative reality*. Thousand Oaks, CA: Sage.

Heath, H., and Cowley, S. (2004). Developing a grounded theory approach: A comparison of Glaser and Strauss. *International Journal of Nursing Studies*, 41(2), 141–150.

Heritage, J. (2011). Conversation analysis: Practices and methods. In D. Silverman (Ed.), *Qualitative research* (3rd ed., pp. 208–230). London: Sage.

Heritage, J. (2005). Conversation analysis and institutional talk. In K. Fitch and R. Sanders (Eds.), *Handbook of language and social interaction* (pp. 103–149). Mahwah, NJ: Lawrence Earlbaum.

Hoggett, P., Beedell, P., Jimenez, L., Mayo, M., and Miller, C. (2010). Working psychosocially and dialogically in research. *Psychoanalysis, Culture & Society*, 15, 173–188.

Holmes, J. (2013). A comparison of clinical psychoanalysis and research interviews. *Human Relations*, 66, 1183–1199.

Hollway, W. (2011). Psycho-social writing from data. *Journal of Psycho-Social Studies*, 4(2). http://www.psychosocialstudies-association.org/wp-content/uploads/2017/01/writingfromdata.pdf.

Hollway, W., and Jefferson, T. (2013) *Doing qualitative research differently: A psychosocial approach* (2nd ed.). London: Sage.

Hutchby, I., and Wooffitt, R. (2008). *Conversation analysis* (2nd ed.). Cambridge: Polity Press.

Jefferson, G. (2004). Glossary of transcript symbols with an introduction. In G. H. Lerner (Ed.), *Conversation analysis: Studies from the first generation* (pp. 13–31). Amsterdam: John Benjamins Publishing Company.

Kiyimba, N., Lester, J., and O'Reilly, M. (2019). *Using naturally occurring data in health research: A practical guide*. Cham, Switzerland: Springer.

Lam, G., Holden, E., Fitzpatrick, M., Raffaele Mendez, L., and Berkman, K. (2020). "Different but connected": Participatory action research using Photovoice to explore well-being in autistic young adults. *Autism*, 24(5), 1246–1259.

Lapping, C. (2011). *Psychoanalysis in social research: Shifting theories and reframing concepts*. Abingdon, Oxfordshire: Routledge.

Lester, J., and O'Reilly, M. (2019). *Applied conversation analysis: Social interaction in institutional settings*. Thousand Oaks, CA: Sage.

Lester, J., O'Reilly, M., Kiyimba, N., and Wong, J. (2018). Discursive psychology: Implications for counselling psychology. *The Counseling Psychologist*, 46(5), 576–607.

Lester, J., O'Reilly, M., and Steele, C. (2023). Promoting the value of discursive psychology for human resource development: A pedagogical guide for qualitative researchers. *Human Resource Development Review*, 22(2), 229–250.

McAdams, D., and McLean, K. (2013). Narrative identity. *Current Directions in Psychological Science*, 22(3), 233–238.

Murray, M. (2003). Narrative psychology. In J. A. Smith (Ed.), *Qualitative psychology: A practical guide to research methods* (pp. 111–131). London: Sage.

Potter, J., and Hepburn, A. (2012). Eight challenges for interview researchers. In *The Sage handbook of interview research: The complexity of the craft* (2nd ed., pp. 555–570). London: Sage.

Riessman, C. (2008). *Narrative methods for the human sciences*. London: Sage.

Russell, G., Kapp, S. K., Elliott, D., Elphick, C., Gwernan-Jones, R., and Owens, C. (2019). Mapping the autistic advantage from the accounts of adults diagnosed with autism: A qualitative study. *Autism in Adulthood*, 1(2), 124–133.

Sacks, H. (1992). *Lectures on conversation* (Vols. I & II, G. Jefferson, Ed.). Oxford: Basil Blackwell.

Sacks, H., Schegloff, E., and Jefferson, G. (1974). A simplest systematics for the organization of turn-taking for conversation. *Language*, 50(4), 696–735.

Sandberg, J. (2005). How do we justify knowledge produced within interpretive approaches? *Organizatonal Research Methods*, 8(1), 41–68.

Schegloff, E. (1997). Whose text? Whose context? *Discourse & Society*, 8, 165–188.

Schegloff, E. (1987). Analyzing single episodes of interaction: An exercise in conversation analysis. *Social Psychology Quarterly*, 50(2), 101–114.

Schegloff, E., Jefferson, G., and Sacks, H. (1977). The preference for self-correction in the organization of repair in conversation. *Language*, 53(2), 361–382.

Seedhouse, P. (2004). Conversation analysis methodology. *Language Learning*, 54(s1), 1–54.

Sidnell, J. (2013). Basic conversation analytic methods. In J. Sidnell and T. Stivers (Ed.), *The handbook of conversation analysis* (pp. 77–100). Chichester, West Sussex: Wiley-Blackwell.

Sidnell, J., and Stivers, T. (Eds.). (2013). *The handbook of conversation analysis*. Chichester, West Sussex: Wiley-Blackwell.

Silverman, D. (1998). *Harvey Sacks: Social science and conversation analysis*. Cambridge: Polity Press.

Smith, B. (2016). Narrative analysis. In E. Lyons and A. Coyle (Eds.), *Analysing qualitative data in psychology* (2nd ed., pp. 202–221). London: Sage.

Smith, J. A. (2004). Reflecting on the development of interpretative phenomenological analysis and its contribution to qualitative research in psychology. *Qualitative Research in Psychology, 1*, 39–54.

Smith, J., Flowers, P., and Larkin, M. (2009). *Interpretative phenomenological analysis: Theory, method and research*. London: Sage.

Starks, H., and Trinidad, S. (2007). Choose your method: A comparison of phenomenology, discourse analysis, and grounded theory. *Qualitative Health Research, 17*(10), 1372–1380.

ten Have, P. (2001). Lay diagnosis in interaction. *Text, 21*(1/2), 251–260.

Thorne, S. (2000). Data analysis in qualitative research. *Evidence Based Nursing, 3*(3), 68–70.

Tileaga, C., and Stokoe, E. (2016). *Discursive psychology*. London: Routledge.

Tomkins, L. (2017). Using interpretative phenomenological psychology in organisational research with working carers. In J. Brooks and N. King (Eds.), *Applied qualitative research in psychology* (pp. 86–100). London: Palgrave Macmillan.

van Dijk, T. (2008). *Discourse and power*. Basingstoke, Hampshire: Palgrave.

Wetherell, M. (2007). A step too far: Discursive psychology, linguistic ethnography and questions of identity. *Journal of Sociolinguistics, 11*(5), 661–681.

Wiggins, S., (2017). *Discursive psychology: Theory, method and applications*. London: Sage.

Willig, C. (2008). *Introducing qualitative research in psychology* (2nd ed.). Milton Keynes: Open University Press.

Wooffitt, R. (2005). *Conversation analysis and discourse analysis: A comparative and critical introduction*. London: Sage.

CHAPTER 20

Dissemination and translating research into practice

> **Learning objectives**
>
> This chapter enables the reader to:
>
> - Identify reasons for dissemination.
> - Recognise ethical considerations in the dissemination of research.
> - Explore the benefits and challenges of writing in teams.
> - Critically assess different methods of dissemination.
> - Assess the importance of translation and the impact of research.
> - Conceptualise knowledge exchange, transfer, mobilisation, and sustainability.

Introduction

Disseminating research brings challenges for inexperienced researchers as they make decisions as to where and how to reach different audiences. In this chapter, we discuss different aspects of dissemination. Of central relevance is impact and the translation of research into practice. For health research there tend to be practical objectives that hold real-world value. Yet, this is not easy. The translation of knowledge yielded through research into implications for practice is far from a straightforward process. This chapter seeks to guide the reader through those challenges.

Based on our experiences as clinician-researchers and in supporting professionals engaged in research, we hold the view that in engaging in research as a practising professional, one views practice differently (it may also be said that engaging in research whilst practising clinically, one views research differently). One can become more critically reflective about one's practice, perhaps, for example, less consumed by anxieties about getting things "wrong", able to engage more thoughtfully with what it means to practise in an ethical way, and more independently minded in identifying principles of best practice for a particular situation. For us, research can be a great tonic to practice, and vice versa. The direct delivery of care, leading care services, and managing others can be highly rewarding, but it is also emotionally taxing, and "progress" in clinical care can follow quite lengthy trajectories. In research, there can, equally, be challenges. Yet, with aspects of the research task, for instance, developing an understanding of issues or the practical mastery of a specific analytical approach, there can be a more immediate sense of gratification. As such, we believe that it is important for practitioners engaged in research to share their learning through various forms of dissemination. Moreover, the process of disseminating research provides a means of learning for practitioners engaged in research.

Reasons for dissemination
Put simply, dissemination is an active strategy to inform audiences of the evidence of an intervention or other research, using planned strategies of communication (Rabin, Brownson, Haire-Joshu et al., 2008). This general definition of dissemination notwithstanding, in the case of qualitative research, many interpretations apply. As such, whilst we present a fairly traditional overview of dissemination and related concepts in this chapter, we invite the reader to take a critical perspective throughout. It has long been recognised that orthodox models of dissemination privilege a narrow set of meanings and can limit the ways in which we convey knowledge (Barnes, Clouder, Pritchard et al., 2003). Indeed, Barnes et al. argued that there are ethical, political, and communicative challenges at the centre of research dissemination, particularly in applied fields like health. Dissemination and implementation of findings for practice are needed as part of the research enterprise to improve outcomes in health and promote equity (Silver, Colditz, and Emmons, 2023).

Putting aside critical arguments about how knowledge is generated, and who has access to and control over the narratives, i.e. how this process can involve exclusionary practices, there are reasons for clinician-researchers to share what they have discovered in their research. First, the ethical process of conducting research relies heavily on weighing the costs to participants of engaging in a study against the potential benefits to many others through an understanding of the findings. Consequently, it is to the participants themselves that we owe the greatest responsibility to use the research as a platform to showcase their voices. Ideally, participants will have some say in where the research is disseminated and how they are represented.

Second, research findings often form the bedrock of decisions made by funders of service providers. Many providers rely on grants or tenders to finance the running of their organisations. Peer-reviewed research publications are the "currency" of academic research often utilised by funders to make hard choices about where their money will be most effectively allocated. Research can demonstrate the effectiveness of therapeutic models, which agencies are delivering the "best" care, and what kinds of services clients and patients find most helpful. At a more micro level, qualitative health research can illuminate the lived experiences of patients/clients in ways that brings a level of insight and understanding for service providers. In this way, set in a wider context of resource and funding constraints, there is a lot at stake in considering (the value of) dissemination and why it should be engaged in by practising health and care professionals engaged in research activity.

Different methods of dissemination
There are many ways you might choose to disseminate your research, and decision-making will largely depend on identifying the audiences you want to reach. Whilst you may want to be a bit creative or innovative in your dissemination, there are several more conventional ways:

- Organisational reports.
- Journal articles and books.
- Conferences and workshops.
- Web pages, blogs, social media.
- To colleagues and practitioners.
- To participants.

Organisational reports
It is likely, especially in the field of health, that your own organisation or the organisation through which you recruited your participants will have asked for, indeed expect, feedback regarding the project, and this is usually in the format of an organisational report. When developing the report, think carefully about who will be reading that report and what kind of messages you want to convey. It may be that there will be multiple audiences for your report, and so you should be mindful of the language you use and the style of writing you develop. A useful way to think about a report is to consider it in two parts: a shorter, initial part which functions as an executive summary of the project, primarily for those readers with limited time who simply want to be made aware of key findings and considerations, and a second, more detailed part that contains the level of detail needed for integrity and transparency.

Journal articles and books
Journals and books are the most common ways in which academic researchers disseminate their work, and writing for publication via these means is a core skill developed during their careers (see, e.g. Thyer, 2008). Publishing journal articles, monographs, and books means the findings of research can reach a national or international audience. Peer-reviewed journal articles are a cornerstone of academic work, and through these individual papers you can focus on specific aspects of the research that you want to report. Depending on the scope of a project, a researcher may write a single article to capture the key findings or write several articles to convey different aspects and publish these in different journals to focus on different points/findings, as long as these do not duplicate each other (Jackson, Walter, Daly, and Cleary, 2014). When selecting a journal to submit an article manuscript to, there are things to consider. You will need to:

- Look at the aims and objectives section of the journal on their webpage. Make sure your work and proposed article are relevant to the journal.
- Read the guidelines for authors carefully. Each journal has its own set of guidelines in relation to formatting, referencing, and structure, as well as its own word count. This is not always easy, and care needs to be taken to consider how much space to

dedicate to different sections of the article (see, e.g. Burnard, 2004). You should plan this well and not exceed the word count, or the journal editorial team is likely to return the article to you.
- Select a journal appropriate to your field and likely to reach the audience you intend to reach.
- If you are based in a university or academic institute, consider the impact factor and ranking of the journal, as universities have metrics for quality and expectations about how research is judged externally.
- For clinician-researchers working outside an academic environment, the journal impact factor may be less important than the reach of the journal to the readership that would benefit most from learning about your findings. There are some journals that are more orientated to practitioner readers (as well as researchers), and these may be most suitable for practice-based research inquiries.

You may also decide to write a book based on your research. A monograph or book with one focus can serve as a valuable way of pulling together the whole project and all the nuanced detail within it. You can develop a book to show the nature of the research and do justice to the participants' narratives. As a significant undertaking, if you are considering writing a book based on your research, you should be mindful that:

- It can be helpful to research different publishers and make sure that you are pitching your book idea to an appropriate place.
- It is a good idea to reach out to commissioning editors representing your discipline within that publishing house and have an email exchange about your book idea before you start developing a proposal.
- If a commissioning editor is interested in your book idea, they will send you the template for the book proposal with guiding headings to help you. Ensure that you give as much detail as possible in the proposal, as this will be reviewed.
- It is a good idea to find someone with book writing experience to read your book proposal before you send it to the publisher, as they will be able to give you some feedback and support during the process.
- Consider if you want to write the book alone or with other authors. We discuss team writing later in this chapter.
- Self-publishing is an alternative route that gives you more control over the process and the end price, and there are advantages. This can be valuable if you wish to produce a book that is affordable for colleagues or clients. However, in academic circles it is worth noting that the self-publishing route tends to be viewed less favourably because of the possibility of a less rigorous quality assurance process. Indeed, with the self-publishing route, it is advisable to have help with proofreading, reviewing, and formatting, so that the finished product is professional.

Conferences and workshops
Conferences are a valuable way of disseminating health research as they bring together collectives of like-minded people to share their research and network. These events are considered valuable activities for researchers, enabling them to hear about the latest

research developments in their field. If you decide to attend a conference, it can be a valuable opportunity to present your own work, and this usually requires the submission of an abstract to the conference organisers. Some people may be perfectly confident and comfortable standing on a stage and presenting their work, but for others this can induce some anxiety. If you are anxious about presenting, then it can be helpful to start with a conference with smaller delegate numbers, and there are some that are designed for early career scholars and students which can make for an ideal point of entry. Hopefully your organisation will see the value of investing in supporting you financially to attend conferences to share your findings with colleagues in this format, as the attendance fee, travel and accommodation costs can be prohibitive for individuals to finance. Even if you are presenting a paper, you will likely still be required to register at the conference as a delegate.

Workshops are also a useful way of disseminating research. They tend to be smaller and more focused than conferences, and this might be something you decide to lead yourself. Alternatively, partnering with others in your organisation to set up a workshop may be valuable, as others may have different complementary skill sets, such as in poster design, website advertising, and event planning. If you are taking bookings, then having someone with administrative skills to handle liaison with the venue, refreshments, delegate resources, and ticket sales will be useful. Generally, practitioners attending workshops expect to go away with some tools, ideas, or skills they can implement in practice. Workshops should, thus, provide a balance of networking opportunities over coffee breaks or lunch, didactic presentations of material, and opportunities for small group discussions or practice.

Webpages, blogs, and social media

The digital world has created new mediums for disseminating research and provides researchers with opportunities to have asynchronous (or synchronous in some cases) dialogue with audiences. The use of the internet for dissemination means that researchers can present their work using audio, audio-visual, stories, photographs, internet graphics, and drawings in creative ways (Cleary and Walter, 2004; Ravinetto and Singh, 2023). Social media, digital technology, and internet-mediated communication are now ubiquitous, and this affords interesting and cost-effective ways for researchers to present their work. Video recordings can be created and uploaded on websites like YouTube™, and social media, as well as visuals on Instagram™ posts, WhatsApp™ groups, X™ (formerly known as Twitter), and so on. Of course, in making use of digital technology, the ethics of dissemination are especially important as these are a global public platform, and additional steps to maintain confidentiality may be necessary.

You may decide to combine an in-person workshop setting with an online recording of the event provided afterwards via your organisation's website. In addition to sharing knowledge, combining dissemination modalities can reach a wider audience and potentially provide a complementary source of revenue for your organisation. If you video record a live workshop, you need to ensure the sound, lighting, and video quality are excellent. Take care to separate out the "teaching" parts of the workshops from question and answer or small group activities, where people may share more personal information that would not be appropriate to reproduce. You might also combine some written forms of dissemination with presentations of your findings. For instance, if you present at a conference or workshop, you could also provide delegates with a booklet or handout summarising your findings and the key applicable messages for their clinical practice.

Sharing findings with colleagues and practitioners

As a clinician-researcher, sharing your research findings with your colleagues in the field and other practitioners in and beyond your own networks can be a practical component of dissemination. Whilst you may do this through workshops and conferences, there are other ways too. To reach practitioners nationally and internationally, you may opt to pursue publishing in academic journals, as outlined above. To reach practitioners you will, though, want to ensure you are identifying journals that target healthcare practitioners in your discipline, and as noted there are some journals specifically designed to reach them. These journals often also publish quality improvement work and service evaluations as well as opinion pieces, which can be an appropriate outlet for shorter practice-based accounts.

More locally, it may be beneficial to organise events within your healthcare organisation or across a region of healthcare organisations to bring together interested practitioners. You could include a training element to this and ensure the event is pedagogical in style to contribute to their learning from your research. Depending on your field of practice, some practitioners are expected to complete a certain number of Continuing Professional Development (CPD) hours each year. You can serve your colleagues by providing certificates of attendance that indicate the number of hours CPD your training involved.

Sharing findings with your participants and/or other service users

Writing for lay audiences is a skill that may present a challenge for some researchers who are more familiar with an academic style to adapt to a different writing style. However, from the perspective of research ethics, dissemination should not be exclusionary, and the people who participated in your research should be provided with an opportunity to hear about the findings. In doing so, you may also want to extend this out to reach other service users of the organisation or more widely, as well as other stakeholders.

Giving feedback about the findings of the research to your participants is not always easy, and there are some tensions in terms of when and how to do this (see Dixon-Woods et al., 2011), particularly as not all participants necessarily want to hear from you again after they have made their contribution (Fenandez, Gao, Strahlendorf, et al., 2009). The problem is that there is limited empirical evidence about participants' preferences related to whether they want findings reported to them, how they want them when they do, and what they do with those findings once they have them (Long, Stewart, and McElfish, 2017). Some researchers have further reported that participants do not always share their experiences because of concerns about participants' health literacy or various logistical barriers to sharing (Long et al., 2019).

When you disseminate findings – or summaries of them – to your participants, or other service users and stakeholders, you should endeavour to engage these groups effectively and use a style and language that will be comprehensible to them without being patronising. Building partnerships with your participants and other stakeholders is necessary to effectively translate the findings of research into practice and thus it is beneficial to treat those involved as partners in the work (Cargo and Mercer, 2008). Sharing your findings with those participants is therefore a vital aspect of the partnership. Studies have identified that, in health research, researchers are not commonly or routinely sharing findings with participants and therefore over time a collaborative approach between researchers is needed to create evidence-based guidelines for ethical and effective sharing (see, for example, Long et al., 2017). Facilitating discussions with participants regarding the findings of the work, the outcomes, and any change or decisions made because of the work is an essential part of partnership working (O'Reilly and Kiyimba, 2015).

An element of sharing research findings with participants used by some researchers is called member checking. This is when researchers send the transcript and findings (usually) to a participant to check the accuracy of what was said. This is somewhat contentious in qualitative research as it reflects a particular epistemological position on cognition and truth which is not shared by all approaches. For example, member checking is likely congruent with critical positions or constructivist ones, but less so with constructionist or relativist stances (Motulsky, 2021). Nonetheless, where epistemologically congruent, some researchers (e.g. Hoggett et al., 2010; Koelsch, 2013) argue that member checking is advantageous, as the researcher returns to the participants with their interpretations, analytical findings, and explanations to ascertain if those constructs resonate with the participants.

We encourage you to carefully consider the appropriateness of member checking when making decisions as to whether it is suitable for your work. Goldblatt, Karnieli-Miller, and Neumann (2011) identified different challenges and problems with member checking, and these are outlined in Box 20.1.

Box 20.1

Things to consider when using member checking (Goldblatt et al., 2011)

There are some concerns with member checking outlined by Goldblatt et al. (2011) and these are:

- **The challenge of privacy** – when engaging in member checking, you should balance the credibility of the research interpretations with the need for privacy for the participants. By returning with the data or analysis to the participants, those narratives may not sit entirely comfortably with them.
- **People's views and experiences are not static** – during the time between data collection and member checking, there may be changes in the participants' views. This may lead to questions from the participants regarding the interpretations of the researcher.

- **Risk of deductive disclosure** – in some research projects, participants are known to each other, and this may mean that by sharing the findings with participants, especially in-depth explanations, they may recognise people they know.
- **Risk of iatrogenic consequences** – there may be a risk that participants find it difficult to challenge your interpretations, and they may perceive you as having greater expertise than them. This experience may leave them feeling disempowered.

When disseminating your work there are some general things to think about practically, and we discuss these in Box 20.2.

Box 20.2
Disseminating to different audiences

There are some issues to consider during the dissemination of your work using the modalities we have described in this chapter:

- **Dealing with rejection** – in academic dissemination, this happens a lot. As a researcher attempting to publish your work in academic journals, you will likely experience desk rejections (where the editor decides the article is not appropriate for their journal) and rejections post-peer review (where the reviewers recommend rejection). Reviewers write in different ways, and they are not always as courteous or constructive. We have experienced a wide range of different kinds of reviews. Some have been critical but constructive and have helped us improve our work, others have been unkind, and some have even been entirely incorrect. For example, we have been asked by reviewers to talk about saturation for sampling adequacy in a conversation analysis project where saturation is an inappropriate marker, and we were asked for coding reliability measures on a reflexive thematic analysis paper, which again is inappropriate. This type of experience is typical, rather than atypical, in working and writing to publish as a researcher.
- **Dealing with open access** – often funding bodies and other institutions require you to publish your work open access. This means that the work is available to others without charge or subscriptions. Some journals now are entirely open access. Be mindful of the quality of some of these and what are referred to by some academic researchers as 'profit-driven' publishers. Often if you work for a healthcare organisation or university, there will be an institutional publishing agreement which means you can select the open access option on publishing. Do check with your organisation and more experienced researchers about suitable target journals for reporting the research.
- **Accessibility and language** – think about who your audience is and what kind of writing style you need to adopt. The work should be accessible to the intended audience and written in a way they can understand and use. It is also necessary to write in a clear way that conforms to integrity standards and expectations and does not include language that might be deemed offensive.

Ethics of dissemination

Before you engage with this section of the chapter, we invite you to reflect on your current beliefs and knowledge about the ways in which ethics are important to dissemination; see Box 20.3.

> **Box 20.3**
> **Reflective activity on dissemination and ethics**
>
> Before you read through this section of the chapter, we encourage you to make a list of what you see as the main ethical issues that might arise in relation to disseminating qualitative health research generally, and more specifically to your own research project.

As we noted earlier in the book, ethical research practice is iterative and there are many ways in which ethics become relevant and applied in qualitative health research. This holds true for the dissemination process where specific ethical concerns are raised. We have previously outlined three main ethical areas in the context of dissemination (O'Reilly and Kiyimba, 2015). The first relates to the moral obligation of researchers and their respective institutions to ensure that the burden placed on participants is worth their time by ensuring that the findings are disseminated. Second, for health research there is an imperative to disseminate beyond reaching other academic scholars in an accessible way. Third is involving participants in the dissemination process and ensuring they know what has happened to their data and how those data are used. If the way that the findings from the data collectively have been analysed and interpreted may be possibly upsetting, then researchers need to consider carefully how this is fed back to participants.

> **Key point!**
> Researchers have an ethical obligation to recognise the power of academic writing in shaping thoughts and knowledge about the world.
> (Reason, 2010)

Researchers have an obligation to disseminate the findings of their research, as participants have invested time and effort into supporting the project, and their voices ought to have a platform to be heard. In presenting the work to different audiences, the researcher will need to demonstrate the legitimacy of the research and show that the work met the quality parameters of the approach. In so doing, the researcher needs to consider how those findings may be perceived by general audiences, including representatives of the media.

When disseminating qualitative research, it is customary to use direct quotations from the data, segments of the transcripts which represent the original recorded data (or excerpts from the textual data) (White, Woodfield, Ritchie, and Ormston, 2014). However, you need to take care to act responsibly and ethically when using quotations. A concern is that quotations can be misused in ways designed to support the interpretation of the researcher (Sandelowski and Leeman, 2012). That is, quotes are used selectively to support a particular argument, rather than the researcher finding a way to organise and articulate the findings. In this way, some qualitative researchers may "cherry-pick" certain quotations to support their position (Morse, 2010). Further, there is a risk that certain phrases or details within the quotations result in a process of deductive disclosure (discussed in Chapter 8) to those persons known to the participants (Stein, 2010). In presenting quotations from participants within different dissemination modalities, the quotations and contextual narratives should be presented in a way that is accessible to the intended audience whilst also bearing in mind the possible risk of deductive disclosure.

> **Key point!**
> Researchers can sometimes struggle to reconcile a wish to communicate their research findings to a wide audience with a concern that the methodological integrity and robustness of their design are diluted in efforts to disseminate to non-expert audiences.
> (O'Reilly and Kiyimba, 2015)

Benefits and challenges of writing in teams

Most researchers opt to work (or find themselves working) as part of a research team. Practitioners (or trainees) undertaking an educational qualification are more likely to be working independently, albeit with supervision, but even then, during dissemination, they may choose to write and publish with others, their peers, supervisors, or wider networks. Writing as part of a team is often rewarding and enjoyable; it can also bring challenges.

- Consider the composition of your team

When writing as part of a team, a key decision is to think about who you want to work with and the reasons for doing or not doing so. Whereas some researchers write in large teams, others may author papers with just one other researcher or two. When deciding who should be involved as a co-author on a paper or series of papers, you need to think about what contribution they bring to the writing. Individuals have different strengths, and it can be valuable to have a team of writers that complement each other in terms of knowledge and skills. It may be that there are different areas of topical knowledge, methods-based knowledge, or disciplinary backgrounds, as well as different levels of experience. It is also useful to consider who qualifies for authorship. Typically, for this, there are expectations, and the Committee on Publication Ethics (COPE) guidelines (2024) can be useful here as:

- It is helpful to discuss authorship during the planning of research and agree on authorship order early on. This may be revisited as the writing project progresses.
- If disputes arise, use facts and guidelines to resolve them.
- Journals often specify the expected minimal contribution for authors, and if these are not met, the individual can be acknowledged for what they have given to the project. The order of authors needs to be agreed upon between the authors, and reasons may be provided to the editor.
- Individuals should not be authors if they have not contributed significantly to the project and the writing process.

Thus, to be an author in a piece of dissemination, the individual should have made a considerable contribution to the research project in terms of conception, data collection, and/or data interpretation. They should have made an intellectual contribution to the writing, and all authors have accountability for the work and its reporting. This relates to the integrity and accuracy of the work.

> **Key point!**
>
> Do not underestimate how important it is to work with people with whom you can collaborate effectively and whom you consider to be professional.

- Consider the author order

Ideally, if you are undertaking a research project as part of a team, then each individual member of the team will have key roles in conducting the research. However, be mindful not to forget to develop some kind of written agreement about what kinds of dissemination you will engage in, who will lead which elements of that dissemination, and what responsibilities each team member will have in relation to the dissemination activities. One decision regarding dissemination, especially for reports and published papers, is who is going to lead the writing and who will be the lead author. The lead author on a report or paper should ideally be the person who does most of the writing or leads the research. As part of the agreement, it also needs to be clear who the co-authors will be and what kind of tasks constitute authorship, as noted above. Traditionally, collecting the data is not usually enough to warrant co-authorship as there is an expectation that each author will have contributed substantially to the reporting of the research activity.

> **Key point!**
>
> Some journals now ask the corresponding author to outline the extent of the writing contribution of each author.

- **Time management and writing routines**

Writing takes time and effort, and disseminating your research via academic journals especially can entail considerable investment in this regard. Typically, work will require multiple drafts before the article is ready to submit and likely be redrafted following the process of peer review. When working as part of a team, it is advantageous to have some discussions in advance about the time commitments each member has so that a plan of action can be made, and a collaborative production of the article can be realised. If you are leading the writing of an article or report, you may want to block out chunks of time in your calendar, rather than trying to undertake the task in shorter periods. It can take a while to focus and get your mind back on the task, and so longer sections of time can be especially helpful to assign to the writing task.

In relation to time management, consider the practicalities of writing in terms of space, i.e. physical and psychological space in having a place to write and (head)space to do so, and process, i.e. a writing routine with steps. Silvia (2007) explained productive academic writing in terms of a range of steps, so a researcher can be productive without writing dominating their life. As part of this, he warned against specious barriers, i.e. waiting for inspiration, lacking time, and not having internet access. He emphasised that such barriers need to be grappled with and set to one side. Writing is most productive when routinised and time is dedicated on a regular basis, involving clear steps through which work will be developed from initial ideas and data through to a manuscript suitable to submit for publication. Putting aside regular time to sit at a keyboard (or with a pen and paper), with no distractions is essential as without this one will struggle to be productive. Indeed, it can be said that as a clinician-researcher, there are many good reasons *not* to write, not least more pressing work demands, which occupy your time and energy clinically. As well as this, as a practitioner, developing an identity as a researcher takes time and one can feel somewhat like an imposter in this role to begin with.

In developing an article, an initial plan, following ideas, and brainstorming mean you have a structure to work with. The initial drafting is the most creative step, and the focus should be on volume writing, i.e. getting words on the page. It can be easier to start with the more descriptive aspects of a piece of work, so, for example, with a standard research report, starting with the method or methodology section. Some researchers advise that you do not revise any writing until you have a full draft completed, not doing so being viewed as akin to trying to decorate a house before it has been fully built. Once the first full draft is complete with references and properly formatted, you may want to take a break so you can return to the work with fresh eyes. At this stage, you can start to consider the format/flow in more depth and refine and revise the writing, whilst keeping in mind the anticipated reader of the work. At this point, you may find that you have more reading to do and need to go back over your sources. You will also likely identify aspects that need to be developed which you can work on incrementally.

Once these are addressed and you either think you have got something good or something that is refined and you are now not sure whether you are making it better or worse by continuing to work on it, it is best to send the draft to co-authors/supervisors for feedback. After this, you can revise it some more (perhaps with their involvement) based on what they feed back. If they say that certain parts do not make sense, it probably will not make sense to others. Working on these aspects, you will be getting closer to a "good" full draft of the work and be in the process of finetuning that should be suitable for peer review. Prior to submission, you and your co-authors will need to concentrate on ensuring the article reads well.

> **Key point!**
>
> Do not underestimate how long it takes to organise the article and undertake the formatting requirements of the journal.

- Finding a mentor or supervisor with experience

As writing up your research, whether it be for a report or journal article, can be quite a daunting experience, it can be helpful when writing as part of a team to find someone who is willing to provide mentorship to you in helping you lead the team and lead on the writing tasks. This way, you can learn from their experience and be supported in the role of writing, as well as having someone you can ask questions to about the dissemination experience. This can be particularly helpful when your work is reviewed. Thus, having a mentor or supervisor, or just a supportive team behind you, is a good idea in the early stages of your academic development. We asked Dr Sewanu Awhangansi about his experience of this and point to his view in Box 20.4.

> **Box 20.4**
>
> **View of being supported in research – Dr Sewanu Awhangansi**
>
> > Dr Sewanu Awhangansi is a Consultant Child and Adolescent Psychiatrist with Leicestershire NHS Partnership Trust. He works for the Child and Adolescent Mental Health Service and conducts research in a range of areas related to global mental health.
>
> As an early career researcher trying to navigate the complex world of academia, the importance of having supportive mentors, working collaboratively as part of a research team, and learning from people who have gone before you cannot be overstated. Drawing from my own experience over the past few years, I can attest that these elements have played a crucial role in shaping my fledgling academic development, particularly as it pertains to writing, publishing, and disseminating academic work.
>
> For one, I have been fortunate to have supportive mentors who have helped nurture my research skills, provided constructive feedback, and given me a broader perspective on my writing. This has helped me navigate the complex challenges of the publication process, and the strategic advice on the best ways to disseminate my work effectively has been appreciated. I have also benefited from the guidance of these mentors, whose advice to be intentional about expanding my research network and collaboration has been invaluable. Their

mentorship has not only improved the quality of my research output but has also instilled in me a sense of self-belief and confidence, which every early career researcher needs a lot of, especially when the journey becomes tough.

Moreso, working as part of a research team has also been instrumental in my academic development so far. Collaborating with colleagues who share similar research interests has allowed me to exchange ideas and engage in stimulating discussions about various short-, medium-, and long-term projects. Through such teamwork, I have been able to appreciate and learn from diverse perspectives, harness collective expertise, and leverage the strengths of each team member to produce not just high-quality research outputs, but also a good number of research publications in a short period of time. Working collaboratively has not only enriched my research career but has also fostered a sense of camaraderie among my research colleagues.

Overall, having supportive people to learn from has broadened my horizons and enriched my academic skillsets. My proficiency in using both quantitative and qualitative research methods has grown. I feel empowered and challenged now to think critically and creatively about various ongoing projects (that I am leading or collaborating with others on). Seeing and learning from others has helped me to continuously strive for excellence in my academic endeavours.

- **Organise writing retreats or writing days**

When writing as part of a team it can be beneficial to come together in person and engage in writing as a collaborative process. This is especially useful when planning the report or article that you want to develop. To safeguard designated time for the task, some teams organise a writing retreat and spend a whole week away somewhere where they can write together every day and have collaborative dialogue in the evenings. Others organise writing days where they spend the day together and map out the dissemination plan, responsibilities, structure of the paper, content, etc., which may be more realistic given other demands on people's time.

Knowledge exchange, transfer, mobilisation, and sustainability

As a clinician-researcher, you are likely to be engaging in applied research with hopes or intentions to realise some kind of impact or change because of the work you have undertaken. This is an endeavour widely written about, with a range of terminology used, including implementation science, impact, and knowledge transformation (amongst others). Before any kind of impact is possible, you first need to exchange and mobilise the knowledge created through the research. Considering this, it is helpful to note some of the different concepts in the literature regarding the translation of (research-based) knowledge into practice. Nutley and Davies (2016) described these as including:

- **Knowledge transfer** – denotes knowledge considered generalisable across different health contexts with the goal to improve the ways of using that knowledge in practice within those contexts.

- **Knowledge exchange** – also considered to be knowledge interaction, where knowledge is viewed as context-linked and the process of knowing is constructed as a social process. Knowledge exchange involves developing effective social and interpersonal relationships which support collaborative learning.
- **Knowledge integration or knowledge intermediation** – refers to when knowledge is interconnected with cultures, local priorities, contexts, and structures, and the goal is to explore the embedded nature of that knowledge. This is realised by people working collaboratively so that they can develop effective systems to understand and articulate the ways in which knowledge and context are interconnected.

The drive for evidence-based healthcare has contributed to debates about how knowledge produced through research is reliably transferred to policymakers, managers, and practitioners who can make changes in practice (Gabbay, le May, Pope et al., 2020) and a greater emphasis on bringing in the voices of those who benefit from the knowledge, such as experts by experience or service users (Davies, Nutley, and Walter, 2008; Swan et al., 2012). This process of transferring knowledge across the research–practice gap is complex (Greenhalgh, 2018), not least because knowledge uptake is more than the direct transfer of knowledge and more than the translation of knowledge, and in fact requires the active engagement of a range of stakeholders with different kinds of knowledge and expertise (Davies et al., 2008).

Knowledge mobilisation is a commonly used term in healthcare research in the UK (Grindell, Sanders, Bec et al., 2022) and we encourage you to consider the meaning of this concept for your research. It is defined as a process of optimising the use of knowledge generated through research (Davies, Powell, and Nutley, 2015), consisting of dissemination, knowledge transfer, and knowledge exchange (Ferlie, Crilly, Jashapara, and Peckham, 2012). To transform knowledge into practice, knowledge mobilisation is necessary for inclusive participation. This begins with knowledge attending to the problem and acknowledges that different kinds of knowledge integrate and engage on a continuum extending from assessing the contribution of research up to co-researching (Sales, Farrández-Berrueco, Sanahuja, and Moliner, 2024). Thus, knowledge mobilisation refers to a process of creating and sharing knowledge so that evidence can be utilised in both practice and policy development (Powell, Davies, and Nutley, 2017).

> **Key point!**
>
> Knowledge mobilisation is a complex concept with various frameworks and theories that can underpin or integrate within it.
>
> (Ward, 2017)

If knowledge mobilisation is to be effective, then knowledge produced through research must be viewed by those in practice as relevant and usable (Chinnery, Dunham, van der Linden et al., 2018). The setting to which the knowledge is to be applied is therefore highly important in the context of knowledge exchange and mobilisation. Researchers must refocus attention on how knowledge exchange and mobilisation might occur practically so that it can be used by decision-makers, accounting for the complex environment where any research-based insights will be applied (Ward et al., 2012).

Translation, transformation, and impact of research
Anchored to notions of knowledge exchange, knowledge mobilisation, and applied dissemination are the concepts of translation, transformation, and impact. For knowledge exchange and mobilisation to be translated into the practical context, it needs to be translated and transformed to be applied, and only then can the knowledge have an impact on practice. These ideas are important in relation to health research as the translation of research findings into changes or improvements in practice is reportedly impeded by considerable time lags, of anything from 10 to 25 years (Morris, Wooding, and Grant., 2011). Transforming knowledge is a complex and challenging endeavour (Gabbay and le May, 2011) and there are fields that have sought to explore how this occurs in research and practice realities. Two of these fields are referred to as translational research and implementation science. Translational research is a rigorous research process where evidence-based interventions are translated to real-world clinical settings (Melnyk and Fineout-Overholt, 2023). Implementation science is the scientific study of methods designed to facilitate the uptake of evidence-based practices and research into the day-to-day practice of practitioners and policy makers (Melnyk and Fineout-Overholt, 2023).

Translation is an essential aspect of health research as the work needs to be interpreted as relevant by practitioners (Fox, 2003), and yet there is little work that explores how this knowledge translation and transformation takes place (Shaw, Gagnon, Carson et al., 2022). Moreover, there are questions raised regarding whose responsibility it is to translate the empirical evidence produced through research for practitioners to utilise that evidence in their practice (O'Reilly and Kiyimba, 2015), which is essential in fields that rely on evidence-based practice. Thus, health research evidence typically sees knowledge in relation to cognition, that is it is viewed as "true knowledge" and perceived as an accurate representation of how things are; however, in research-based evidence, it is not always the case that the knowledge can be used in practice due to gaps between professional personal knowledge and professional practical knowledge (Biesta, 2007). In healthcare, the evidence-based medicine movement has been a prominent influence on how we view knowledge translation and transformation. This movement was influential for implementation science in promoting the value of the work of health and social services being grounded in the best evidence available (Greenhalgh, Raftery, Hanney, Glover, 2016; Straus, Tetroe, and Graham, 2013). For health research, then, researchers and practitioners need to be encouraged to work together through interprofessional collaboration, as the implementation of research needs epistemically diverse teams to develop questions and promote interdisciplinary solutions (Portney, 2020), involving a direct application of science to practice.

To have application for practice means that there is a need for research impact, and this is a commonly used metric for ascertaining quality in research (Webster, Gastaldo, Durant et al., 2019). Impact can be a nebulous concept. In research, impact is conceived of as a process, and one requiring communication and translation of research findings to audiences who can mobilise the knowledge so that practice or policy may be changed (Nardon et al., 2021). Early work distinguished different kinds of impact, and Bhola (2000) delineated three distinct types:

1. **Impact by design** – where impact is a result of the specific intervention or piece of research.
2. **Impact by interaction** – where outcomes of a specific intervention interact with other concurrent interventions and thus there may be an enhancement or inhibition of the effects.
3. **Impact by emergence** – whereby the outcomes that emerge from an original intervention also interact with cultural processes and those from history.

> **Key point!**
>
> The growth of expectations to achieve impact can create some difficulties for those undertaking qualitative research, especially those working from critical epistemologies.
> (Cann and DeMeulenaere, 2020)

As we can see from the three types of impact offered in Bhola's (2000) typology, they have intervention at the centre and positivism as a framework which is not (necessarily) congruent with many qualitative approaches. Indeed, as Ross (2022, n.p.) observed:

> the methodological conceptualization of impact has been construed much more narrowly, in association with positivist epistemologies, causal, (uni)directional relationships between variables, experimental (or quasi-experimental) research, and, therefore, primarily with quantitative techniques for data analysis.

Ross argued, therefore, that the qualitative community needs to "reclaim impact" and conceptualise the term differently to show what can be known through approaches alternative to positivism in a way that moves beyond such narrow epistemological positioning. Based on this standpoint, Ross advocated that a broader frame of reference for impact is needed in the academic world, consistent with how the term is conceived in social science inquiry, which is especially important given the emphasis on policy and practice and impact as a central decision indicator in funding for research support. With this frame of reference, there is the benefit of a "dialogic conceptualisation of impact" where participants' views on their engagement with transformation are centralised.

We are now witnessing a subtle shift in the conceptualisations of impact and there is a growing evidence base around qualitative research findings and their applicability to practice (Ellis and Clark, 2015). With this, there is some recognition that impact is not unidirectional or passive but requires iterative and active reflection as well as engagement between participants, researchers, and community members (Ross, 2022). However, the timescale taken to achieve impact in any meaningful way can be a considerable challenge to all researchers, including those practising qualitative approaches (Marti, Flecha, Rodriguez, and Bosch, 2020). Part of the ongoing challenge to making meaningful impact for qualitative researchers is that the perceived value of qualitative evidence for clinical decision-making and policy is not always recognised by practitioners or some scholars (Ellis and Clark, 2015). Creating impact in a meaningful way, and in ways that are sustainable, must broach the gap between research, translation, mobilisation, and change, as we have demonstrated in this chapter.

Author reflections and concluding remarks

As this is the last chapter, all three of us reflect here on the dissemination of research and the translation of findings into practice.

From Michelle

The process of writing this book has been an interesting point of reflection. I have been teaching qualitative methods in health for many years, and so many of my mentees, supervisees, and students have been healthcare practitioners from various disciplinary backgrounds. In developing the chapters, I have critically challenged myself to examine the evidence in an inquisitive way and to think about how to translate vast amounts of methodological argument and knowledge into meaningful and practical ways of working for those in busy clinical roles trying to make a difference in practice. This dissemination and knowledge chapter has captured some of the complexities and realities of qualitative health research well and hopefully is a chapter that makes the reader stop and think about the purpose of their work.

From Philip

Compared to Michelle, I have been involved in teaching qualitative methods to health professionals for a much shorter period of time. In fact, it was a privilege to be supported by Michelle to undertake research when practising in a CAMHS team as a mental health practitioner. In my own work and writing as a researcher, the issue of how to translate complex issues relating to methodology into practical implications has very much been a live consideration for some time. Consistent with what was said in this chapter regarding the importance of mentors (in research but particularly writing as a researcher), I feel fortunate to have worked with several colleagues who have helped me learn (a lot) as a practitioner researcher. This experience has meant that writing for publication was not as daunting as it could have been.

Working with practitioner colleagues in shared evaluation and research projects, I have, at times, ruminated about reporting what I worry is "basic" (or even banal) applied research. By this, I do not mean that it did not add something to a wider body of evidence or help other professionals in some way and is not worth communicating the findings of. Rather, I worried that I needed to pursue research and writing projects that are, in some way, more substantial, weightier in terms of theory used and methodological matters engaged with.

Yet, over time, my experience has been that engaging in many, relatively small team-based projects has been instructive in the real-world value of such applied work, especially in the influence it can have in a local context to the benefit of the communities served. Indeed, now having less time to personally pursue this type of work, as a supervisor and teacher of research, I find I miss being as engaged as I was in such projects and the close interface there was with practice. Indeed, it is something that I cannot see myself *not doing*. I've also found there are avenues for "weightier" work in theorising and thinking about the interface between practice and research and how ideas about research are altered in qualitative inquiries led by practitioner researchers whose minds are, invariably, shaped by their everyday experience in practice.

I hope that this book is of use to other clinician-researchers who engage in research, that they are not discouraged by the challenges this entails, and that they find networks that can support them in their work.

From Nikki

In my field of work as a clinical psychologist, I am acutely aware of the importance of research findings being available to practitioners on the ground, as well as to clients themselves. I have noticed a gradual shift in my dissemination practices away from academic conferences specialising in research techniques, towards smaller conferences, workshops, and publications that are delivered in collaboration with practitioners. It is a challenge as a clinician-researcher to maintain professional credibility in both the academic and practitioner spaces. In my experience, academics tend to prefer high-impact, peer-reviewed technical journals for dissemination, whereas practitioners generally prefer face-to-face small group workshop settings where they can really get to grips with how to apply the findings in their own work. I still straddle both worlds – a little uncomfortably at times – but try to both maintain professional credibility as an academic and to have the language and real-world experience to be a trustworthy trainer in the space of practitioner workshops.

These reflections conclude *Qualitative Health Research: A Practical Guide for Clinical Practitioners*. Our hope is that you have learned something about doing qualitative health research as a clinician-researcher – hopefully in relation to different aspects of the research endeavour. At the very beginning of the book, we said we take the value of research for improving clinical practice as a foundational assumption for the book. With this mind, we will end by wishing you all the very best with your project.

References

Barnes, V., Clouder, D., Pritchard, J., Hughes, C., and Purkis, J. (2003). Deconstructing dissemination: Dissemination as qualitative research. *Qualitative Research*, 3(2), 147–164.

Bhola, H. (2000). A discourse on impact evaluation: A model and its application to a literacy intervention in Ghana. *Evaluation*, 6(2), 161–117.

Biesta, G. (2007). Why "what works" won't work: Evidence-based practice and the democratic deficit in educational research. *Educational Theory*, 57(1), 1–22.

Burnard, P. (2004). Writing a qualitative research report. *Accident & Emergency Nursing*, 12(3), 176–181.

Cann, C., and DeMeulenaere, E. (2020). *The activist academic: Engaged scholarship for resistance, hope and social change*. Gorham, ME: Myers Education Press.

Cargo, M., and Mercer, S. (2008). The value and challenges of participatory research: Strengthening its practice. *Annual Review of Public Health*, 29, 325–350.

Chinnery, F., Dunham, K., van der Linden, B., Westmore, M., and Whitlock, E. (2018). Ensuring value in health-related research. *The Lancet, 391*, 836–837.

Cleary, M., and Walter, G. (2004). Apportioning our time and energy: Oral presentation, poster, journal article or other? *International Journal of Mental Health Nursing, 13*(3), 204–207.

COPE Guidelines. (2024). How to handle authorship disputes: A guide for new researchers. https://publicationethics.org/resources/guidelines-new/how-handle-authorship-disputesa-guide-new-researchers

Davies, H., Nutley, S., and Walter, I. (2008). Why "knowledge transfer" is misconceived for applied social research. *Journal of Health Services Research & Policy, 13*(3), 188–190.

Davies, H., Powell, A., and Nutley, S. (2015). Mobilising knowledge to improve UK health care: Learning from other countries and other sectors—a multimethod mapping study. *Health Services & Delivery Research, 3*, 1–190.

Dixon-Woods, M., Tarrant, C., Jackson, C., Jones, D., and Kenyon, S. (2011). Providing the results of research to participants: A mixed-method study of the benefits and challenges of a consultative approach. *Clinical Trials, 8*(3), 330–341.

Ellis, R., and Clark, A. (2015). How to improve knowledge translation of qualitative research into clinical practice. *International Journal of Nursing Student Scholarship, 2*(4), 27–31.

Ferlie, E., Crilly, T., Jashapara, A., and Peckham, A. (2012). Knowledge mobilisation in healthcare: A critical review of health sector and generic management literature. *Social Science & Medicine, 74*, 1297–1304.

Fernandez, C., Gao, J., Strahlendorf, C., Moghrabi, A., Davis Pentz, R., Barfield, R., Baker, J., Santor, D.,Weijer, C., and Kodish, E. (2009). Providing research results to participants: Attitudes and needs of adolescents and parents of children with cancer. *Journal of Clinical Oncology, 27*(6), 878–883.

Fox, N. (2003). Practice-based evidence: Towards collaborative and transgressive research. *Sociology, 37*(1), 81–102.

Gabbay, J., and Le May, A. (2011). *Practice-based evidence for healthcare: Clinical mindlines.* London: Routledge.

Gabbay, J., le May, A., Pope, C. et al. (2020). Uncovering the processes of knowledge transformation: The example of local evidence-informed policy-making in United Kingdom healthcare. *Health Research Policy & Systems, 18*, 110.

Goldblatt, H., Karnieli-Miller, O., and Neumann, M. (2011). Sharing qualitative research findings with participants: Study experiences of methodological and ethical dilemmas. *Patient Education & Counseling, 82*(3), 389–395.

Greenhalgh, T. (2018). *How to implement evidence based healthcare.* Oxford: Wiley Blackwell.

Greenhalgh, T., Raftery, J., Hanney, S., and Glover, M. (2016). Research impact: A narrative review. *BMC Medicine, 14*(1), 78–16.

Grindell, C., Sanders, T., Bec, R., Tod, A., and Wolstenholme, D. (2022). Improving knowledge mobilisation in healthcare: A qualitative exploration of creative co-design methods. *Evidence & Policy, 18*(2), 265–290.

Hoggett, P., Beedell, P., Jimenez, L., Mayo, M., and Miller, C. (2010). Working psychosocially and dialogically in research. *Psychoanalysis, Culture & Society, 15*, 173–188.

Jackson, D., Walter, G., Daly, J., and Cleary, M. (2014). Multiple outputs from single studies: Acceptable division of findings vs. "salami" slicing. *Journal of Clinical Nursing, 23*(1–2), 1–2.

Koelsch, L. (2013). Reconceptualising the member check interview. *International Journal of Qualitative Methods, 12*, 168–179.

Long, C., Purvis, R., Flood-Grady, E., Kimminau, K., Rhyne, R.., Burge, M., Stewart, M., Jenkins, A., James, L. and McElfish, P. (2019). Health researchers' experiences, perceptions and barriers related to sharing study results with participants. *Health Research Policy & Systems, 17*, 1–11.

Long, C., Stewart, M., and McElfish, P. (2017). Health research participants are not receiving research results: A collaborative solution is needed. *Trials, 18*, 1–4.

Marti, T., Flecha, R., Rodriguez, J., and Bosch, J. (2020). Qualitative inquiry: A key element for assessing the social impact of research. *Qualitative Inquiry*, 26(8–9), 948–954.

Melnyk, B., and Fineout-Overholt, E. (2023). *Evidence-based practice in nursing and healthcare: A guide to best practice* (5th ed.). USA: Lippincott Williams & Wilkins.

Morris, Z., Wooding, S., and Grant, J. (2011). The answer is 17 years, what is the question: Understanding time lags in translation research. *The Journal of Social Media in Society*, 104(12), 510–520.

Morse, J. M. (2010). "Cherry picking": Writing from thin data. *Qualitative Health Research*, 20(1), 3–3.

Motulsky, S. (2021). Is member checking the gold standard of quality in qualitative research? *Qualitative Psychology*, 8(3), 389–406.

Nardon, L., Hari, A., and Aarma, K. (2021). Reflective interviewing – increasing social impact through research. *International Journal of Qualitative Methods*, 20, 1–12.

Nutley, S., and Davies, H. (2016). Knowledge mobilisation: Creating, sharing and using knowledge. In K. Orr, S. Nutley, S. Russell, R. Bain, B. Hacking, and C. Moran (Eds.), *Knowledge and practice in business and organisations*. London: Routledge.

O'Reilly, M., and Kiyimba, N. (2015). *Advanced qualitative research: A guide to contemporary theoretical debates*. London: Sage.

Portney, L. (2020). *Foundations of clinical research: Applications to evidence-based practice*. Philadelphia, PA: F.A Davis Company.

Powell, A., Davies, H., and Nutley, S. (2017). Missing in action? The role of the knowledge mobilisation literature in developing knowledge mobilisation practices. *Evidence & Policy*, 13(2), 201–23.

Rabin, B., Brownson, R., Haire-Joshu, D., Kreuter, M., and Weaver, N. (2008). A glossary for dissemination and implementation research in health. *Journal of Public Health Management & Practice*, 14(2), 117–123.

Ravinetto, R., and Singh, J. A. (2023). Responsible dissemination of health and medical research: Some guidance points. *BMJ Evidence-Based Medicine*, 28(3), 144–147.

Reason, M. (2010). *Mind maps, presentational knowledge and the dissemination of qualitative research*. NCRM working paper series: ESRC National Centre for Research Methods.

Ross, K. (2022). Reclaiming impact in qualitative research. *Qualitative Social Research*, 23(2), Art 5.

Sales, A., Farrández-Berrueco, R., Sanahuja, A., and Moliner, O. (2024). Knowledge mobilisation strategies for responsible and inclusive academic research. *European Journal of Higher Education*, 14(1), 20–39.

Sandelowski, M., and Leeman, J. (2012). Writing usable qualitative health research findings. *Qualitative Health Research*, 22(10), 1404–1413.

Shaw, J., Gagnon, M., Carson, A., Gastaldo, D., Gladstone, B., Webster, F., and Eakin, J. (2022). Advancing the impact of critical qualitative research on policy, practice, and science. *International Journal of Qualitative Methods*, 21, 1–11.

Silvia, P. (2007). *How to write a lot: A practical guide to productive academic writing*. Washington, DC: American Psychological Association.

Silver, M., Colditz, G., and Emmons, K. (2023). The promise and challenges of dissemination and implementation research. In D. Chambrers (Ed.), *Dissemination and implementation research in health: Translating science to practice* (pp. 3–26). Oxford: Oxford University Press.

Stein, A. (2010). Sex, truths, and audiotape: Anonymity and the ethics of public exposure in ethnography. *Journal of Contemporary Ethnography*, 39(5), 554–568.

Straus, S., Tetroe, J., and Graham, I. (2013). *Knowledge translation in health care: Moving from evidence to practice*. Hoboken, NJ: John Wiley & Sons.

Swan, J., Clarke, A., Nicolini, D., Powell, J., Scarbrough, H., Roginski, C., Gkeredakis, E., Mills, P., and Taylor-Phillips, S. (2012). *Evidence in management decisions: Advancing knowledge utilisation in healthcare management*. NIHR Health Services and Delivery Programme.

Thyer, B. (2008). *Preparing research articles*. Oxford: Oxford University Press.

Ward, V. (2017). Why, whose, what and how? A framework for knowledge mobilisers. *Evidence & Policy, 13*(3), 477–497.

Ward, V., Smith, S., House, A., and Hamer, S. (2012). Exploring knowledge exchange: A useful framework for practice and policy. *Social Science & Medicine, 74*, 297–304.

Webster, F., Gastaldo, D., Durant, S., Eakin, J., Gladstone, B., Parsons, J., Peter, E., and Shaw, J. (2019). Doing science differently: A framework for assessing the careers of qualitative scholars in the health sciences. *International Journal of Qualitative Methods, 18*.

White, C., Woodfield, K., Ritchie, J., and Ormston, R. (2014). Writing up qualitative research. In J. Ritchie, J. Lewis, C. McNaughton Nicholls, and R. Ormston (Eds.), *Qualitative research practice: A guide for social science students and researchers* (pp. 367–400). London: Sage.

Index

Note: Page numbers in **bold** reference tables.

academic scholars, partnerships with 339
accessibility, dissemination 396
acknowledging positionality 173
action research 110–112
adjacency pairs 382
Adkins, T. 60
adults 4; *see also* older adults
advisory boards, Public Patient Involvement and Engagement (PPIE) 134
aims 73–74
analytic approaches, choosing 384
analytic framework **355**
analytic memo **355**
anonymity 156–157
Aotearoa, New Zealand 176
applying for institutional ethical review approval 163–166
appraising research evidence 62
art, participatory techniques 266–267
articles, critiquing 89
asymmetric relations, clinician-researchers 183–186
atypical communication 333
audio recording 320–322
auditability 114
audits 12; clinical audits 18
author order, when writing in teams 399
autism, female autism 23
auto gatekeepers **137**
autoethnography 106–107

autonomy, deontological principles **152**
Awhangansi, S. 401–402
axiology 36–37

base size saturation 201
beneficence, deontological principles **152**
blogs, for dissemination 393–394
Boston Medical Centre 20
boundary drift 179
bricolage 24
burnout 230–231

CA *see* conversation analysis
cafe convenor **264**
cafe host **264**
cafe-style approach 262–264
cancel culture 213
case studies 257–259
categories, framework analysis **355**
charity settings, physical safety 237
charting, framework analysis **355**
child advisory board 145
child protection 158
childhood 4
children 4; participation levels 212; World Awareness for Children in Trauma (WACIT) 306–307
Children Act (1989, 2004 England and Wales) 158
Children's Act (2014 New Zealand) 158

411

INDEX

Chrisostomou, Leanne 383
Clarke, Dave 166
classical ethnography 106
clients 3; versus clinicians 184
clinical academic careers 339–340
clinical audits 12; quality improvement (QI) 18
clinical experience 53–54
clinical leader, quality improvement (QI) 13
clinical skills: building rapport 334–335; communicating with participants 333–334; (quasi-)therapeutic qualities of research participation 335–336; value of 337
clinician-researchers 3–4, 6, 170–171, 187–189; asymmetric relations and power 183–186; dual roles 176–181; evidence 64; positionality 172–175; practitioner profiles 187; reflexivity 181–183; value of 339–340
clinicians, versus patient/client/service users 184
Cochrane, A. 55
Cochrane group 85
code 362
code labels 362
code saturation 199
codebook approaches to thematic analysis 349–356, **348**
codebook thematic approaches 96–97
codes of conduct *see* ethics
co-design 138–140, 143
coding, thematic analysis 361–362
coding reliability, thematic analysis 96, 347–349
coercion 179; risk of 186
collaboration, partnerships 340–343; with academic scholars 339
communicating with participants 333–334
community settings, physical safety 237
conceptual codes 200
concrete codes 200
conducting pilot studies 90–91
conferences, dissemination 392–393
confidentiality 156–158
consent, informed consent 152–155, 314
consent-based vulnerability 220
consequentialism **151**
contextual questions 70
convenience sampling 193–194
conversation analysis (CA) 103–104, 381–383
co-production 140–141
core competencies 56
COREQ (COnsolidating criteria for REporting Qualitative research) 113
co-researching 142–143, 145
COVID-19 pandemic, digital methods 305–307
credibility 114
critical discourse analysis 101–102

critical ethnography 106
critical position 37
critical realism **38**
critical reviews 84
critical theory 40
critical thinking 61–63, 160–163
criticisms of interviewing **292**
critiquing articles 89
crystallisation 121

data collection 235, 251, 270–271; case studies 257–259; diaries as data 259–261; digital methods 304–305; documents 261–262; methods 252–253; naturally occurring data 251–255; observations 256–257; online data collection 307–312; participatory techniques 264–268; practical steps for 337; secondary data analysis 268–270; World Café approach 262–264
data management 160, 162, 323–324
data ownership 313–314
data privacy 323–324
data protection 160; management, storage and privacy 323–324
data saturation 199–202
data storage 323–324
data triangulation 118–119
decisions, research diaries 9
deductive codes 200
deductive disclosure 156–157
deductive research 31
denaturalism, transcripts 325
dentists, as researchers 172
deontological principles **152**
deontology 151
depth, qualitative research 161
description, objectives 74
descriptive questions 70
descriptive research **21**
design team, World Café roles **264**
designing research questions 68–73
designing schedule of questions for interviews and focus groups 296–297
developmental evaluations **20**
DFSS method, Six Sigma approach 17
dialectical pluralism 40
dialogic interviews 288–289
dialogic narrative analysis **373**
dialogic narrative approach **105**
diaries *see* research diaries
differentiating aims, objectives, outputs, and outcomes 73–77
digital capital 304
digital communication methods 304–305
digital divide 304, 307
digital environment 302–303; COVID-19 pandemic 305–307

INDEX

digital ethics of care 145
digital literacy 304
digital media 303
digital methods 304–305; COVID-19 pandemic 305–307; internet-mediated research 312–315; online data collection 307–312
digital spaces, determining public and privates spaces 313–314
digital video-conference platforms 309
discourse analysis 101, 379–380
discursive approaches 100–101
discursive psychology 101, **102**, 379–380
dissemination: blogs 393–394; conferences 392–393; to different audiences 396; ethics 397–398; journal articles 391–392; knowledge exchange 402–404; organisational reports 391; reasons for 390; sharing findings with participants/service users 394–395; sharing with colleagues and practitioners 394; social media 393–394; translation 404–406; webpages 393–394; workshops 392–393; writing in teams 398–402
diversity, research teams 143–144
documents, as data 261–262
Dogra, Nisha 46–47
domain gatekeepers **137**
domains of quality improvement **13**
drawing, participatory techniques 266–267
Drewett, A. 104
dual roles 176–181; mitigating challenges of 179–180

Eddy, D. 55
email 310–312
emancipatory interviews 287–288
emancipatory questions 70
emic approach 32
emotional burnout 230–231
emotional safety 229–232
emotional well-being 232–233
empathy 230
empathy interviews 280–282
empiricism 31, 40
empowerment 289
encryption 322
engagement in research 138; co-design 138–140, 143; co-production 140–141; co-researching 142–143; overlaps 143
epistemological reflexivity **182**
epistemology 30, 35, 39–45
Equality Act (UK) 218
ethical governance 163–166
ethicality 114
ethics 151–152, 166–167; anonymity 156–157; confidentiality 156–157; data protection 160; of dissemination 397–398; domains of ethical interest 162–163; informed consent 152–155; institutional ethical review approval 163–166; in internet-mediated research 312–315; privacy statements 160; right to withdraw 152–155; safeguarding 157–159; secondary data analysis 270
ethics applications: developing 164; things to remember 165
ethics committees(Institutional Review Boards) 163
ethics of care, power and 185–186
ethnographic approaches 106; video reflexive ethnography 106–107
ethnographic interviews 282–284
ethnography 106; autoethnography 107
etic approach 32
evaluations: developmental evaluations **20**; formative evaluations **20**; impact evaluations **21**; process evaluations **21**; rapid cycle evaluations **20**; service evaluations 18–19; summative evaluations **20**
evaluative questions 70
evidence 51–53, 64–65; clinical experience 53–54; critical thinking and 61–63; implementing in practice 62–63; local context 54–55; patient/service-user and family experiences 54; practice-based evidence 63–64; qualitative evidence 58–60; research evidence 53
evidence hierarchies 57–58; criticisms of 61
evidence-based medicine 55
evidence-based practice 55–57; criticisms of 60–61
excessive disclosure 179
exclusion criteria for participants 197
executive sponsors, quality improvement (QI) 13
existentialism 40–41
experiential knowledge and expertise 54
experts by experience 3, 133–134
explanation, objectives 74
explanatory questions 70
explanatory research **21**
exploration, objectives 74
exploratory research **21**
extreme or deviant cases sampling 193

face-to-face interviewing 313
face-to-face meetings 308
factual information, research diaries 8
fairness-based vulnerability 220
familiarisation, template analysis 351
family experiences 54
FANIM *see* free association narrative interview method
female autism 23

413

feminism 41
feminist interviews 289–290
fieldwork 235–237
focus groups 275; building rapport 334–335; designing schedule of questions 296–297; general guidance for 297–298; and group interviews 293–296; videoconferencing 309
formative evaluations 20
framework analysis, codebook approaches to thematic analysis 354–356
free association narrative interview method (FANIM) 108, 290, 378
funding, writing proposals for 82
funding bodies 81

Gadamer, H. 98
gatekeepers 136–138
gender, and autism 23
generative questions 70
grant applications, developing 80–83
grassroots 64
grounded theory analysis 109–110, 371–372
group interviews 293–296
guardian gatekeepers 137

hard-to-reach 215–216
harms 157–158
health inequity 352
Heidegger, M. 98–99
hermeneutics 41
heterogeneity 115–116, 205
hidden populations 216
Homan, L. 206
homogeneity 112–115
homogenous sampling 193
hospitals/hospice, fieldwork 236
humanism 41
Hunt, S. 352–354
Husserl, R. 98–99

ICT *see* Information and Communication Technologies
idealism 37, 41–42
ideological questions 70
idiographic approach 32
impact evaluations 21
impact of research 404–406
impaired capacity 185
improvement advisers, quality improvement (QI) 13
inappropriate disclosure 179
incentives for participants 196
inclusion criteria for participants 197
incompatibility of expectations 179
indexing, framework analysis 355
inductive codes 200
inductive research 31

influence, objectives 74
Information and Communication Technologies (ICT) 303
information literacy 303–304
information power 202–203
informed consent 152–155; internet-mediated research 314
inherent vulnerability 220
insider positions 176–181
insider status 219
instant messaging 310–312
institutional ethical review approval, applying for 163–166
institutional gatekeepers 137
Institutional Review Boards 163
integration 120–121
integrative themes 353
interactional narrative analysis 373
interdisciplinary research, quality improvement (QI) 23–24
internet 303
internet-mediated data collections 312
internet-mediated methods 304–305; ethical considerations 312–315
inter-paradigmatic methods 122
interpretative phenomenological analysis (IPA) 99–100, 369–371
interpreters, transcription 327–328
interpretivism 37, 42
intersubjectivity 33
interventionist interviews 285–286
interventions 64–65
interviews 275–277; building rapport 334–335; criticisms of interviewing 292; designing schedule of questions 296–297; dialogic interviews 288–289; emancipatory interviews 287–288; empathy interviews 280–282; ethnographic interviews 282–284; feminist interviews 289–290; general guidance for 297–298; group interviews 293–296; interventionist interviews 285–286; narrative interviews 277–279; naturally occurring interviews 284–285; phenomenological interviews 290–291; problems with 291–293; psychoanalytic interviews 290; reflective interviews 279–280; therapeutic interviews 286–287; transformative interviews 285–286; *see also* focus groups
intra-paradigmatic mixed methods 122
IPA *see* interpretative phenomenological analysis
iterative process 161

joint contributors 142
journal articles, dissemination 391–392
justice, deontological principles 152

INDEX

Kaupapa Māori research framework 176–177
knowledge 30, 35; *see also* evidence
knowledge exchange 403
knowledge integration 403
knowledge intermediation 403
knowledge mobilisation 403
knowledge transfer 402
knowledge-making 212

ladder of participation 211
Lean Model approach 16
levels of participation 211–213
limitations of quality improvement (QI) 17–18
listening, therapeutic style of 333
literature review 83–88
Little, S. 132–133
local context, evidence 54–55
locations for fieldwork 235–237
logic models: planning projects 78–80; typology of **80**
lone worker policies 234
LOSST LIFFE project 247

macro-social constructionism 44
majority world 5
Majumder, P. 6
managing risk 244–245
mapping positionality 175
mapping reviews 84–85
marginalised populations 217
materialism 37, **38**, 42
meaning saturation 199
media literacy 304
member checking 395–396
mental health 5
mental health in-patient hospital or outpatient clinic, fieldwork 236–237
mentors 401
meta-analysis 85
metaphysics 35
methodological obligation 172
methodology 30; theory in qualitative research 45
methods: mixing qualitative methods 116–118; theory in qualitative research 45
micro-social constructionism 44
minority world 5
mixed-studies/mixed-methods reviews 85
mixing intra-paradigmatic research 117
mixing qualitative approaches 116–118
Model for Improvement approach (PDSA cycle approach) 15–16
monological knowledge 24
Moore, I. 22–23

naive realism **38**
narrative analysis 372–375
narrative approaches 104–106

narrative interviews 277–279
narrative reviews 84; developing 88
National Research Ethics Service (NRES) 166
naturalism 31; transcripts 325
naturally occurring data 251–255
naturally occurring interviews 284–285
new information threshold, saturation 201
next-turn-proof-procedure 382
NHS England, safeguarding 159
nomothetic approach 32
non-maleficence, deontological principles **152**
non-solicited diaries 260
Noweisser, T. 100
NRES *see* National Research Ethics Services

objectives 74–75
objectivism 32
observations 256–257
observer roles 256
older adults 4
oncologists, as researchers 171
online data collection 307–312
online safeguarding 314–315
ontology 30, 37–38, 44
open access, dissemination 396
opportunistic sampling 193
organisational gatekeepers **137**
organisational reports for dissemination 391
outcomes 76–77
outputs 75–77
outsider positions 176–181
overlaps 143
overview literature reviews 85

paradigms 30–33, 35
participants: communicating with 333–334; fieldwork in homes 235–236; recruiting 195–197; versus researchers 184; sharing findings 394–395
participation, (quasi-)therapeutic qualities of research participation 335–336
participation levels 211–213
participatory action research 112
participatory research 112
participatory techniques 264–265; drawing and art 266–267; photography 267–268; PhotoVoice 267–268; vignettes 265–266
partnerships 306, 340–343; with academic scholars 339
pathogenic vulnerability 220
patients 3; versus clinicians 184; experiences 54
PDSA cycle approach 15–16
peer researchers 306–307
Peerally, M. F. 132–133
personal narrative analysis **373**
personal reflexivity **182**
phenomenological approaches 98–99

415

INDEX

phenomenological interviews 290–291
phenomenology 42, 98
philosophy 34–35
photography, participatory techniques 267–268
PhotoVoice, participatory techniques 267–268
physical safety 233–238
physical threats 233–234
physical well-being 238
PICOT model 73
pilot studies, conducting 90–91
planning projects 68; conducting pilot studies 90–91; designing research questions 68–73; differentiating aims, objectives, outputs, and outcomes 73–77; literature review 83–88; quality improvement (QI) projects 13–15; writing research proposals 77–83
policies for researcher safety 241–243
positionality, researcher positionality 172–175
positivism 37, 39
post incident, researcher safety 245–246, **245**
post-modernism 42
post-positivism 39
post-structuralism 43
power: clinician-researchers 183–186; information power 202–203; knowledge-making 212
power dynamics 184–185; researcher-participant relationships 289
power hierarchies, action research 112
PPIE *see* Public Patient Involvement and Engagement
practice-based evidence 63–64
practice-near research 338
practices, conversation analysis (CA) 382
practitioner perspective 5
practitioner profiles 187
pragmatism 43
prediction, objectives 74
preference organisation, conversation analysis (CA) 382
preliminary coding, template analysis 351
preventing harm, researcher safety 242–244
primary analysis 269
privacy statements 160
private online spaces 313–314
privilege, clinician-researchers 185
PRNs (PbRNs) 64
process evaluations 21
processes of informed consent 155
professional transformation 338
promoting participation 211–213
pseudo-anonymity 156
psychiatrists, as researchers 171
psychoanalytic interviews 290

psychoanalytic therapy 107
psychoanalytically informed analysis 376–379
psychoanalytically informed approaches 107–109
psychoanalytically informed methods 109
public online spaces 313–314
Public Patient Involvement and Engagement (PPIE) 130–136; advisory boards 134; child advisory board 145; experts by experience 133–134; reasons for using **132**; steering groups 134; tokenism 134–136; videoconferencing 309
purposeful random sampling 193
purposeful sampling 192–193

QI *see* quality improvement
qualitative approach 30–31
qualitative evidence 58–60
qualitative evidence synthesis 85
qualitative health research 21–22
qualitative research, quality improvement (QI) 19–23
qualitative systematic review 85
quality assurance 65; grounded theory analysis 371–372
quality improvement projects 11–12
quality improvement (QI) 11–13, 25–26, 112; clinical audits 18; doing projects 15–17; domains of **13**; interdisciplinary research 23–24; limitations of 17–18; planning a project 13–15; qualitative research 19–23; service evaluations 18–19; teams 13
quality indicators in qualitative research **113**
quality markers 112
quantitative approach 30–31
quantitative research 122
(quasi-)therapeutic qualities of research participation 335–336

Randomised Controlled Trials (RCTs) 53, 57, 73, 90
rapid cycle evaluations **20**
rapid reviews 85
rapport, building in interviews and focus groups 334–335
rationalism 31
RCTs *see* Randomised Controlled Trials
reading research articles critically 88–89
realism 37; variants of **38**
recording: audio/video 319–320; practical issues with 322–323
recruiting: participants 195–197; vulnerable populations 215–221
recruitment process 195–196
reflection 7–8; self-reflection 181–183
reflection-in-action 8, 181
reflection-on-action 8

INDEX

reflective activity, research diaries 9
reflective interviews 279–280
reflexive thematic analysis 97, **348**, 356–360, 365; themes 363–364
reflexivity 7, 114, 173, 280; clinician-researchers 181–183; Public Patient Involvement and Engagement (PPIE) 131
rejection, dealing with 396
relationship building 336
relativism 38
reliability, coding reliability 347–349
repair, conversation analysis (CA) 382
research articles, reading critically 88–89
research diaries: as data 259–261; importance of 8–9
research evidence 53; appraising 62
research philosophy 34–35
research proposals, writing 77–83
research questions, designing 68–73
research teams 143–146, 238; writing together 398–402
researcher involvement 161
researcher positionality 172–175
researcher safety 225–227, 246–247; emotional safety 229–232; managing 241–246; physical safety 233–238; and sensitive research 227–229; transcriptionist safety 238–241
researcher-generated data 251–252, 255; benefits of **256**
researcher-participant relationships 176
researchers, versus participants 184
re-use/re-analysis 269
rhetorical narrative analysis **373**
right to withdraw 152–155
risk 226; managing in the moment 244–245
risk assessment 226–227
risk of coercion 186
risk of harm from others 157
risk of harm to others 157
risk of harm to self 157
routine practice 63
rumination 230
run length, saturation 201

safeguarding 157–159; online 314–315
safety *see* researcher safety
sample sizes 197–199, 204–206
sampling 192; convenience sampling 193–194; purposeful sampling 192–193; saturation 199–202; theoretical sampling 194–195
sampling adequacy 114, 197–206
saturation 199–202
SCALE ENDO project 132–133
scientific method 53
scoping reviews 85; developing 87–88
secondary analysis 269

secondary data analysis 268–270
secondary traumatic stress 230–232
Secondary Traumatic Stress Scale (STSS) 231–232
seldom-heard 216
self-publishing 392
self-reflection 181–183
semi-structured interviews 276
sensitive research, and researcher safety 227–229
sensitive topics, doing research on 213–214
sensitivity 214
sequence organisation, conversation analysis (CA) 381
service evaluations 12, 18–19
service users 3; versus clinicians 184; experiences 54; sharing findings 394–395
sharing findings with colleagues and practitioners 394
sharing findings with participants/service users 394–395
simultaneous analysis 269
situational vulnerability 220
Six Sigma approach 16–17
SMART, objectives 74–75
snowball sampling 193
social constructionism 43–44
social constructionist paradigm 366
social constructivism 44
social identity maps 174
social justice, transformative interviews 285–286
social media 303, 313–314; for dissemination 393–394
socially disadvantaged populations 216
solicited diaries 260
Sommantico, Massimiliano 378
specialist gatekeepers **137**
stakeholder mapping 14–15
standardised artefacts, documents as 261
stanzas 374
state-of-the-art reviews 85
steering groups, Public Patient Involvement and Engagement (PPIE) 134
STEPS model 72
stopping criterion 205
storytelling 278
stratified purposeful sampling 193
strophes 374
structural narrative analysis **373**
structural narrative approach **105**
structured interviews 276
STSS *see* Secondary Traumatic Stress Scale
subjectivism 32
subtle realism **38**
Swords, C. 228–229
symbolic interactionism 43
system leaders, quality improvement (QI) 13

417

INDEX

systematic reviews 85–87
systematic search and review 85
systematised review 85

table host **264**
team leads, quality improvement (QI) 13
teams 143–146, 238; quality improvement (QI) 13; writing in 398–402
technical experts, quality improvement (QI) 13
telephone meetings 308–309
template analysis, codebook approaches to thematic analysis 350–354
text-based methods 310–312
thematic analysis 346–347; codebook approaches to thematic analysis 349–356; coding 361–362; coding reliability 347–349; creating themes and doing analysis 363–365; reflexive thematic analysis 356–360; theory 360–361
thematic approaches 95–97
thematic narrative analysis **373**
thematic narrative approach **105**
thematic reviews, developing 88
thematic saturation 199–202
themes, creating 363–365
theoretical sampling 194–195
theoretical saturation 199–202
theory 29, 45–47; axiology 36–37; epistemology 39–45; methodology and method 45; narrative approaches 105; ontology 37–38; paradigms 30–33; role of 33–34; thematic analysis 360–361
therapeutic interviews 286–287
therapeutic qualities of research participation 335–336
therapeutic style of listening 333
thick descriptions **21**, 369
threats 233–234
time management, when writing in teams 400–401
Tobacco Treatment Consult service **20**
tokenism, Public Patient Involvement and Engagement (PPIE) 134–136
transcription 319–320; considerations in commissioning 328; as interpretive activity 324–327; technology as an aid 326–327; transcriptionist safety 238–241; translation 327–328
transcripts, anonymity 156–157
transferability 114
transformative interviews 285–286
transforming knowledge 404–406
transition relevance place 382
translation 404–406; in transcriptions 327–328
transparency 33, 114; secondary data analysis 270

triangulation 118–119
Tromans, S. 180–181
trustworthiness 114
turn construction unit 382
turn design, conversation analysis (CA) 382
turn-allocation 382
turn-sharing 382
turn-taking 382
types of qualitative research: action research 110–112; conversation analysis (CA) 103–104; critical discourse analysis 101–103; discourse analysis 101; discursive approaches 100–101; discursive psychology 101; ethnographic approaches 106; grounded theory approaches 109–110; integrated approach 120–121; interpretative phenomenological analysis (IPA) 99–100; mixing qualitative approaches 116–118; narrative approaches 104–106; phenomenological approaches 98–99; psychoanalytically informed approaches 107–109; thematic approaches 95–97
typical case sampling 193
typology of logic models **80**

umbrella reviews 85
under-privileged 185
underserved populations 216–217
universal quality checklists 115
unstructured interviews 276

validity 114
value theory 35
vicarious traumatisation 230–231
video recording 320–321; encryption 322
video reflexive ethnography (VRE) 106–107
video-conference platforms 309
videoconferencing 309–310
vignettes 265–266
virtue ethics **151**
visibility 162
visual narrative analysis **373**
visual narrative approach **105**
volunteer settings, physical safety 237
Vostanis, P. 306–307
VRE see video reflexive ethnography
vulnerability 215–221
vulnerable adults 158–159
vulnerable populations, recruiting 215–221

WACIT see World Awareness for Children in Trauma
WAD see work as done
WAI see word as imagined
webpages, dissemination 393–394
Wellcome Trust 145
whakawhanaungatanga 188

word as imagined (WAI) 107
work as done (WAD) 107
workshops, dissemination 392–393
World Awareness for Children in Trauma (WACIT) 306–307
World Café approach 262–264
World Café roles **264**

writing: research proposals 77–83; research questions 70–73; in teams 398–402
writing retreats/days, research teams 402
writing routines, for teams 400–401

young people 4; *see also* children
YouthCan IMPACT project **20**

For Product Safety Concerns and Information please contact our
EU representative GPSR@taylorandfrancis.com Taylor & Francis
Verlag GmbH, Kaufingerstraße 24, 80331 München, Germany